A Textbook of Orthodontics

W. J. B. Houston
FDS RCS(Edin), PhD, DOrth
Professor of Orthodontics
United Medical and Dental Schools of Guy's and St Thomas Hospitals, London

W. J. Tulley
PhD, BDS, FDS RCS, DOrth
Emeritus Professor of Orthodontics
United Medical and Dental Schools of Guy's and St Thomas Hospitals, London

With contributions by
A. C. Campbell BDS FDS RCS MRCS LRCP DOrthRCS
Emeritus Consultant, Guy's Hospital, London

D. Poswillo DDS DSc MDhc FDS FIBiol FRCPath
Professor of Dental Surgery,
United Medical and Dental Schools of Guy's and St Thomas Hospitals, London

M. E. Foster MB ChB, MScD, FDS FFD
Consultant Oral Surgeon
North Manchester General Hospital
Crumpsall, Manchester

WRIGHT

London   Boston   Singapore   Sydney   Toronto   Wellington

Wright is an imprint of Butterworth Scientific

PART OF REED INTERNATIONAL P.L.C.

All rights reserved. No part of this publication may be reproduced in any material form (including photocopying or storing it in any medium by electronic means and whether or not transiently or incidentally to some other use of this publication) without the written permission of the copyright owner except in accordance with the provisions of the Copyright, Designs and Patents Act 1988 or under the terms of a licence issued by the Copyright Licensing Agency Ltd, 33–34 Alfred Place, London, England WC1E 7DP. Applications for the copyright owner's written permission to reproduce any part of this publication should be addressed to the Publishers.

Warning: The doing of an unauthorised act in relation to a copyright work may result in both a civil claim for damages and criminal prosecution.

This book is sold subject to the Standard Conditions of Sale of Net Books and may not be re-sold in the UK below the net price given by the Publishers in their current price list.

First published by John Wright and Sons Ltd 1986
Reprinted 1989
© Butterworth & Co. (Publishers) Ltd, 1986.

British Library Cataloguing in Publication Data
Houston, W.J.B.
A Textbook of Orthodontics
1. Orthodontics
I. Title II. Tulley, W.J.
617.6'43 RK521

ISBN 0 7236 0747 8

Photoset by Apek Typesetters, Avon House, Blackfriars Road, Nailsea, Bristol BS19 2DJ
Printed and bound by Page Bros Ltd, Norwich, Norfolk.

A Textbook of Orthodontics

Preface

This book is the successor to 'A Manual of Practical Orthodontics' by Tulley and Campbell, which is now outdated. There have been many developments in the theory and practice of orthodontics over the past few years and the undergraduate student is now expected to have a much wider understanding of the subject. The requirements of the undergraduate course and the basis of more advanced postgraduate studies are covered by the text when supplemented by clinical and practical experience. The need for an understanding of biological principles in orthodontic diagnosis and treatment planning is stressed. Many topics within orthodontics are still controversial, and an attempt has been made to provide a coherent and clinically sound theoretical framework to the subject, without the distraction of too many debatable concepts that are at present outside the mainstream of orthodontic thought.

Mr A. C. Campbell, co-author of the predecessor to this text, has contributed to Chapter 20 on Craniofacial Anomalies, and Professor David Poswillo has written Chapter 19 with Mr. Murray Foster, as well as contributing to the content of Chapter 8 and 20. We are grateful for their collaboration.

Publication has come at a time when the Dental Schools of the Royal Dental Hospital and of Guy's Hospital have merged and we were able to draw upon the extensive experience available in the two orthodontic departments. We are indebted to the many colleagues who have helped us in innumerable ways, particularly in the discussion of ideas and in help with illustrative material. It is not possible to mention everyone by name, but we particularly wish to acknowledge the following:—

Mrs Mary Calvert
Miss Sue Farrant
Mrs Liz Jones
Mr Des McElroy
Mr Mike Mars
Mr Robert Mordecai
Mr D. A. Plint
Mr Allan Thom
Miss Cheryl Tracey
Mr David Ramsey
Mr Laurence Usiskin

who have helped us in many ways, particularly with illustrative material.

Miss U. Desai prepared prints from slides of the clinical cases, and we greatly appreciate her skill and helpfulness. Miss Ann Taylor undertook the great majority of the secretarial work in the preparation of the text and we are very grateful for her work and forbearance in preparing a number of drafts.

W. J. B. H
W. J. T. T

Contents

Chapter 1

Introduction

Orthodontics is the branch of dentistry concerned with growth of the face, development of the occlusion and the prevention and correction of occlusal anomalies. Thus the study of orthodontics includes factors such as variations in facial development and growth and in orofacial function that may influence occclusal development; it also includes the effects of occlusal variations on facial appearance and on the health and function of the masticatory system.

The Place of Orthodontics in General Dental Practice

The general dental practitioner has the responsibility of monitoring the dental status of his child patients and so it is important for him to have a thorough understanding of occlusal development, of the factors that may influence it and of the indications for and timing of treatment.

A number of common simple occlusal problems can be treated with removable appliances and these should be within the scope of the general practitioner with the appropriate skills and training. However, it is important for him to appreciate the limitations of his own experience and of the appliances he is competent to use. What seems superficially to be simple irregularity may in reality be much more complex, and ill-advised attempts to treat such problems with extractions and removable appliances may only make things much worse.

The general practitioner should have some knowledge of the potentials and limitations of fixed appliances, but although modern materials and equipment have simplified some aspects of fixed appliance treatment, their effective use requires extended training and the practitioner must not embark on a technique in which he is not competent.

OCCLUSAL VARIATION

Central to the the study of orthodontics is occlusal variation, and so it is convenient to start with the concept of ideal occlusion. Ideal occlusion in man is seldom, if ever, found: it is a hypothetical concept based upon the anatomy of the teeth and is useful as a benchmark by which occlusal irregularities and treatment objectives can be judged. While all the possible approximal and occlusal contacts required to satisfy ideal occlusion can be described in detail, this would be of limited value from a clinical point of view and it is sufficient to specify a number of general principles.

Ideal Occlusion in the Permanent Dentition

1   Each arch is regular with the teeth at ideal inclinations and the correct approximal relationship at each interdental contact area.
2   The arch relationships are such that each lower tooth (except the central incisor) contacts the corresponding upper tooth and the tooth anterior to it (*Fig.* 1.1). The upper arch overlaps the lower anteriorly and laterally. In particular:
a   Labial segments: The lower incisor edges occlude with the cingulum plateau of the upper incisors and their inclinations are such that the overjet is 2–3 mm and the overbite is between one-third and one-half of the height of the lower incisor crowns. The midlines coincide.
b. Buccal segments: Both anteroposteriorly and transversely the upper and lower teeth have the correct intercuspal relationships. In particular, note that the upper canine occludes in the embrasure between the lower canine and first premolar, and that the mesiobuccal cusp of the upper molar may not occlude directly with the anterior buccal groove of the lower first permanent molar, as described by Angle, but slightly distal to it (*see Fig.* 1.2).
3   When the teeth are in maximum intercuspation, the mandible is in a position of centric relation, i.e. both condyles are in symmetric, retruded, unstrained positions in the glenoid fossae.
4   During mandibular excursions, functional relationships are correct. In particular during lateral excursions there should be either group function or a cuspid rise on the working side with no occlusal contact on the contra-lateral side (*Fig.* 1.3); and in protrusion the occlusion should be on the incisor teeth but not on the molars.

Normal Occlusion (see Fig. 1.1)

This term encompasses minor deviations from the ideal that do not constitute aesthetic or functional problems. It is not possible to specify precisely the limits of normal occlusion and so there can be disagreement even between experienced clinicians about the categorization of borderline cases. For example, a minor

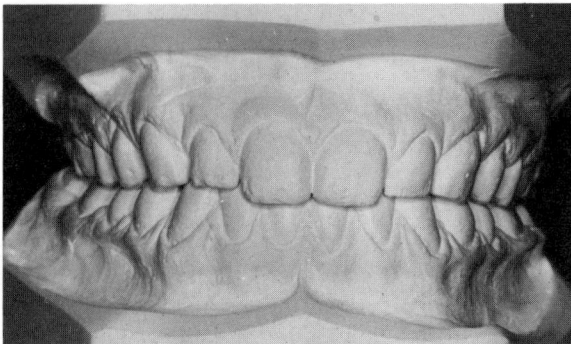

Fig. 1.1. Normal occlusion in the permanent dentition.

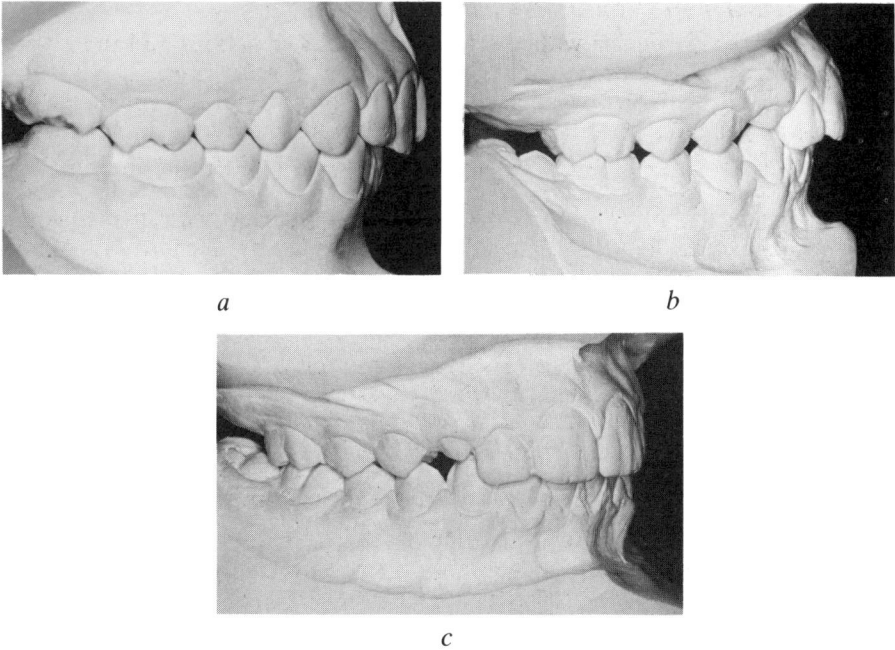

Fig. 1.2. *a*, A Class I buccal segment relationship. There is full intercuspation of all the bucccal teeth. Note that the distobuccal cusp of the upper first permanent molar occludes with the embrasure distal to the lower molar. In this case the anterior buccal cusp of the upper first permanent molar occludes with the buccal groove of the lower molar, but in some cases, it lies behind the groove. *b*, A pseudo Class I molar relationship. The anterior buccal cusp of the upper first permanent molar occludes with the buccal groove of the lower molar. However the upper first permanent molar does not occlude with the lower second permanent molar. Note that this molar relationship does not allow a correct intercuspation of the premolars and canines, and that the buccal segment relationship is fundamentally Class II. *c*, When the occlusion in (*b*) is viewed obliquely, as is normally done when examining the occlusion in the mouth, the buccal segment relationship appears to be Class I.

irregularity of the lower incisors might be considered acceptable by one but not by another. Where there is no evidence that an irregularity is or could be disadvantageous to the patient, the occlusion should be classified as normal.

Malocclusion

Appreciable deviations from the ideal that may be considered aesthetically or functionally unsatisfactory are called malocclusions. It is important not to equate the possession of a malocclusion with the need for treatment. A malocclusion that is considered to be unsightly by one patient may be acceptable to another, depending upon other facial features, personality and attitudes. A potentially traumatic occlusal relationship (*Fig.* 1.4) merits treatment in the well-motivated patient but may be best left alone in the patient with a neglected mouth.

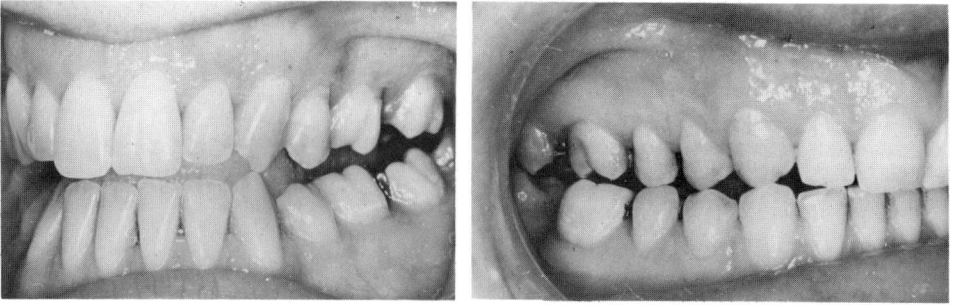

a   b

Fig. 1.3. In the lateral excursion there should be either (a) cuspid rise where only the canine teeth on the working side are in contact, or (b) group function where most of the teeth on the working side are in contact. Note that the teeth on the non-working side should be out of contact.

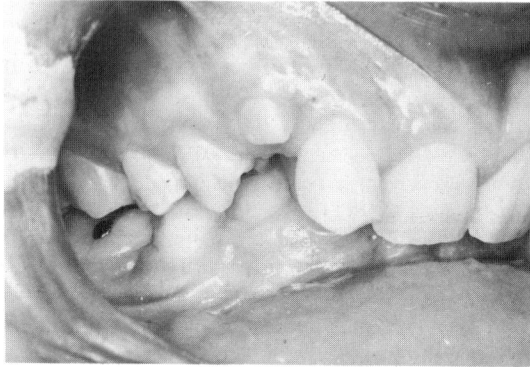

Fig. 1.4. A potentially traumatic occlusion. The lower incisor edges occlude with the gingiva palatal to the upper incisors. This type of occlusion is often associated with gingival trauma in the long term.

INDICATIONS FOR ORTHODONTIC TREATMENT

Aesthetic Criteria

By far the most common reason for a patient to seek orthodontic treatment is dissatisfaction with the appearance of the teeth. Facial appearance can be very important to an individual's self image, well-being and success in society. Dental irregularities can be facially handicapping and thus merit orthodontic treatment on these grounds alone. The social acceptability of a particular occlusion depends not only on the arrangement of the teeth but on other facial features such as nose, lips and cheeks, on the personality of the patient and on the attitudes of the society in which he or she lives. Minor and inconspicuous irregularities do not merit treatment on aesthetic grounds even though the occasional patient may be worried by them.

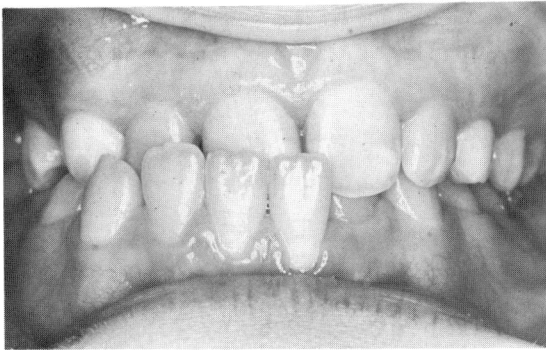

Fig. 1.5. A traumatic relationship with gingival recession at one lower incisor. The reverse overjet must be corrected urgently.

Functional Criteria

A number of occlusal irregularities, such as instanding upper incisors, labial crowding of a lower incisor and a very deep overbite, can be associated with periodontal damage in an appreciable proportion of cases with these conditions (*Fig*. 1.5). Functional mandibular displacements, associated with anterior and lateral crossbites, lead to both muscular and joint dysfunction which give rise to facial pain in certain cases. Thus early correction of these malocclusions is indicated.

Gross irregularities of the teeth are associated with caries and periodontal disease as a result of food stagnation and plaque accumulation. However, where plaque control is good, there is no evidence that dental irregularity by itself leads to periodontal breakdown. The control of established periodontal disease may be more difficult in the presence of certain tooth malpositions, for example, where there is root approximation of adjacent teeth so that the bony septum between them is very thin.

Table 1.1. Prevalence of malocclusion (per cent)

	Gardiner[1] 5–15 yr	Todd[2] 11–12 yr	Foster and Day[3] 11–12 yr
Class I (including normal)	65·7	63·0	44·3
Class II			
division 1	3·0 ⎫	18·5 ⎫	27·2 ⎫
division 2	0·8 ⎬ 8·1	4·5 ⎬ 33·5	17·7 ⎬ 52·2
indefinite	4·3 ⎭	10·5 ⎭	7·3 ⎭
Class III	0·4	3·0	3·5
Some treatment required	74·2	41·5	59·9

[1]Gardiner J. (1956) A survey of malocclusion and some aetiological factors in 1000 Sheffield schoolchildren. *Dent. Practit.* **6**; 187–98.
[2]Todd J. E. (1975) *Children's Dental Health in England and Wales*, 1973. London, HMSO.
[3]Foster T. D. and Day A. J. W. (1974) A survey of malocclusion and the need for orthodontic treatment in a Shropshire school population. *Br. J. Orthodont.* **1**; 73–8.

Prevalence of Malocclusion

Estimates of the prevalence of malocclusion vary widely, even for the one population, in part at least because of lack of agreement between different investigators (*Table* 1.1). The problem of the assessment of malocclusion is discussed at greater length in Chapter 5.

Chapter 2

Development of Normal Occlusion

Since the beginning of this century, many studies have been made of the developing occlusion by the laborious collection of serial models.[1,2] Some have concentrated on describing the ideal development of occlusion, while others have also described acceptable variations.[3-10]

Few adults achieve a dentition that approaches the ideal, with 32 teeth in good alignment. One study[11] revealed that less than 10 per cent of a group of adults had a full complement of teeth without third molar impactions or late incisor crowding and only 5 per cent had anything approaching an ideal occlusion.

The dental practitioner must have an understanding of the normal milestones in the development of the occlusion and the variations that are functionally and aesthetically acceptable. This will enable him to appreciate where there is a deviation from the normal which is likely to require treatment and the age at which this could be most effective.

The neonate is without teeth for approximately the first 6 months of life and the gum pads in which teeth are developing are covered with dense fibrous periosteum and are divided into segmented elevations (*Fig.* 2.1). The segments relating to the second deciduous molars are not well defined until 5 months of age. The upper gum pad is horseshoe-shaped and the lower is U-shaped and

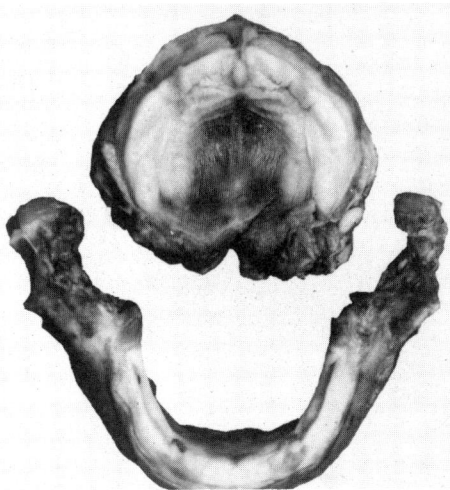

Fig. 2.1. Occlusal view of gum pads at birth.

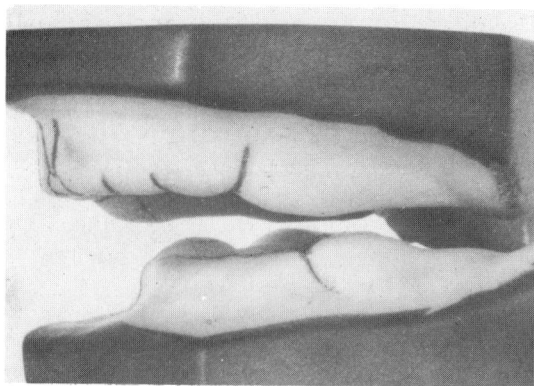

Fig. 2.2. Lateral view of gum pads at birth showing the relationship of the lateral sulci.

somewhat flattened anteriorly. There is a well-defined groove distal to the crypts of the deciduous canines in both arches, which is known as the 'lateral sulcus'. The arch of the upper gum pad is both wider and longer than that of the lower and the palatal vault is almost flat. The alveolar process is separated on the palatal side by a horizontal groove known as the 'dental' or 'gingival groove' and the labial crest of the lower gum pad is slightly everted.

The gum pads are not brought together in function as the mouth at this stage is designed for suckle feeding. Although attempts have been made to define a true relationship between the upper and lower gum pads, any position of contact is artificial and difficult to record with accuracy. It has been shown that, despite considerable variation in the anteroposterior relationship of the gum pads, a normal occlusion may still develop. At birth the lower gum pad lies distal to the upper to a variable degree. This position is judged by the relationship of the lateral sulci (*Fig.* 2.2).

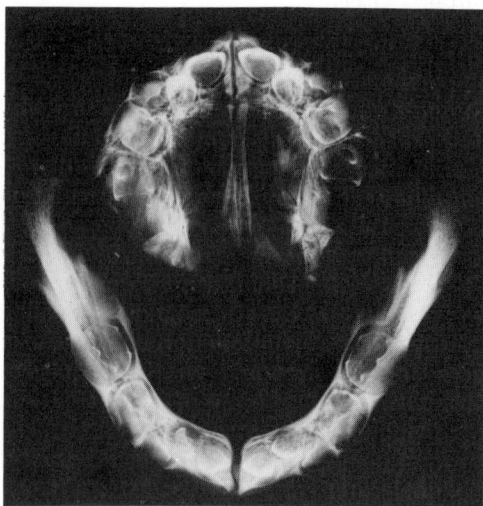

Fig. 2.3. Radiograph of gum pads shown in *Fig.* 2.1 demonstrating positions of the unerupted teeth in their crypts.

At this stage the tongue is blunt and quite large relative to the size of the jaws and it rests between the gum pads in contact with the lower lip, which forms the principal boundary to the anterior part of the oral cavity. The fraenum of the upper lip is attached to the crest of the gum pad and there is fibrous continuity with the incisal papilla in the palate.

An occlusal X-ray of the gum pads at birth shows there to be some crowding of the upper and lower deciduous teeth in their crypts (*Fig.* 2.3). This does not necessarily indicate that they will be crowded when they erupt.

DEVELOPMENT OF DECIDUOUS DENTITION

During the first year, the gum pads enlarge and the arches widen slightly to accommodate all the teeth. There is some adjustment in jaw relationship. The lower gum pad is only slightly distal to the upper by the time the deciduous incisors erupt.

The timing of incisor eruption is variable (*Table* 2.1) and may begin at any time within the first year. Parents often need to be reassured about this variation as they may have been told that teeth should start to appear by 6 months. Usually the lower central incisors erupt first, followed shortly by the upper central incisors. The deciduous incisors are smaller, whiter and more upright than their successors and at first the overbite tends to be rather deep. This is not an indicator of the eventual overbite as it will reduce over the next 3–4 years. The first deciduous molars are the next teeth to erupt, at between 1 year and 18 months, followed by the deciduous canines and finally the second deciduous molars (*Fig.* 2.4).

Table 2.1. Typical ages of eruption and mesiodistal widths of the deciduous teeth.

	Time of eruption (mth)	Mesiodistal width (mm)
Maxillary teeth		
Central incisor	8	6·5
Lateral incisor	9	5·0
Canine	18	6·5
First molar	14	7·0
Second molar	24	8·5
Mandibular teeth		
Central incisor	6	4·0
Lateral incisor	7	4·5
Canine	16	5·5
First molar	12	8·0
Second molar	20	9·5

Eruption times vary considerably. Up to 6 months earlier or later than the times given is not unusual.
Mesiodistal widths vary by up to 20 per cent on either side of the figures given.
Calcification of the deciduous teeth begins between 4 and 6 months *in utero*.
Root formation is complete between 12 and 18 months after eruption.

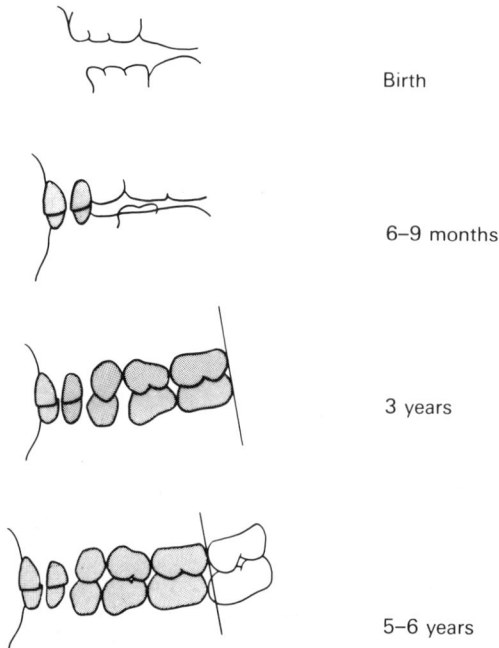

Birth

6–9 months

3 years

Fig. 2.4. Development of the dentition from birth to 6 years.

5–6 years

In some instances the incisors erupt with spaces and these tend to close; but there is often space distal to the lower canine and mesial to the upper canine. This may be referred to as the 'primate space' named after an equivalent space found in the primate dentition.

The deciduous dentition is rarely complete before the age of 3 years. At this time the incisors are upright and the overbite is rather deep but not traumatic. The anteroposterior relationship of the arches is as shown in *Fig.* 2.4, with the distal edges of the upper and lower second deciduous molars flush in the same vertical plane. At this stage there are some common variations that do not necessarily indicate any gross abnormality in the permanent dentition. There may or may not be spacing in the deciduous dentition and the overbite may be quite variable. Where there is digit-sucking there may be a frank open bite which disappears with the withdrawal of the habit before the permanent teeth erupt. In other cases the overbite may be excessively deep, but this again may not reflect the future pattern in the permanent dentition.

There is some doubt as to whether there is any appreciable lateral or anteroposterior increase in arch size during the next 3 years but there is a definite change in the anteroposterior relationship. It is not clear whether this is due to the lower teeth moving forwards in relation to the upper teeth, or an actual change in jaw relationship. Attrition of the deciduous teeth is necessary to allow the occlusal change. By the time the first permanent molars are due to erupt the distal edges of the second deciduous molars may no longer be flush in the vertical plane (*Fig.* 2.4) because of the change in arch relationship or because the lower primate space has closed.

By 5 years of age, the deciduous teeth have suffered some attrition and the incisors often have an edge-to-edge relationship and show varying degrees of

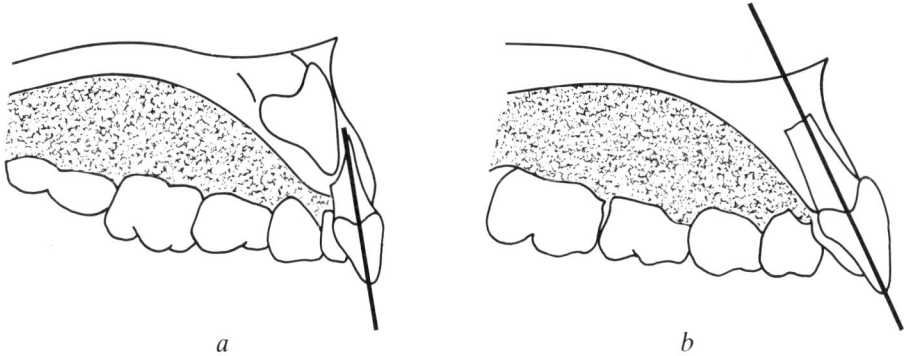

Fig. 2.5. *a*, Position of the upper central incisors prior to eruption. *b*, After eruption, the inclination of the upper central incisors may change under the influence of the lips and tongue.

spacing. It has been found that if the primary teeth erupt with spacing and this increases, there is a good chance of avoiding crowding in the permanent dentition, but this is by no means always true.[12]

The mixed dentition phase begins with the eruption of the first permanent molars at approximately 6 years of age. The first permanent molars may be guided into a cusp-to-cusp relationship by the distal surfaces of the deciduous second molars if they are flush at this stage. If the lower arch has moved forwards relative to the upper, the permanent molars may erupt more nearly into full intercuspation.[13]

The upper first permanent molars develop in the maxillary tuberosity with the occlusal surfaces facing distally and buccally as well as occlusally. Growth in maxillary length is necessary to allow them to erupt into the line of the arch. The mandibular molars develop under the anterior border of the ascending ramus of the mandible and growth in mandibular length is necessary if these teeth are to have room to erupt.

The permanent incisors are larger than their predecessors and are accommodated by erupting into a more proclined position and in a wider arc. There is also some increase in intercanine width. Teeth in the lower labial segment usually erupt before their upper counterparts. They may appear lingually and then move forwards, due to pressure from the tongue, into their correct position as their predecessors are shed. Teeth in the upper labial segment develop on the palatal aspects of the roots of their predecessors and erupt downwards, outwards and forwards (*Fig.* 2.5). It is important to recognize this pre-eruptive position because it explains why the teeth may be deflected from the normal path of eruption (*see* Chapter 9).

When the upper central incisors first erupt, a midline diastema is normally present. The upper lateral incisors develop in a more palatal position than the central incisors and are overlapped by them, but become free to move labially as the central incisors erupt. Their apices always remain slightly more palatal than those of the central incisors. It is this phase in the development of the upper labial segment which concerns parents and they may seek advice. It was described by Broadbent as the 'ugly duckling' stage, a term which has gone out of fashion because it may not be appropriate to use to parents or children. This

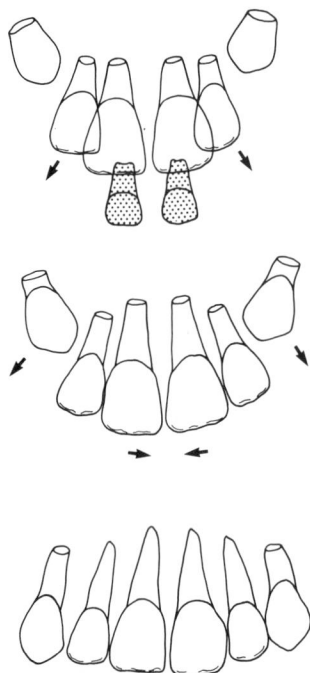

Fig. 2.6. Pattern of eruption of the upper incisors and canines showing the change in inclination of the teeth and the closure of the midline diastema.

natural developmental stage should not be mistaken for a malocclusion and treatment is not indicated to close the diastema (*Fig.* 2.6), which will normally close completely on eruption of the upper permanent canines (*Fig.* 2.7).

The crowns of the upper lateral incisors have a slight distal inclination and there is partial closure of the midline space as they erupt. The distal inclination of the lateral incisors reflects the fact that the developing permanent canines are high and closely associated with the roots of the lateral incisors at this time. As development proceeds, the canines move buccally and should be palpable high in the buccal sulcus, and the lateral incisors become more upright. The upper labial fraenum should no longer be attached to the crest of the alveolar process but to its labial surface, quite clear of the incisors. If a low attachment persists it may cause interference with space closure (*see* Chapter 9).

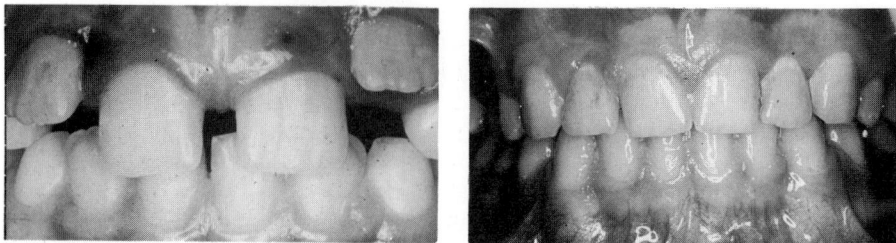

a *b*

Fig. 2.7. *a*, A marked example of the 'ugly duckling' stage at seven and a half years of age. *b*, By 12 years of age, the upper permanent canines have erupted and the incisor spacing has closed naturally.

Table 2.2. Typical ages of eruption and mesiodistal widths of the permanent teeth

	Time of eruption (yr)	Mesiodistal width (mm)
Maxillary teeth		
Central incisor	7·5	8·5
Lateral incisor	8·5	6·5
Canine	11·5	8·0
First premolar	10·0	7·0
Second premolar	11·0	6·5
First molar	6·0	10·0
Second molar	12·0	9·5
Mandibular teeth		
Central incisor	6·5	5·5
Lateral incisor	7·5	6·0
Canine	10·5	7·0
First premolar	10·5	7·0
Second premolar	11·0	7·0
First molar	6·0	11·0
Second molar	12·0	10·5

The figures given both for eruption times and for mesiodistal widths commonly vary by up to 20 per cent on either side of the figures given.

Calcification dates are variable but the permanent teeth have usually started to calcify as follows:

At birth $\frac{6}{6}$ by 6 months $\frac{1\ 3}{123}$ Between 8 and 14 years $\frac{8}{8}$

by 2 year $\frac{2\ 4}{4}$ by 4 years $\frac{5\ 7}{5\ 7}$

Root formation is normally completed 2–3 years after eruption.

The overbite is little more than one-third the length of the crowns of the lower central incisors, but over the next few years it tends to reduce.

At this stage there are a number of common variations. The size of the diastema and the degree of distal tilt of the lateral incisors both vary considerably (*Fig.* 2.7). The overbite may be reduced or incomplete, particularly if there is a residual digit-sucking habit. If a diastema is not present and the lateral incisors are slightly palatally displaced, this is a strong indication that crowding may remain and may even get worse with the eruption of the permanent canines.

The replacement of deciduous teeth by their successors in the buccal segments may begin as early as 7 years of age and is not always complete by the age of 12 (*Table* 2.2). There is a discrepancy in the total space occupied by the deciduous cheek teeth compared with that required for their successors. Although the permanent canines are wider than their predecessors, particularly in the upper arch, premolars are narrower than deciduous molars. Thus the combined mesiodistal width of the permanent canines and premolars is usually less than that of the deciduous canines and molars. The surplus space, or 'leeway space' as it is called, is greater in the lower jaw than in the upper (*Fig.* 2.8). This means that when all deciduous teeth have been replaced the upper first permanent molar will have drifted forwards to a lesser extent than the lower first molar. The normal cuspal relationship may not be established until this time.[14]

The sequence of eruption is variable. In the lower buccal segment the first tooth to erupt is either the lower first premolar or the lower canine. The lower

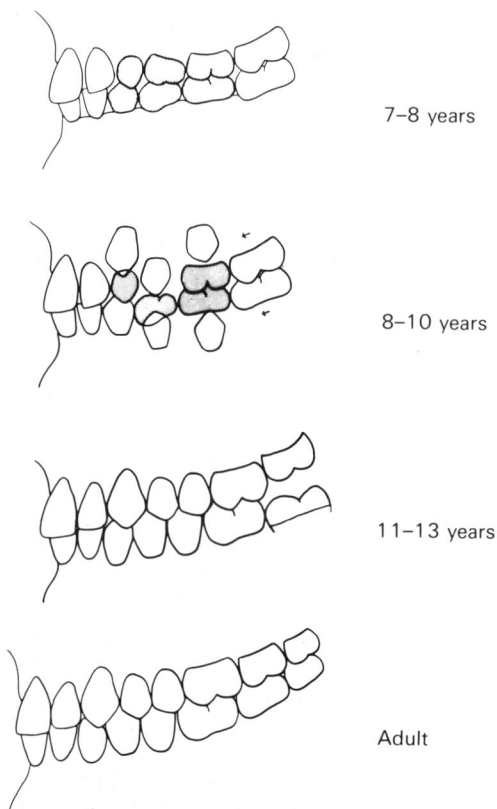

7–8 years

8–10 years

11–13 years

Fig. 2.8. Changes from the mixed to the permanent dentition between 7 and 18 years of age.

Adult

second premolar sometimes erupts after the second permanent molar. In the upper buccal segment the first premolar usually erupts first, followed by the canine. This tooth has a long path of eruption from its developmental position and this is one of the factors contributing to its frequently aberrant position. The canine erupts into a wider arc in the same way as the upper incisors and any remaining space between the upper central incisors should close. The upper second premolar erupts a little before its lower counterpart.

The usual sequence of eruption of permanent teeth in the buccal segment is particularly significant if extractions for the relief of crowding are contemplated. The emergence of the upper first premolar well before the canine usually allows this tooth to be extracted in good time to allow natural canine alignment.

In the lower arch, plans for the extraction of the first premolar may be delayed if the canine erupts first. Planned extraction of the second premolar is usually accompanied by the use of a fixed appliance to align the teeth. The fact that it is the last tooth of the series to erupt dictates a later start to active treatment.

To complete the full adult dentition the second molars erupt between 12 and 14 years, followed by the third molars whose eruption dates are between 16 and 20 years. These molars follow a similar path of eruption to that described for the first permanent molars. In the full dentition the upper buccal segments are tilted slightly outwards and the lower buccal segments tilted slightly lingually. The occlusal plane has a distinct upward curve (curve of Spee). The mandibular teeth are set one inclined plane in advance of the maxillary teeth because the mandibular incisors are smaller mesiodistally than the maxillary incisors *(See Fig. 2.8)*.

The maxillary teeth are half a cusp to the buccal of the mandibular teeth (i.e. they are not cusp-to-cusp) and the mesiobuccal cusp of the upper first permanent molar occludes with the anterior buccal groove of the lower first permanent molar *(see Fig. 1.2)*.

A more reliable indicator of a normal arch relationship is that the upper permanent canine occludes in the embrasure between the lower permanent canine and first premolar. The lower incisors should occlude with the cingulum plateau of the upper incisors so that the overbite is about a third of the height of the lower incisor crowns and the overjet is approximately 2 mm.

Three aspects of this later stage of development should be noted. First, there may be an increase in incisor crowding, particularly in the lower arch; secondly, there is usually an increase in the interincisal angle; and thirdly, there may be a slight increase in mandibular prognathism.[15, 16] The increase in incisor crowding is not found in every case, but a dentition that shows a slight slipping of the contact points of upper and lower incisors, at the time of eruption of the second molars, is likely to show an increase in crowding by 18–20 years of age.

Many factors may contribute to late incisor crowding. The tendency to increased prognathism and forward mandibular rotation described in Chapter 4, together with restricting forces from the lips, prevents any increase in arch perimeter.[17] As the apical regions move downwards and forwards with growth, the soft tissue influence may be one of the factors responsible for the increase in interincisal angle.[18]

Another factor that may contribute to incisor crowding is continuing mesial drift of buccal teeth. The cause of mesial drift is not fully understood, but due to the mesial inclination of upper and lower teeth the vertical occlusal forces of occlusion produce an anterior component of force. Added to this, the erupting third molars may exert a forward pressure on the other teeth as they attempt to gain the arch; but late incisor crowding can still occur where third molars are missing.

REFERENCES

1. Friel S. (1954) The development of ideal occlusion of the gum pads and the teeth. *Am. J. Orthodont.* **40**; 196.
2. Chapman H. (1935) The normal dental arch and its changes from birth to adult. *Br. Dent. J.* **58**; 201.
3. Sillman J. H. (1951) Serial study of good occlusion from birth to twelve years. *Am. J. Orthodont.* **37**; 481.
4. Leighton B. C. (1968) Some observations on vertical development and the dentition. *Proc. R. Soc. Med.* **61**; 1273–7.
5. Leighton B. C. (1969) The early signs of malocclusion. *Trans. Eur. Orthodont. Soc.* pp. 353–68.
6. Leighton B. C. (1971) The value of prophecy in orthodontics. *Dent. Practit.* **21**; 359–72.
7. Foster T. D. and Hamilton M. C. (1969) Occlusion in the primary dentition. *Br. Dent. J.* **126**; 76–9.
8. Foster T. D., Hamilton M. C. and Lavelle C. L. B. (1969) Dentition and dental arch dimensions in British children at the age of 2 to 3 years. *Arch. Oral Biol.* **14**; 1031–40.
9. Clinch L. M. (1954) Analysis of serial models between three and eight years of age. *Dent. Rec.* **71**; 61–72.

10. Moorrees C. F. A. (1959) *The Dentition of the Growing Child*. Cambridge, Mass., Harvard University Press.
11. Tulley W. J. (1962) Electromyographic study of the orofacial muscles in relation to the occlusion of the teeth and the form of the jaws. PhD Thesis, University of London.
12. Baume L. J. (1950) Physiological tooth migration and its significance for the development of occlusion. *J. Dent. Res.* **29**; 123.
13. Bonnar M. E. (1956) Aspects of the transition from deciduous to permanent dentition. *Dent. Practit.* **7**; 42.
14. Angle E. H. (1898) *Malocclusion of the Teeth*. Philadelphia, S. S. White Dental Manufacturing Co.
15. Björk A. (1951) Discussion on the significance of growth changes in facial pattern and their relationship to changes in occlusion. *Dent. Rec.* **71**; 197.
16. Lande M. J. (1952) Growth behaviour of the human bony facial profile as revealed by serial cephalometric roentgenology. *Angle Orthodont.* **22**; 78.
17. Brodie A. G. (1940) Some recent observations on the growth of the face and their implications to the orthodontist. *Am. J. Orthodont.* **26**; 471.
18. Tulley W. J. (1957) Observations on the path of eruption of the incisors. *Trans. Eur. Orthodont. Soc.* pp. 279–89.

Chapter 3

The Normal Development of Oral Function

The mouth performs a wide range of functions and recent research has highlighted the complexity of these even in the newborn. In textbooks describing the detailed physiology and anatomy of the oral cavity there is little reference to the development of the various oral functions as the child grows and matures. The dental practitioner needs to know something of these milestones in development if he is to appreciate where oral function deviates from the norm to the point of being a problem in the treatment of a malocclusion.

Oral and related functions are discussed under eight headings: (1) Breathing—airway maintenance and mandibular posture. (2) Mechanisms of obtaining an anterior oral seal. (3) Exploration of objects. (4) Feeding: suckle feeding; spoon feeding; mastication; swallowing. (5) Speech. (6) Facial expression. (7) Mandibular positions and paths of closure. (8) Occlusal function.

BREATHING—AIRWAY MAINTENANCE AND MANDIBULAR POSTURE

The newborn infant is essentially a nasal breather. The lips may be just together or slightly parted. The upper lip and facial musculature are rather flaccid and immobile compared with the more active lower lip. Breathing is evoked spontaneously at birth and, if the infant is to survive, a posture of the mandible and hyoid bone must be established to ensure that the airway is maintained well before full development of the reflexes that enable the child to orientate its head in space. Some children born with so-called 'micrognathia' may not in fact have a very small mandible, but the reflex mechanism required to establish this essential postural position is immature and the tongue can fall back and obstruct the airway if the child is not carefully nursed and safeguarded.

The laryngeal skeleton is high in the neck and there is a close relationship between the dorsum of the tongue, the soft palate and the epiglottis, which makes oral breathing extremely difficult (*Fig.* 3.1). The newborn baby has to learn to mouth breathe. Any temporary stoppage of the nasal airway embarrasses respiration and if this happens the majority of newborn infants will only gasp irregularly or cry. A small percentage fail to breathe through their mouth at all; this may be a factor in the Sudden Infant Death Syndrome (Cot Death).

The infant's tongue fills most of the oral cavity and is in contact laterally with the cheeks and anteriorly with the lower lip. The tongue is blunt and the tip develops later coincident with the need for increasing mobility. The tongue has a

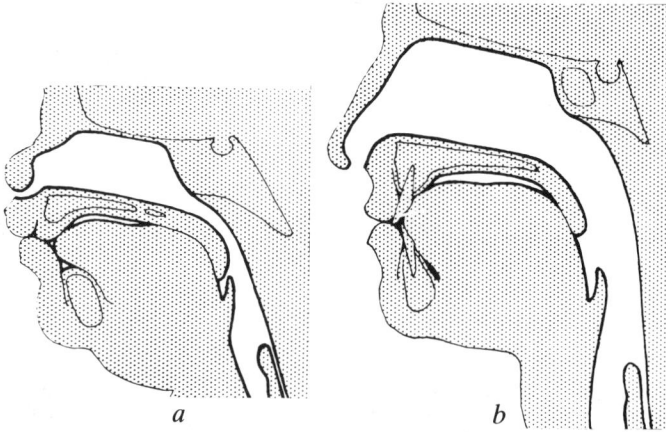

Fig. 3.1. Sagittal section of the head of an infant compared with that of an adult showing how the epiglottis descends relative to the soft palate with growth. Note the posterior oral seal between tongue and soft palate.

strong sensory affinity for the lower lip—if the lip is drawn forwards, the tongue follows.

As the child grows, the laryngeal skeleton descends in the neck and although the tongue remains in contact with the soft palate the glottic opening is no longer in close proximity to the uvula (*Fig.* 3.1).

The mandible takes up a definite postural position in relation to the maxilla in the first 6 months of life, as the child gains control over the muscles supporting its head and back and sits up. The gum pads at this stage are separated widely at rest. With eruption of deciduous teeth and development of the alveolar processes, the space between the jaws is taken up until the teeth come to lie 2–3 mm apart when the mandible is in the rest position.[1]

Mandibular posture changes with the position of the head and the true resting posture should be examined when the subject is looking straight ahead while sitting or standing upright. Movements of the mandible are described as starting from the 'rest position', and closure from rest into a fully occluded position of the teeth should be a simple hinge movement.

Normal mandibular posture is referred to as the 'innate' or 'inbuilt posture' to distinguish it from habitual postural positions which may develop to compensate for skeletal and dental variations.

The facial and lingual musculature take no active part in normal breathing. The lips should be together at rest without conscious contraction of the orbicular sphincter and the tongue and soft palate are in contact. Many children have lips that are too short or flaccid to achieve lip seal without conscious effort (*Fig.* 3.2), but they do not necessarily breathe through the mouth, as contact of the tongue and palate forms a secondary sphincter which closes off the airway (*Fig.* 3.1), and there may also be an adaptive anterior oral seal.

The term 'lip incompetence' is used to describe lips that are anatomically too short to effect a seal without circumoral contraction when the mandible is in the rest position. In cases where a patient is a true mouth breather, the lips may not be 'incompetent' but merely habitually held apart. When nasal obstruction is relieved, a lip seal may or may not be established immediately.[2] Where the lips

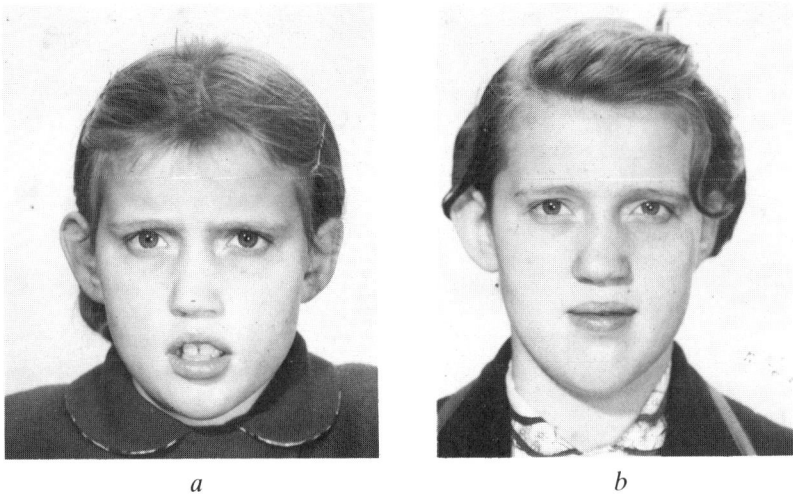

a   b

Fig. 3.2. a, This patient has incompetent lips which are habitually parted. She does not mouth breathe because there is an adaptive anterior oral seal and the posterior oral seal is patent. b, This girl has a Class II skeletal pattern and incompetent lips but postures the mandible forwards to obtain a lip seal.

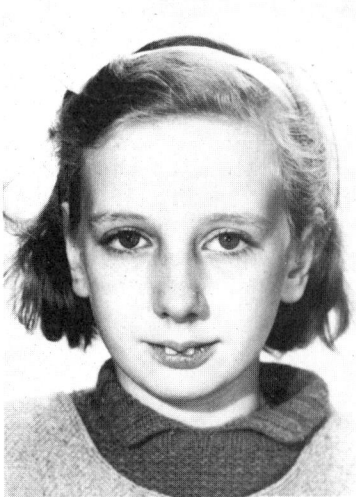

Fig. 3.3. The lips are potentially competent, being separated by the teeth. When the overjet is reduced, a lip seal will be obtained.

are separated by the incisor teeth, but will come together at rest when the dental interference is removed, they may be described as 'potentially competent' (Fig. 3.3). Approximately 50 per cent of English children at the age of 11 years have some degree of lip incompetence.

Mouth breathing can have some effects on the occlusion. The mandible is postured downwards and the tongue is lowered, affecting the muscular balance of the teeth. Thus the upper arch tends to be narrow and the upper incisors to be proclined. Quite dramatic malocclusions occur in monkeys when the nasal airway is blocked[3] but in children with chronic nasal obstruction it has been

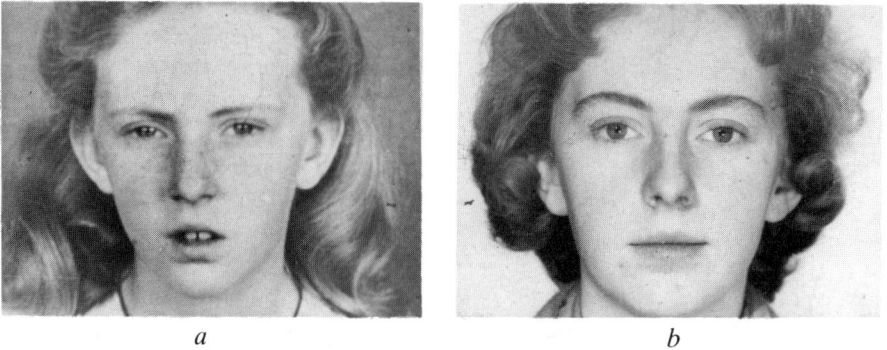

Fig. 3.4. a, A patient with so-called 'adenoidal' facies; in fact she does not breathe through her mouth. b, With increasing age, the facial musculature has matured and there is a habitual lip seal.

found that there are only minor changes in the occlusion and these can be reversed when the obstruction is relieved. There seems to be little effect on facial growth. In fact, chronic nasal obstruction is not very common and most children with habitually parted lips breathe through their noses. An adaptive anterior oral seal is formed between tongue and lower lip and there is usually a posterior seal between tongue and soft palate. Too much importance has been attached to mouth breathing as an aetiological factor in maldevelopment of the face and occlusion (*Fig.* 3.4.)

MECHANISMS OF OBTAINING AN ANTERIOR ORAL SEAL

Most adults and many children maintain a lip seal with little or no circumoral contraction. Habitually parted lips are more common in young children than in adults. This may be due in part to differential growth in lip length and lower facial height, but can also be attributed to a greater self-awareness in adults who achieve a lip seal as a matter of habit, even though some muscular effort is required.

Where the lips are parted, either because they are too short or because the incisal overjet is large, an adaptive oral seal will usually be produced by contact of the lower lip with the tongue or with the mucosa palatal to the upper incisors. In some cases with an increased overjet the mandible is postured forwards to facilitate a lip seal (*see Fig.* 3.2b).[4, 5]

EXPLORATION OF OBJECTS

In the infant, mouthing is one of the main methods of exploration. Objects are placed in the mouth to gain a sense of size and shape in what is known as the 'hand-to-mouth behaviour' and which continues for most of the first year; harmful objects must thus be kept out of the child's reach. How the child learns to appreciate shapes and how coordination of eyes and hands takes over is shown in *Fig.* 3.5. Mouth exploration remains important even after quite skilful coordination is attained.[6]

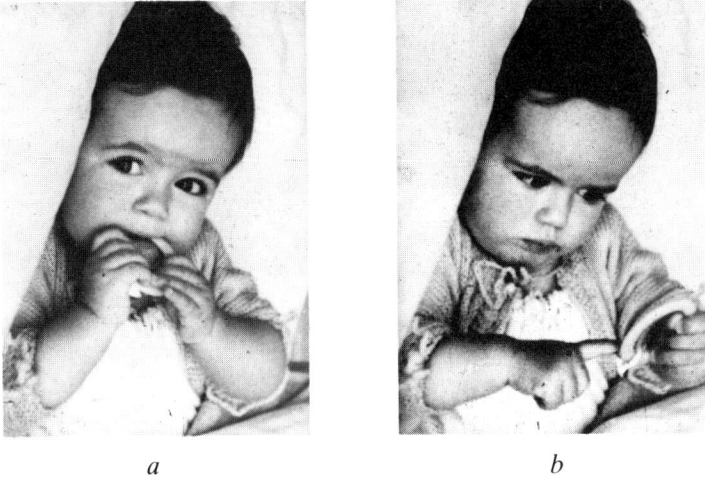

a   *b*

Fig. 3.5. The young infant explores objects with mouth, hands and eyes.

Sucking of a finger or thumb is very common in the infant, who appears to derive comfort and pleasure from the habit. It is of little importance at this age and its role in the aetiology of malocclusion has been overemphasized in the past.

Although the deciduous dental arches may be malformed by persistent sucking, reflecting the way in which the force is exerted (*Fig.* 3.6), many children give up the habit before the eruption of permanent teeth—and many habits do not have the intensity or duration to cause malformation. Sucking habits are only one of the factors that may deflect the permanent incisors from their path of eruption. It is better to regard them as a normal feature of infant behaviour, certainly up to the age of 3 years. Chapter 9 contains more detailed discussion of

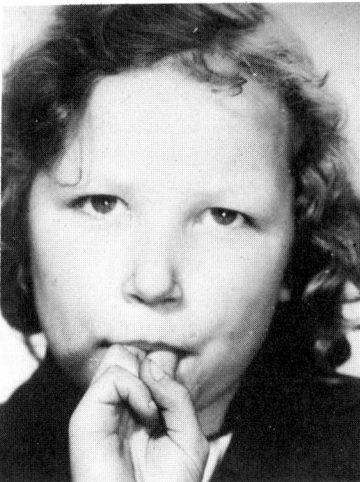

Fig. 3.6. A typical finger-sucking habit.

the clinical significance and methods of treatment of malocclusions resulting from prolonged sucking habits.

FEEDING

Suckling

Infant feeding takes place by the rhythmic pumping action known as 'suckling'. In the first few days after birth the lips are not readily poised, but a primitive rooting reflex exists and when the child is nursed it turns its head naturally to the breast. When a child is fed naturally, the nipple and areola are grasped between the upper gum pad and the dorsum of the tongue, which comes forwards over the lower gum pad. The lips form a seal and the mouth cavity is enlarged as the jaw is lowered. The central portion of the tongue is deeply grooved anteroposteriorly and its edges are everted. When the tongue is raised anteriorly this groove is obliterated from before backwards, followed by firm elevation of the jaws. The nipple is considerably extended and taken well back into the mouth and the squeezing action is completed by contraction of the floor of the mouth. This action is called 'suckling' to differentiate it from 'sucking' which is the creation of an intra-oral negative pressure.[7] In suckling, an intra-oral negative pressure is created by the depression of the mandible at one stage of the cycle, but there is also a pumping and squeezing action which is typical of 'milking'.

There is no evidence that the jaws and dental arches of the bottle-fed child will be smaller or less well related than those of the breast-fed child. Post-normal occlusion is equally common among breast- and bottle-fed children and the adverse mechanical effects of artificial feeding have been greatly exaggerated.

Spoon Feeding and Weaning

Mixed feeding begins at between 4 and 6 months of age. At this time the lips are becoming more active. Lip activity manifests itself in a spluttering kind of lip play, which delights the parents.

The lips are not poised when first presented with a spoon. The tongue movements are still primitive and the infant tries to suckle food from the spoon (*Fig.* 3.7). The lips are not able to keep food entirely within the mouth and the food leaks out and runs down the chin. Between 4 and 6 months of age coordination of lip movements brings about a change in feeding pattern. The child soon begins to pout and smack the lips and the upper lip is drawn over the spoon. The child learns to suck in semi-solid food and to sip from a cup. The lower lip also becomes more active and is drawn in to prevent escape of food. This makes the mother's task in feeding the child considerably easier. Swallowing takes place with the gum pads widely separated.

Mastication

This complex pattern of movements is used to move food about the mouth, to break it up and insalivate it preparatory to swallowing. Premasticatory movements of the mandible can be seen before the eruption of teeth. These are at first mainly vertical but protrusive movements occur with the eruption of deciduous

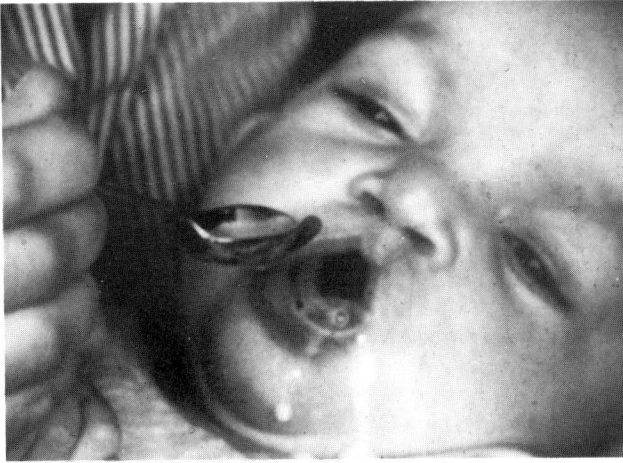

Fig. 3.7. Weaning. Note the primitive sucking action of the tongue when first presented with a spoon. Lip activity facilitates spoon feeding.

canines and lateral movements follow, becoming more purposeful with the eruption of the deciduous molars. The infant pattern of chewing becomes well defined by the end of the first year. By 18 months the child is able to enjoy meat and tougher foods and lateral excursions of the jaw are more marked. Chewing is a complicated process which requires effortful attention. The 2-year-old child chews more automatically, and by 3 years the pattern is comparatively mature.

There is considerable variation in mastication from one individual to another. It is modified according to the particular occlusion of the teeth, to the relationship of the jaws and to the form of the articular surfaces of the temporomandibular joint. Mastication requires practice, but is probably built up on an underlying innate coordinating pattern which once established does not require concentrated attention.[8]

Mastication can be divided into two main phases: the biting or incision of food, and its comminution.

Soft foods are taken into the mouth by the action of the lips. In eating tougher foods that have not been artificially prepared, portions are bitten off, using the incisor teeth as shears. Two processes are at work: holding food by the incisors and canines and tearing a portion away, and an incisive stroke which bites the food cleanly. The tearing of food is reminiscent of our animal ancestry.

The portion of food taken into the mouth is further comminuted before being subjected to the complex milling process of chewing. The dorsum of the tongue acts as a conveyor belt and pushes the food towards the occlusal surfaces of the premolar and molar teeth. The food is at the same time insalivated and prepared for swallowing.

The cheeks and lips contract rhythmically to scoop food from the buccal sulcus and to keep it between the teeth. During chewing the supporting tissues of the teeth are protected from undue stress by a reflex mechanism involving receptors in the periodontal tissues. Occlusal disharmonies bring about a change in the masticatory pattern and major adaptations may occur without serious loss of efficiency.

Swallowing

In the infant the peristaltic type of action during suckling produces a stream of milk which passes down lateral channels on either side of the larynx and is prevented from entering it by a flap valve mechanism operating between the soft palate and dorsum of the tongue. The high position of the epiglottis behind the soft palate may enable suckling to occur without cessation of breathing. However, some authorities have described a discrete swallow with nasopharyngeal closure after two or three suckling movements.

Swallowing in the weaned infant does not follow the same pattern as in the older child or adult. Teeth are not yet present or are just erupting and the gum pads are widely separated. Food is scooped directly on to the dorsum of the tongue. The tip has developed and this facilitates the movement of food about the mouth. As food is passed back into the oropharynx, the gum pads do not come together and the lips and cheeks contract to meet the spread tongue.

As deciduous teeth erupt and the alveolar processes develop, the mouth becomes divided into the vestibule and the oral cavity proper. Alveolar bone and teeth now form the anterior and lateral rigid boundaries to the oral cavity when the teeth are occluded. Occlusion of the teeth during swallowing becomes more frequent and the lips usually play a progressively less important part in the swallowing of masticated food and saliva.

Swallowing action can be divided into three phases:[9, 10] first, the intra-oral mechanism by which the food is transferred from the anterior to the posterior part of the mouth; secondly, the passage of food through the isthmus of the fauces into the oropharynx; and thirdly, the movement of food down the oesophagus. The intra-oral phase of swallowing is of particular interest to the orthodontist and differs in detail according to the type of food and the state in which it is swallowed.

The term 'basic swallow' refers to the swallowing of saliva, an activity which occurs at frequent intervals through the day and night.[11, 12] The intra-oral phase of swallowing may be divided into two stages: the first is the action that moves the substance to be swallowed posteriorly and the second, or 'mylohyoid phase', transfers the food into the oropharynx. Fluids taken into the mouth are swept on to the dorsum of the tongue and held in a groove formed by the eversion of the lateral margins and depression of the centre. This trough is obliterated from before backwards by progressive contraction of the transverse muscle fibres and the fluid is thus moved into the swallow–preparatory position on the posterior aspect of the dorsum of the tongue. For the 'mylohyoid phase' or second stage of swallowing the teeth are normally occluded to fix the mandible, allowing a firm base for the contraction of the mylohyoid muscles elevating the floor of the mouth. The tongue is compressed against the palate and the lateral and anterior rigid walls of the cavity formed by the teeth and alveolar processes.

Semi-solid food is usually insalivated to a paste and so rarely is there a true bolus. This paste is collected on the dorsum of the tongue and massaged against the palate.

During sipping from a cup, the teeth are not occluded and the tongue acts as a simple conveyor belt in the floor of the mouth; fluid is sucked on to the tongue by the creation of an intra-oral negative pressure.

The teeth are not firmly occluded when swallowing soft and succulent foods. The pattern of swallowing here is similar to that used by the infant: the lips and cheeks contract to resist the spread of the tongue and the swallow is more in the nature of a gulp. Although swallowing is usually accompanied by firm occlusion of the teeth, there are wide variations.

Atypical Swallowing Patterns

Various atypical swallowing actions have been described and related to different forms of malocclusion.[13–15] It was thought that the 'tooth-apart swallow', where lip activity is increased, was a factor restricting the development of the dental arches during growth. This view is no longer tenable because it is the interplay of the lingual, labial and buccal tissues, both in form and in resting posture, that dictates the arch perimeter.

Two principal atypical swallowing patterns are of clinical importance— adaptive and endogenous.

Adaptive patterns of swallowing are particularly common where the lips are incompetent and there is a Class II, division 1 incisor relationship. The anterior oral seal is formed by contact between the lower lip or the tongue and the palatal mucosa. Swallowing takes place with the teeth parted and if the tongue habitually lies over the lower incisor edges, the overbite will be incomplete, but only to a small extent. In some cases with a Class II, division 1 incisor relationship the mandible is postured forwards to enable a lip seal to be obtained, and again swallowing will take place with the teeth parted.

Other adaptations of swallowing behaviour are found when there is an incomplete overbite or anterior open bite due, for example, to a digit-sucking habit or to skeletal factors. The tongue will generally ooze forwards to fill the gap and may contribute to the anterior oral seal. These many variations of swallowing behaviour are interesting and should be noted during orthodontic case assessment, but in general they do not impose limitations on the treatment of the malocclusion.

Endogenous atypical swallowing behaviour is an unusual condition associated with a rather forcible primary tongue thrust. This is not a habit activity and cannot be modified effectively. The thrusting of the tongue results in upper incisor proclination and a substantially incomplete overbite. Recognition of a true primary tongue thrust is important because overjet reduction will relapse under its influence. There are no definite guidelines but the tongue seems to be particularly active in speech, circumoral contraction during swallowing is greater than would be expected from the degree of lip incompetence and the overbite is incomplete to a substantial extent, usually without any other obvious explanation such as digit-sucking or a large lower facial height.

SPEECH

The first sounds made at birth are those of a 'baby cry'. At 1 month throaty noises are produced and by 2–3 months vowel sounds start to be used in 'conversations' which have many of the rhythms and pacing of normal speech. Between 6 and 7 months of age babies of different language groups start to show distinguishable differences in sound usage. Syllables with plosive consonants preceding vowels are made, coincident with increased lip play in feeding. These are soon collected together to give the typical 'dada', 'baba', etc. Although these sounds bring delight to fond parents, they have no meaning. By repetition and by copying parents and older children sounds begin to take on a meaning. By 1 year the infant may use several simple words and understand many more. Similarly, articulation may precede understanding by 'parrotting' of words or phrases. At between 15 months and 2 years a child has his own jargon, and by 2 years can put several words together. He talks incessantly and is quick to imitate.

Speech may be an acquired skill, but is none the less built up on underlying coordinating patterns of motor activity. It is a complicated process involving the production of basic notes in the larynx, known as 'phonation', and modification of these by changing the shape of the cavities in the mouth, nose and throat, which is known as 'articulation'. Although there are classic descriptions of the position of the tongue and other articulating elements in various speech sounds, there is considerable individual variation, particularly when taking into consideration the variations in the shape and size of the oral cavity. The different ways in which sounds are put together in connected speech determine the articulatory movements,

Speech, being an acquired behaviour, is susceptible to the influence of bad habits. For normal speech it is important to have normal receptor mechanisms (good hearing), normal central connections and normal effector mechanisms. The special case of cleft palate is one problem that comes within the sphere of influence of the orthodontist (see Chapter 20).

Some children have a degree of tongue-tie which is not a problem in the development of speech. Most paediatricians recommend that this should be ignored, except when the ability to cleanse the mouth naturally is markedly impaired.

It has been shown that a malocclusion is rarely the primary cause of a speech defect and conversely that speech defects are rarely the cause of a malocclusion. From the practical viewpoint an interdental lisp will disappear if it is merely an immature behaviour associated with a transient sucking habit.[16-19]

Some children appear to have a tongue that is less agile in performing the delicate movements required for certain speech sounds, of which the 'S' sound is one of the more precise. Children with difficulties in coordinating speech may also have difficulties in coordinating other body movements.

FACIAL EXPRESSION

It has already been pointed out that in the newborn infant the facial musculature, particularly that of the middle third of the face, is rather flaccid; the lips may be just resting together or slightly parted and the upper lip is everted. Lip posture at this time does not relate closely to the future situation as the child grows and develops. Quite early expressive movements become meaningful and the face becomes more animated. Facial expression depends to some extent on the shape and configuration of the soft tissues.

The muscles of facial expression, varying as they do in anatomical configuration, also relate to the underlying bony structure. For example, where there is a retrusive mandible there may be a rather taut lower lip musculature, so that in

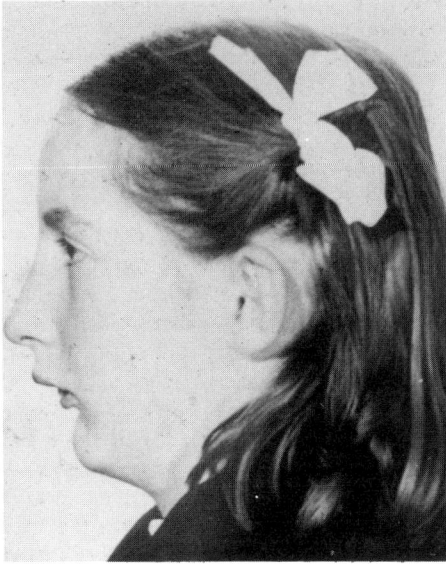

Fig. 3.8. The very tight lower lip with a sling-like action under the upper incisors makes orthodontic correction of the associated Class II, division 1 incisor relationship problematic.

expressive behaviour this may be drawn up in the form of a tight sling under the upper incisors (*Fig.* 3.8). Such activity may make for considerable difficulty in correcting the overjet.

MANDIBULAR POSITIONS AND PATHS OF CLOSURE

When the mandible is habitually postured forwards there may be an upwards and backwards path of closure into centric occlusion, rather than simple hinge closure. This is a mandibular deviation. It is important to distinguish mandibular deviations from displacement, because the former are not associated with muscle or joint pain, whereas the latter may be.

Mandibular displacements are caused by premature contacts of the teeth which enforce a shift of the mandible to obtain a position of maximum occlusion. With a lateral displacement such as is produced by a unilateral crossbite (*see Fig.* 10.5) the position of maximal intercuspation is not one of centric relation. An anterior displacement may be caused by one or more instanding upper incisors. When all the incisors are instanding, the displacement is often associated with overclosure of the mandible, because the control of muscular contraction is disturbed and the occlusion is established with an overclosed position of the mandible. Posterior mandibular displacements are quite rare in an unmutilated dentition but can be found in Class II, division 2 cases where posterior teeth have been lost.

Mandibular displacements are associated with quite severe disruption of the pattern of activity of the muscles of mastication which will often lead to pain and dysfunction in the long term. Treatment to eliminate the displacement is important.

OCCLUSAL FUNCTION

The occlusion of the teeth, the temporomandibular joints and the muscles of mastication should function harmoniously during mandibular movements. At rest, the mandible should be in a position of centric relation with the condyles in maximally retruded, unstrained positions within the glenoid fossae. Closure from rest to occlusion should be a hinge movement. There is often a slight anterior shift of up to 1 mm between the terminal hinge position and centric occlusion and this is perfectly acceptable. A larger anterior shift or a lateral movement due to cuspal guidance is a displacement that may lead to muscular dysharmony and tenderness.

When the mandible is protruded, with the teeth held lightly in occlusion, it moves downwards: it moves anteriorly as a result of incisal guidance and posteriorly as a result of condylar guidance, and this should result in disclusion of the cheek teeth. An incisor malrelationship may mean that this does not happen smoothly. For example, with a Class III incisor relationship or an anterior open bite incisal guidance is lacking, and with a Class II incisor relationship incisal guidance may be abrupt.

In lateral excursions of the mandible, the condyle on the working side rotates and moves laterally by up to 1 mm—the Bennett movement. The non-working side condyle moves forwards and downwards on the articular eminence. On the working side, there should be either canine guidance or group function (*see Fig. 1.3*) of the occlusion. In an occlusion with canine guidance, all teeth except the canines are out of occlusion in lateral excursion. In an occlusion with group function, all or most of the teeth on the working side are in contact during lateral excursions (the buccal cusps of the lower teeth slide down the palatal surfaces of the buccal cusps of the upper teeth until a cusp-to-cusp relationship is obtained; the lingual cusps do not usually contact). Both canine guidance and group functions are perfectly satisfactory. In some occlusions, for example with a Class II, division 2 incisor relationship, where the overbite is very deep, lateral excursions are very limited due to incisor locking. These patients chew with a chopping movement of the mandible and with little lateral excursion, but this does not seem to be a problem for the patient.

The teeth on the non-working side should not contact in lateral excursion. Non-working side contacts create appreciable occlusal disturbances and may be associated with muscle and joint problems.

For the orthodontist, these simple guidelines will generally suffice for the evaluation of occlusal function before and after treatment. Wear facets or articulating paper can reveal premature or non-working side contacts. Where orthodontic treatment is undertaken in conjunction with occlusal rehabilitation in an adult, a more detailed analysis of occlusal function may be necessary, with the help of models mounted on an adjustable articulator.

It should be remembered that some rebound often follows orthodontic treatment and that long-term minor occlusal changes occur for as long as facial growth continues. Thus orthodontic treatment must be planned to produce an occlusion that will settle well and will be stable. Occlusal objectives may vary with different treatment approaches. With edgewise appliances, for example, rather precise tooth positioning with little need for settling is the objective. Many practitioners using the Begg technique deliberately over-treat arch mal-relationships and deep overbites to allow for rebound and settling. Provided that this has been well judged, the tooth contacts will guide the settling so that an excellent occlusion results, just as happens in a developing normal occlusion where tooth contacts guide the erupting teeth.

REFERENCES

1. Thompson J. R. and Brodie A. G. (1946) The rest position of the mandible and its significance to dental science. *J. Am. Dent. Assoc.* **33**; 151.
2. Gwynne-Evans E. (1951) Organisation of the orofacial muscles in relation to breathing and feeding. *Br. Dent. J.* **91**; 125.
3. Harvold E., Chierici G. and Vargervik K. (1972) Experiments on the development of dental malocclusions. *Am. J. Orthodont.* **61**; 38–44.
4. Ballard C. F. (1962) The clinical significance of innate and adaptive postures and motor behaviour. *Dent. Practit.* **12**; 219.
5. Ballard C. F. (1955) Consideration of the physiological background of mandibular posture and movement. *Dent. Practit.* **6**; 80.
6. Gesell A. (1942) Morphologies of mouth and mouth behaviour. *Am. J. Orthodont.* **28**; 367.
7. Ardran G. M. and Lind J. (1958) A cine-radiographic study of breast-feeding. *Br. J. Radiol.* **31**; 156.
8. Ahlgren, J. (1976) Masticatory movements in man. In: *Mastication.* Bristol, Wright, pp.119–30.
9. Whillis J. W. (1946) Movements of the tongue in deglutition. *Trans. Br. Soc. Orthodont.* pp. 121–9.
10. Ardran G. M. and Kemp F. H. (1951) The mechanism of swallowing. *Proc. R. Soc. Med.* **44**; 1038.
11. Lear C. S. C., Flanagan J. B. jun. and Moorrees C. F. A. (1963) The frequency of deglutition in man. *Arch. Oral Biol.* **10**; 1.
12. Rix R. E. (1946) Deglutition and the teeth. *Dent. Rec.* **66**; 105.
13. Rix R. E. (1948) Deglutition. 25th Annual Congress of the European Orthodontic Society, July 1948. *Trans. Euro. Orthodont. Soc.* p. 191.
14. Rogers J. H. (1961) Swallowing patterns of a normal population sample compared to those of patients from an orthodontic practice. *Am. J. Orthodont.* **47**; 674.
15. Cleall J. F. (1964) Deglutition–a study of form and function. DDS Thesis, University of New Zealand.
16. Hopkin G. B. and McEwen J. D. (1955) Speech and the orthodontist. *Dent. Practit.* **6**; 123.
17. Vig P. S. (1973) Evolutionary concepts relating to language and the morphology of the oral complex. *Trans. Europ. Orthodont. Soc.* p. 527.
18. Fawcus R. (1966) An investigation into lingual sensory motor skills in children and adults with normal speech. *Dent. Practit.* **17**; 70.
19. Subtelny J. G. and Subtelny J. (1962) Malocclusion, speech and deglutition. *Am. J. Orthodont.* **48**; 685.

ADDITIONAL READING

Dubner R., Sessle B. J. and Storey A. T. (1978) *The Neural Basis of Oral and Facial Function.* New York, Plenum Press.
Friel E. S. (1926) An investigation into the relation of function and form (malocclusion). *Br. Dent. J.* **47**; 353.
Huber E. (1931) *Evolution of Facial Musculature and Facial Expression.* Baltimore, Md., Johns Hopkins Press.

Lowe A. A. and Sessle B. J. (1973) Tongue activity during respiration, jaw opening and swallowing in the cat. *Can. J. Physiol. Pharmacol.* **51**; 1009–11.

Luffingham J. K. (1966) Intraoral pressures. PhD Thesis, University of London.

Moss J. P. (1980) The soft tissue environment of teeth and jaws. An experimental and clinical study. Parts 2 and 3. *Br. J. Orthodont.* **7**; 205–16.

Peat J. H. (1968) A cephalometric study of tongue position. *Am. J. Orthodont.* **54**; 339–51.

Perry J. T. (1954) Role of the neuromuscular system in functional activity of the mandible. *J. Am. Dent. Assoc.* **48**; 665.

Sims F. W. (1958) The pressure exerted on the maxillary and mandibular central incisors by the perioral and lingual musculature in acceptable occlusion. *Am. J. Orthodont.* **44**, 64–5.

Tulley W. J. (1963) The development of the orofacial musculature *Clin. Development. Med.,* 13.

Tulley W. J. (1964) The tongue, that unruly member. *Dent. Practit.* **15**; 27.

Chapter 4

Facial Growth

The control of growth of an organism or tissue depends on the interaction between genetic (the genotype) and environmental factors. The result of this interaction is the phenotype. For cells, the environment includes all influences external to them, including tissue fluids and other cells. The genetic control of growth of one organ may influence growth of another and so some genetic factors act indirectly: they are known as epigenetic factors. The extent of environmental influences depends on the tissue under consideration and on the severity of these external effects, while the nature of response of the cells is genetically determined.

Any organ or tissue requires an adequate level of nutrition and an appropriate hormonal balance if growth is to be within normal limits: nutritional deprivation and hormonal deficiencies stunt growth. However, given favourable environmental conditions, many features of the individual are determined largely by genetic factors. For example, the ultimate stature of a child and its general physical constitution are affected little by normal variations in environmental conditions. However, other features (for example fat deposition and muscle growth) are very sensitive to environmental variation, although individual differences in response are under genetic control. Thus the observed characteristics of the individual depend on a complex interplay between genetic and environmental influences.

The elucidation of the relative importance of genetic and environmental factors is difficult and in the field of craniofacial growth many of the problems are still unresolved. Information has been derived from experiments on animals where the external conditions can be varied in a controlled manner and the response observed; from clinical investigations of the effects of different forms of treatment in children; and from studies of families and of twins in an attempt to assess the heritability of different features. A few of the obvious problems of interpreting such information are that findings in experimental animals may not be applicable directly to other species; human variability in growth makes the response to treatment difficult to discern; and in studies of the likeness of related individuals, environmental effects may be underestimated because the conditions within families tend to be rather similar.

The orthodontist is concerned with the interaction between genetic and environmental factors in determining facial growth for a number of reasons. If external factors have an effect on facial growth in general, and on jaw relationships in particular, they could be important in the aetiology of malocclusion and interception and prevention would have to be considered. For example, in the past, the role of bottle feeding of infants and of oral respiration have been considered important in the aetiology of malocclusion. It is now generally recognized that factors such as these have little or no influence on jaw malrelationships. Of equal interest is whether orthodontic treatment, as an environmental factor, is capable of influencing jaw growth or relationships. Clearly if jaw growth could be controlled, the treatment of many malocclusions would be simplified. The question here is not whether jaw and occlusal relationships are normally under genetic control, but to what extent the normal controlling factors can permanently be overridden by orthodontic appliances. The fact that certain occlusal relationships have a high hereditability does not mean that they cannot be changed by orthodontic means and permanence of the induced changes depends on the degree to which the natural controlling factors can adapt to the new tooth positions.

The complexity of the interaction between genetically determined and environmental factors makes discussion of the control of growth confusing except for the simplest circumstances, and it is clearer to talk in terms of intrinsic and extrinsic influences upon growth. The level of interest may be the cell, the structured tissue, the functional region or the entire organism. When speaking of the organism, extrinsic factors include environmental factors such as nutritional availability and exercise. At cellular level, extrinsic factors comprise nutritional and hormonal variations and interaction with other cells, which may in turn be influenced by genetic and environmental factors.

Intrinsic control implies that given common extrinsic factors, variation between individuals or within the one individual are determined at that level. For example, the epiphyses of the short bones of the hand (*see Fig.* 4.3) grow by different amounts and fuse at different times and these variations reflect differences in control intrinsic to the cartilages themselves.

In considering the extent to which a particular feature can be influenced by extrinsic factors, it is convenient to speak of the tightness of intrinsic control. Some features, for example blood groupings, are under tight intrinsic control at cellular level and are unaffected by even the severest environmental variations. At the other extreme are features that are more loosely controlled. Skin colour, at least in the Caucasian races, depends to a large extent on the amount of ultraviolet light to which it is exposed and a tan can be acquired or lost quite rapidly. However, different skin types respond in different manners to the same intensity and duration of exposure to light, and these differences are at least in part the result of intrinsic variation.

In considering craniofacial growth, the tissues of primary interest are bone and muscle.

BONE GROWTH

Bone grows either by replacement of cartilage or by periosteal activity, and these two processes differ in the extent of their intrinsic control at tissue level. Experimental results suggest that the amount of cartilage growth is under rather tight intrinsic control. The most convincing support for this comes from experiments where bones have been transplanted into different sites (e.g. spleen or brain). Noel and Wright[1] reported that when tail vertebrae from very young mice were transplanted, the amount of growth in length was at least as great as would normally have been expected; and Chalmers and Ray[2] found that tibiae from young mice transplanted into immunologically compatible litter mates grew in length to nearly the normal extent. It might have been expected that transplantation would have impeded growth through interference with the blood supply, and so these results indicate clearly that the amount of growth at epiphyseal plates is controlled primarily by factors within the cartilages themselves.

Epiphyseal bone growth is susceptible to some extrinsic influences: hormonal and nutritional deficiencies impair growth and it has been found that tension in the periosteum constrains epiphyseal growth to a small extent.[3] Presumably tensions in muscles, tendons and ligaments could have similar minor effects.

In contrast, periosteal activity is very susceptible to extrinsic influences. Pressure applied to the periosteum stimulates the appearance of osteoclasts and bone resorption occurs; whereas if the periosteum is pulled away from the bone surface, osteoblastic activity and bone formation follow. Control of periosteal activity is not, however, merely a simple matter of pressure and tension. Even under the one muscle attachment, adjacent areas of periosteum may be formative and resorptive. In order to maintain the form of a growing bone, complex patterns of periosteal bone formation and resorption occur and the mechanism of the control of these fields is obscure. Periosteum also responds to bone deformation. It has been known for centuries that a bone that had been fractured and healed in malalignment would gradually remodel towards its original form, and these observations were the basis of Wolff's 'Law of the Transformation of Bone'[4] which stated in abbreviated form that: 'wherever in a bone pressure and tension stresses are caused, bone formation takes place; but wherever relief from pressure or tension occurs, bone substance disappears'.

The link between the physical deformation of the bone and the biological response of the periosteum has been the subject of much speculation. Stress, strain and changes in surface curvature have all been suggested as crucial factors but none of these provides an adequate explanation.[5] More recently it has been suggested that changes in the surface electrical charge of the bone prompt the cellular response.[6] It is known that bone behaves as a piezo-electric material and that changes in surface charge do occur with deformation. A negative charge is associated with bone formation and a positive charge with bone resorption. It has also been found that the application of direct current to bone can promote remodelling and accelerate tooth movement,[7] but whether this is a specific effect or merely the result of perturbation of cellular activity,[8] as is also produced by magnetic fields, is not yet clear.

Sutures and periodontal ligaments can be regarded as periosteal modifications which respond to physical forces in a similar manner to periosteum: tension is associated with bone formation and compression with resorption, a phenomenon upon which orthodontic tooth movement depends.

MUSCLE GROWTH

The diameter of muscle fibres is determined by the work they undertake, and muscular development can be achieved by the appropriate exercises. The length of muscle fibres is affected by the distance through which they habitually have to contract.[9] If the range of action of a muscle is increased experimentally in the growing animal, the number of sarcomeres in the fibres may be increased: sarcomere contraction is determined by their structure and thus the potential range of action of a muscle fibre is determined by their number. Fibres may be arranged in series and so the shortening of the muscle may be greater than that of the individual fibre. Growth in length of a muscle and the separation by growth of its bony attachments must be coordinated. In most muscles, the fibres at one or both ends have a tendinous attachment. This may be a well-defined tendon or aponeurosis, or it may be in the form of discrete connective tissue fibres which are attached to the periosteum. This tendinous attachment provides a means of adjustment during growth between the length of muscle fibre or muscle belly, and the distance between its bony attachments.

GROWTH CHARACTERISTICS OF DIFFERENT TISSUE SYSTEMS

Different tissues and organs exhibit different patterns of growth. The classic work on this topic was undertaken by Scammon[10] who, on a cross-sectional basis, constructed growth curves for neural, lymphoid and general somatic tissues (*Fig.* 4.1). Most somatic tissues increase steadily throughout the period of growth, with a modest acceleration at the time of puberty and levelling off to a plateau soon after this. In contrast, tissues of neural origin such as brain and eyes are relatively advanced at the time of birth and reach a plateau soon after 6 years of age. This is relevant to growth of the calvarium and orbits because skeletal growth at these sites follows the pattern of growth of the neural tissues. Lymphoid tissues reach their maximum size in childhood and regress later. It is quite common therefore to find that partial nasal obstruction associated with adenoid enlargement improves during the adolescent period.

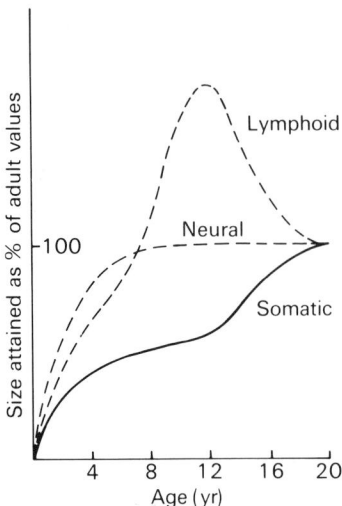

Fig. 4.1. Growth curves for different tissue systems. (After Scammon R. E. (1930) in Harris J. A. et al. (ed.) *The Measurement of Man.* University of Minnesota Press.)

GROWTH IN STATURE

Growth in stature has been investigated more thoroughly than has growth in facial dimensions, which follows a similar pattern; it is therefore useful to consider this first. Stature follows a general somatic curve of growth with a steady diminution in velocity after birth except for a brief reversal during the pubertal growth spurt (*Fig.* 4.2). After the peak of the pubertal spurt, growth declines rapidly. This is relevant to orthodontic treatment in that some aspects, such as overbite reduction, are much simpler while there is still appreciable facial growth than after growth has ceased.

The Pubertal Growth Spurt

On average, the peak of the growth spurt occurs at 12 years in girls and at 14 years in boys.[11] There is, however, appreciable individual variation, with a standard deviation of nearly 1 year. This means that in approximately two children out of three, the growth spurt will occur within 1 year of the average time, and in 19 out of 20 it will occur within 2 years of the average. The growth spurt is a manifestation of physical maturity and attempts have been made to identify other aspects of physical maturity that would give a better guide to the timing of the growth spurt. Skeletal age, estimated from the development stages of the bones of the hand and wrist (*Fig.* 4.3), has proved to be useful in helping to predict adult stature, but the correlation with the timing of the growth spurt

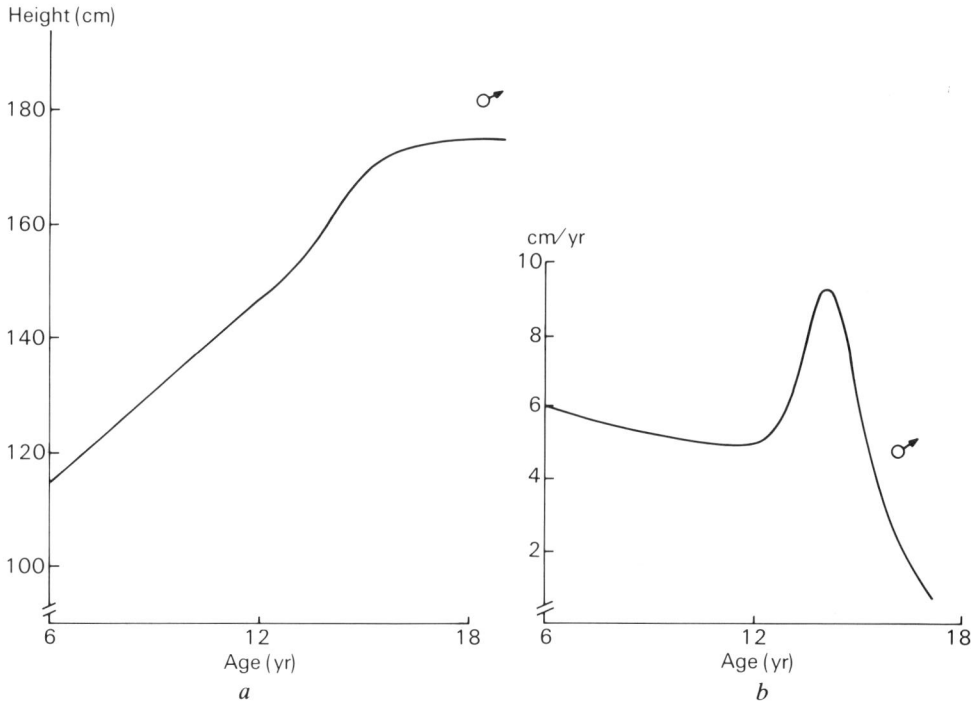

Fig. 4.2. Growth curves for stature. *a*, Height attained; *b*, Velocity.

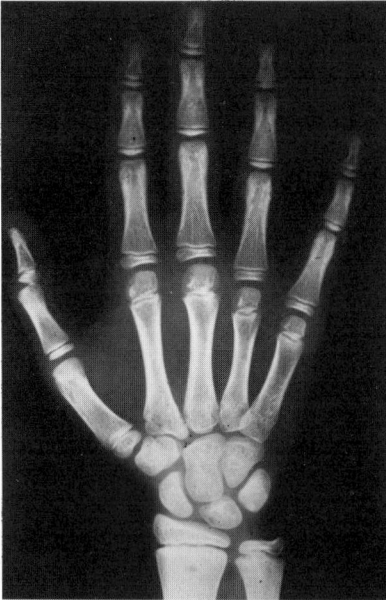

Fig. 4.3. A hand-wrist radiograph.

appears to be rather low and it is doubtful whether this offers a better basis for the timing of the growth spurt than does chronological age.[12] Dental development is not correlated with the timing of the pubertal growth spurt and so it is not of predictive value.[13] The secondary sex characteristics appear at the time of puberty but variations in their timing are not sufficiently well correlated with the timing of the growth spurt to be of practical predictive value. However, it has been found that menarche in girls and the change to adult voice characteristics in boys occur soon after the peak of the growth spurt[14] and so these features can reasonably be used to indicate whether or not this has passed.

It may be considered that there has been too much emphasis on the relationship of the timing of the growth spurt to orthodontic treatment. The relevant question in the treatment of patients where growth is important is whether or not an appreciable amount of growth can still be expected. Where growth would be helpful, such as in Class II cases where a deep overbite has to be reduced and where favourable growth changes might improve the skeletal pattern, it is probably best to proceed with treatment as soon as dental development justifies this. In most cases this will be when the upper permanent canines are just emerging. If dental development is retarded and the child has reached the average age of the peak of the growth spurt, treatment should be commenced in order at least to reduce the overbite while awaiting the eruption of more teeth. This is a problem only in severe Class II cases because milder occlusal problems can be managed without help from growth.

In some circumstances it is important to know that growth is virtually complete. Surgical correction of jaw malrelationships is usually delayed until after the pubertal spurt. In moderately severe Class III cases at the limits of orthodontic treatment it may be best to delay orthodontic intervention in case unfavourable facial growth changes occur which would take the malocclusion beyond the bounds of orthodontic correction. In a patient showing signs of having passed the peak of the growth spurt (adult voice in boys/menarche in girls) and who is gaining height at less than 7 cm per year, it can be concluded that growth is almost complete. This can also be confirmed from hand–wrist radiographs showing fusion of the radial and ulnar epiphyses. Facial growth continues at a very slow rate well into adult life and may be responsible for minor changes in incisor crowding. However, this is not relevant to the timing of orthodontic treatment or of orthognathic surgery.

SKULL GROWTH

The Calvarium

The calvarium comprises the bones and parts of bones that develop from the membranous coverings of the brain—the frontal, parietal and squamous parts of the temporals and occipital. In the fetus, ossification centres appear in the membranes covering the brain and the osseus territories expand until they meet. Some of these forming bones fuse while others remain separated by sutures, which may usefully be regarded as periosteal modifications. At birth the bony covering of the brain is incomplete (*Fig.* 4.4) and the remaining membranous areas are known as fontanelles. The bone margins extend to cover the fontanelles during the first year.

The factors determining the location and timing of fusion of the sutures are still obscure. The calvarial sutures lie over the different reflections in the dura mater and so tension in the membranous coverings of the brain during growth

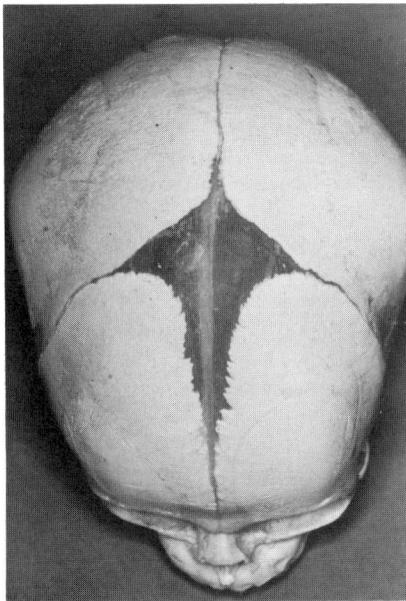

Fig. 4.4. Calvarium of a neonate. The fontanelles are areas where the bony covering is not yet complete.

may determine suture location.[15] Premature sutural fusion occurs in certain developmental abnormalities (e.g. Crouzon's syndrome) and fusion can be precipitated experimentally by transplanting periosteum across the suture or by glueing the adjacent bones together.[16] However, the factors determining normal suture fusion are not clear.

Soon after birth the bones of the calvarium are seen to consist of two plates, the outer and inner tables separated by cancellous bone, the diploae. The inner table follows the contours of the brain while the outer table becomes elevated into ridges according to the functional demands made upon it: the temporal and nuchal crests provide extended sites for muscle attachment, although in man they are not very prominent. The mastoid process similarly provides a site of muscle attachment and the supra-orbital ridges develop, possibly in response to the distribution of stresses in the calvarium generated by mastication and other muscular forces.

The calvarium is of little direct relevance to the orthodontist, but its structural and functional simplicity in comparison with other regions of the skull make it a useful model in which to investigate sutural and periosteal growth; moreover findings from this region have been applied by analogy, though not always wisely, to growth of the facial skeleton.

It is helpful to consider skeletal growth in terms of functional areas rather than anatomically individual bones. The calvarium incorporates the squamous parts of complex bones that also contribute to entirely distinct functional areas and the growth and control of these different parts of single bones is almost completely independent. For example, although the temporal bone has squamous and petrous parts, their functions and patterns of growth are quite distinct. The squamous part is more closely related to the other bones of the calvarium in its origin and control of growth than it is to the rest of the temporal bone.

There is good clinical and experimental evidence that the sutures of the calvarium have little if any independent growth potential:[17] growth at the sutures does not force apart the adjacent bones but rather the suture responds to external forces separating the bones, which in the calvarium are provided largely by the increase in volume of the brain and cerebrospinal fluid.[18] Nature's experiments of hydrocephaly, where the volume of cerebrospinal fluid is increased, and of microcephaly, where brain growth is deficient, demonstrate how sutural growth is augmented or diminished respectively. These conditions have been reproduced experimentally in animals, with similar effects on calvarial growth. It has also been demonstrated that when sutures are transferred to non-functional sites, no growth occurs,[17] while transplantation across an epiphysis results in growth in the suture to match that in the epiphyseal cartilaginous plate.[19] While growth of the sutural tissues may not be sufficient to generate the forces to separate the bones, the bone edges do have a certain independent growth potential: for example, when they are growing towards one another to form sutures, they do so at a rate greater than the separation of the bone edges due to brain growth, otherwise the suture would never be established!

The various ridges and surface modifications of the calvarium are the results of local periosteal activity. This is not a simple matter of muscular tension pulling out processes on the bone surface: the direction of growth is often opposite to that of a muscle pull, and below a single area of muscular attachment both apposition and resorption may be seen. Rather, the expansion of the muscle seems to promote an expansion of the local periosteal area, with the production of crests and ridges accordingly. Where the outer and inner tables diverge appreciably from one another, the intervening area may be pneumatized, as in the frontal sinus and mastoid air cells, which has the effect of maintaining strength without excessive weight.

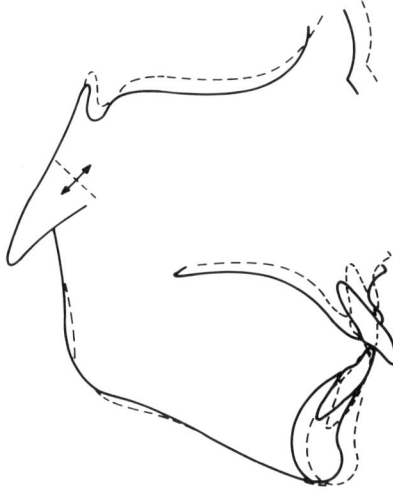

Fig. 4.5. Growth at the spheno-occipital synchondrosis carries the anterior cranial base upwards and forwards. The tracings are superimposed on the basi-occiput. Solid line, age 12 years; broken line, age 15 years.

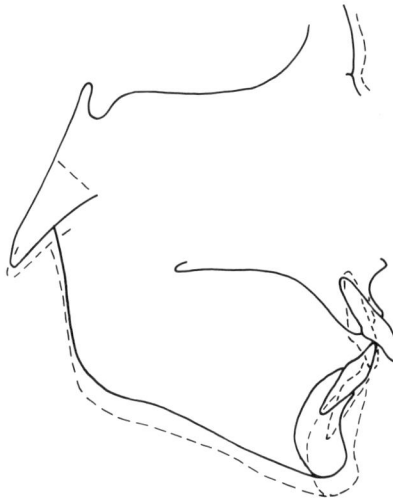

Fig. 4.6. The conventional method of superimposition of lateral skull radiographs on the structures of the anterior cranial base gives the impression that the mandible is displaced downwards and backwards with growth. Compare this picture with the alternative superimposition of the same records in Fig. 4.5. Solid line, age 12 years; broken line, age 15 years.

The Cranial Base

The cranial base comprises the bones that originate from the chondrocranium of the embryo—the plate of cartilage that develops on the ventral surface of the brain. The bones that arise from this cartilage include the ethmoid, body of sphenoid, basiocciput and petrous temporals. The cartilage that remains between these bones, in particular between the body of the sphenoid and the ethmoid anteriorly, and the occipital posteriorly, forms sites at which growth occurs by proliferation of cartilage cells. These cartilaginous joints, or synchondroses, are analagous to the epiphyses of long bones except that the growth plate is symmetrical, with cartilage proliferation and bone growth occurring on both sides.

The extent to which growth of the cranial base synchondroses is under tight intrinsic control is still a matter of controversy, and the relative inaccessibility and complexity of the area makes conclusive experimental investigations difficult. However, the weight of evidence currently available suggests that they are comparable to epiphyses in that growth is under rather tight intrinsic control and they are not very susceptible to extrinsic influences.

The length and growth of the cranial base has an important effect on jaw relationships. The upper facial skeleton is related by its articulations to the anterior cranial fossa while the mandible, through the temporomandibular joint, is related to the middle cranial fossa. Growth at the synchondroses, in particular at the spheno-occipital synchondrosis, carries the maxilla upwards and forwards relative to the mandible and so contributes to the depth and height of the face (*Fig*. 4.5).

The spheno-occipital synchondrosis fuses at about the age of puberty (12–14 years), while the spheno-ethmoidal synchondrosis fuses at 6–7 years of age.[20] This means that the floor of the anterior cranial fossa in the midline is fairly stable from the age of 7 years and so provides an area within the craniofacial complex that can be used as a frame of reference for the superimposition of serial lateral skull radiographs of a child (*Fig*. 4.6). This gives a somewhat distorted view of the pattern of facial growth, for example the temporomandibular joint appears to be displaced downwards and backwards, and this should be remembered when comparing serial radiographs in this way.

The importance of cranial base growth is illustrated well in conditions in which it is deficient. In the disorders known collectively as achondroplasia, the cranial base is short and so the maxilla is retruded. In most individuals with mandibular retrusion, it is found on average that the cranial base is longer than in groups with mandibular protrusion.[21] In these cases, cranial base length is one of a number of factors that may contribute to the overall jaw malrelationship.

The Facial Skeleton

The facial skeleton serves a variety of functional requirements: vision, respiration, olfaction, mastication, deglutition and speech are only some of the functional demands on the facial region and it is not surprising that it is structurally complex. Growth has to be integrated so that none of the functional requirements is encroached upon.

In the neonate the facial skeleton constitutes a smaller proportion of the head than in the adult (*Fig*. 4.7). This reflects the different patterns of growth of the

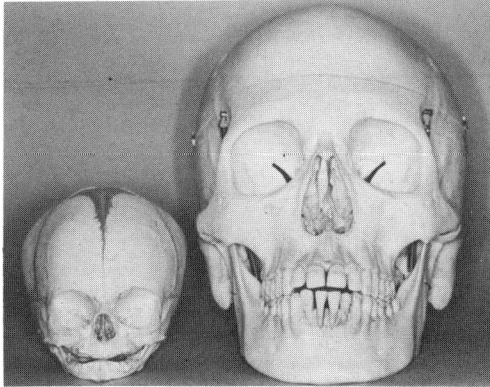

a

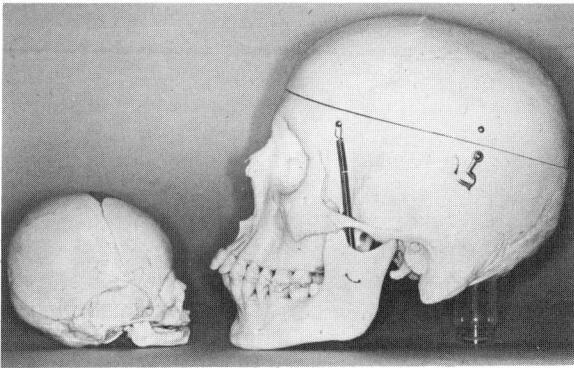

b

Fig. 4.7. Neonate and adult skulls. Note the differences in the skeletal proportions.

calvarium, which follows a neural growth curve, and the facial skeleton, which follows a typically somatic pathway. Thus the face in the adult is considerably more prominent than in the young child. Within the face the proportions change: the greatest amount of growth is in facial depth and the least in width, so that on average, the face becomes relatively longer and narrower. In the neonate the eyes are relatively large as they follow a neural growth curve and will grow less than will the rest of the face. Conversely the young child's nose is small and the adult form of nose is attained only after puberty. Jaw relationships also change with growth and this is discussed below in the section on growth of the intermaxillary space.

Thus, with growth, the character of the face changes in ways that are subtle and complex and that have a bearing on the appearance of the dentition. At the most obvious level, a child of 8 years of age with a good occlusion may appear to have teeth that are too large and prominent relative to the rest of the face. The face will continue to grow, however, and particularly with growth of the nose and chin and maturation of the facial soft tissues, the teeth will become much less dominant.

Lip posture often changes at around the time of puberty. The lips are parted habitually in many young children, but most of them will maintain a lip seal after puberty. This may in part reflect differential growth in lip length and in lower face height and in part a greater self-awareness with age. These changes can well affect the positions of balance of the teeth and this can be relevant when planning orthodontic treatment: for example, for the child with a Class II, division 1 malocclusion, overjet reduction may not be stable at 9 or 10 years of age because the lower lip will not control the retracted upper incisors, but by 13 or 14 years of age the lip posture may have matured sufficiently to ensure stability.

The Upper Facial Skeleton

The maxilla and other bones of the upper facial skeleton are related to one another and to the bones of the cranial base at sutures. The maxilla grows downwards and forwards from the anterior cranial base, in part by displacement with growth at the suture system and in part by drift resulting from periosteal remodelling (*Fig.* 4.8).

The pattern of growth of the upper facial skeleton has been studied extensively by histological methods and by the use of serial radiographs of children where metallic markers have been inserted into the maxilla to act as fixed reference points.[22] Sutural separation continues until facial growth is nearly complete. In general, periosteal apposition of bone occurs on the outer and anterior surfaces of the maxilla, on the oral surface of the hard palate and at the alveolar processes while resorption is seen on the nasal surface of the hard palate and on the walls of the maxillary antrum. This extensive remodelling means that there are no stable natural landmarks that can be used to relate serial radiographs of the one child in order to display the individual pattern of periosteal activity. Björk[22] has reported that the anterior surface of the zygomatic process is

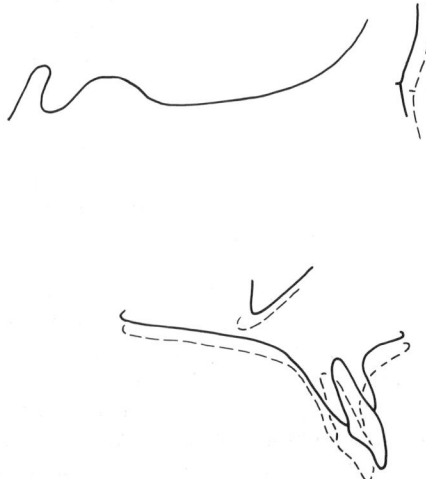

Fig. 4.8. The maxilla grows downwards from the anterior cranial base, in part by displacement (growth at the sutures), and in part by drift (periosteal apposition and resorption of bones). Solid line, 12 years; broken line, 14 years.

relatively stable but this is too limited in extent to form a reliable area for superimposition. Björk's studies with metallic implants have demonstrated that the pattern of maxillary growth may be more complex than had previously been thought. The downward displacement of the maxilla associated with growth at sutures may have a rotational component, which in turn is masked by periosteal remodelling and compensatory drift of the teeth.

The determinants of sutural growth in the upper face have been a matter of much controversy. The classic view was that growth at the suture itself was responsible for the displacement of the maxilla and that in this respect sutures were akin to the epiphyseal plates of long bones. However, the appropriate comparison is with sutures of the calvarium which, as already discussed, have virtually no independent growth potential: they are sites at which growth can occur, not centres of active growth. It is now generally accepted that the facial sutures are sites where growth can occur in response to separating forces generated elsewhere. A major gap in our knowledge is the identification of the primary growth centres. The cartilaginous nasal septum has been implicated by several authors.[23] Early experiments where the nasal septum was removed surgically in animals showed major disturbance of upper facial growth, but there was also scar tissue formation and disruption in blood supply, which in themselves would affect skeletal growth. Subsequent less traumatic experiments demonstrated that when the nasal septum is dislocated or partially removed, suture growth is reduced though not inhibited.[24] In children with clefts of the lip and palate, it is found that the lesser segment which is isolated from the nasal septum exhibits less sutural growth than would be expected normally, but growth is not inhibited.

Growth of the eyeballs is important in growth of the orbit, and if an eye is lost early orbital growth is severely affected. There are probably also effects on the sutural growth of the surrounding bones, including the maxilla. Growth of the eyeball is nearly complete by 7 years of age while sutural growth continues for a much longer period and so it could be a factor only in younger children.

Suggestions have been made that nasal airflow has an important influence[25] but these have no scientific foundation. Indeed, in children with congenital nasal obstruction upper facial growth is nearly normal, and any slight deficiency cannot be attributed to the lack of nasal airflow.[26]

It is probably a mistake to seek a single key factor as being responsible for upper facial growth: growth of the eyeball, of the nasal septum, of the sutural tissues and even tension within the muscles and fascia attached to the maxilla probably all play a part, the importance of which may vary from time to time and from case to case.

One reason why the mechanisms controlling growth of the upper facial complex are of such interest is the possibility of growth being influenced by external factors or by treatment. It has been convincingly demonstrated in experimental animals that growth of the circum-maxillary sutures can be reduced or inhibited by the application of distally directed traction to the maxilla.[27] Provided that the traction is of a sufficient magnitude to override the normal controlling mechanisms and is applied continually it is hardly surprising that sutural growth should be prevented. Anterior traction can accelerate growth at the circum-maxillary sutures and so increase the displacement of the maxilla relative to the cranial base.[28] Unless the growth of the basic controlling mechanisms is altered too, it must be anticipated that maxillary growth will rebound following removal of the appliances and this is indeed found.

Although there is much talk of the orthopaedic effects of extra-oral traction to the maxilla in children, it is difficult to affect maxillary growth permanently to a clinically important extent. The extra-oral appliances would have to be worn continually over an appreciable period of time, which is not generally acceptable socially. In children at the age when orthodontic treatment is usually under-taken, the amount of sutural growth is rather small, and so even if this were inhibited completely, the effects would be minimal. Significant sutural resorp-tion is not likely to be obtained because of the complexity and large surface area of the sutures, and so appreciable retraction or advancement of the maxilla is not obtained, even with the most assiduous wear of the relevant appliances. As mentioned previously, the small changes that are produced may well be lost by rebound unless treatment is continued until growth has ceased. A major practical problem is that the appliances have to be attached to the teeth, which move more readily than do the bones of the facial skeleton, and the amount and duration of extra-oral traction that can be used may well be limited by the risk of unwanted tooth movements, particularly when anterior traction is applied to the maxilla. It has to be accepted that appreciable changes in maxillary position that might be desirable in a number of malocclusions cannot be obtained in a child by orthodontic means. Force systems that could result in unfavourable growth changes, however, should be avoided.

The Mandible

The mandible develops in membrane, in association with but not arising from Meckel's cartilage. Secondary cartilages do appear in the mandible, the most important of these being the condylar cartilage. The classic view was that growth of the mandibular condyle was under tight genetic control and thrust the mandible downwards and forwards from its articulation within the skull. Many investigators disagree, and argue that this cartilage is more like a periosteal modification than a primary growth cartilage, and that growth at this site occurs secondarily to growth elsewhere, carrying the mandible downwards and forwards.[29] It has also been argued that control of growth does not lie within the condylar cartilage itself but that it is influenced by the actions of the adjacent musculature, and in particular by the lateral pterygoid muscle. At the present time no conclusive evidence is available to settle this dispute. What is clear is that normal growth at the condylar cartilage is required if mandibular length and the relationship of the mandible to the upper facial skeleton are to be within normal limits. The greater part of mandibular growth is the result of periosteal activity and much of this occurs in response to the functional demands of the muscles attached to the mandible. The coronoid and angle are muscular proces-ses whose presence and development depend on the presence and development of the temporal muscle, and the medial pterygoid and masseter respectively. In experiments in animals where the muscle is ablated or denervated, the corre-sponding muscular process fails to develop or is vestigial.[30] The presence and growth of the alveolar process is dependent on the development and position of the teeth: in children with anodontia there is no alveolar process and following extraction of teeth, it is resorbed. The alveolar processes grow to keep pace with eruption of the teeth and when the teeth are moved by an orthodontic appliance, it is remodelled accordingly.

The extent to which condylar growth can be modified in amount or direction by extrinsic influences is clearly a matter of clinical orthodontic interest. Destruction of the condylar cartilage as a result of infection or disease results in a very severe facial deformity, because not only does the mandible fail to grow in overall length, but it is attached to the temporal bone by the capsule, which may well be scarred. The facial deformity is much less severe if the mandible can be freed of such ankylosis because it is then carried into a more normal relationship with the upper facial skeleton by the musculature and other soft tissues.[31]

The cartilage of the mandibular condyle has been the subject of extensive study and widespread disagreement. Some authors have maintained that the condylar cartilage is comparable to epiphyseal cartilage of a long bone in that the control of growth lies within the cells themselves. Others have pointed out that developmentally and histochemically the condylar fibrocartilage is very different from the hyaline cartilage of epiphyseal plates: it is a secondary cartilage and it is thus possible that the control of its growth is different.[17]

It has been suggested by some authors that the condylar cartilage is merely a local periosteal modification at the joint surface, and that its growth is controlled in the same way as is periosteum elsewhere. Experimental studies in animals have shown that cellular proliferation in the condylar cartilage can be influenced by appliances that displace the jaw forwards;[32] but it is in fact much more difficult to control its activity than in the case of periosteum, sutures or periodontal ligaments. The evidence suggests that while epiphyseal cartilages (and cartilages of the synchondroses) are under tight intrinsic control and periosteal activity is under rather loose intrinsic control, condylar cartilage lies somewhere between the two. Although claims have been made that condylar growth can be influenced in children by some types of appliance,[25] the average changes reported are small and seem to be of questionable clinical importance. This may be because it is difficult to generate the stimuli that would be most

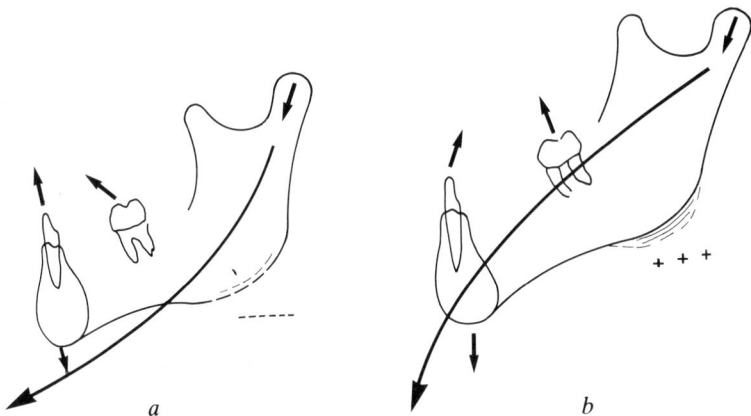

Fig. 4.9. Growth rotations of the mandible occur when there is a discrepancy in the amounts of growth in anterior and posterior facial heights. The amount of rotation is masked by periosteal modelling in the mandible and dento-alveolar adaptation. *a*, anterior growth rotation; *b*, posterior growth rotation.

effective in influencing condylar growth, and because orthodontic treatment is normally undertaken for older children where the major part of growth has already been completed and where the condylar cartilage is less responsive to environmental variation.

Growth Rotations

The classic view of mandibular growth based upon the analysis of lateral skull radiographs is that it grows downwards and forwards relative to the anterior cranial base in a more or less linear fashion (*see Fig.* 4.6). However, Björk[33] has shown that in many children some degree of mandibular rotation occurs during its descent (*Fig.* 4.9). These findings were based upon examination of lateral skull radiographs of children who had metallic implants placed in the bone of the mandible to provide fixed reference points. The extent of rotation is masked by periosteal remodelling so that the mandibular plane appears to descend in a nearly parallel fashion. Anterior rotations are more common than are posterior rotations but in most children they are small in amount.

MECHANISMS OF GROWTH ROTATIONS

A mandibular growth rotation is merely a manifestation of a discrepancy in growth of anterior and posterior facial heights. Where posterior facial height increases more than does anterior facial height there will be an anterior growth rotation and vice versa.

Growth in posterior facial height depends on the vertical components of growth at the condyle and at the spheno-occipital synchondrosis. Anterior facial height growth depends on the relative growth of the muscles of mastication, the suprahyoid muscles and the associated fascia. As the head is carried vertically by growth of the cervical column, the entire chain of muscles and fascia between the cranium and the thorax grows and stretches and the bones forming links in that chain—the mandible and hyoid—descend relative to the cranial base (*Fig.* 4.10).

Mandibular growth rotations are important for their effects on normal occlusal development and because they may influence the ease with which overbite changes are achieved by orthodontic treatment.

OCCLUSAL CHANGES WITH MANDIBULAR GROWTH ROTATIONS

Where there is an anterior growth rotation, and in the absence of compensating tooth movements, the lower incisors would become more retroclined within the face. However, dento-alveolar adaptation under the influence of tongue and lips results in a labial tipping of the incisors so that their inclination to reference lines within the upper facial skeleton is more or less maintained. Full adaptation to the rotation may not occur because of contact with the upper incisors and because at the same time the mandible may be growing forwards relative to the maxilla. When the mandible rotates anteriorly, the posterior teeth have an upwards and forwards pattern of eruption and, particularly if there has been incomplete adaptation of the incisors, crowding will develop in the incisor region owing to the shortening of the arch. With a posterior pattern of mandibular rotation the incisors adapt by tipping back and, although the buccal teeth will

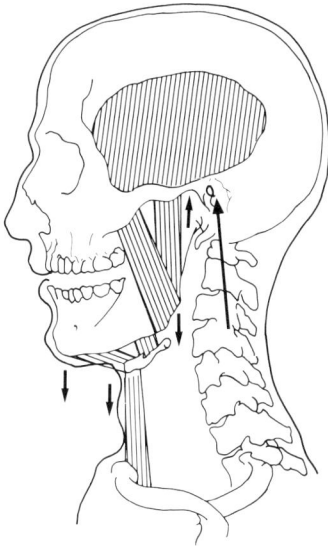

Fig. 4.10. Growth of the cervical column
means that the muscles and fascia between
the cranium and thorax stretch and this
influences the level of the hyoid bone
and mandibular symphysis.

have a posteriorly directed path of eruption, shortening of the arch again tends
to occur, with crowding of the labial segment. Thus mandibular growth rotations
are one of the factors that contribute to the development of incisor crowding in
the permanent dentition.

Growth of the Intermaxillary Space

The intermaxillary space lies between the maxillary and mandibular dental
bases. Its dimensions depend on the relationship between maxilla and mandible.
The teeth and alveolar processes grow vertically to establish an occlusion and
this is maintained by continued dento-alveolar development as the intermaxillary space grows in height. Where the intermaxillary height is excessive,
the teeth and alveolar processes may fail to maintain an occlusion (*Fig.* 4.11).
Skeletal open bites of this sort tend to worsen with facial growth and in the most
severe cases only the last standing molars will meet. Orthodontic correction is
not usually feasible in these cases, because extrusion of the teeth may not be
accompanied by alveolar bone growth, and so the periodontal support of the
teeth would be reduced. In addition, these patients usually have incompetent
lips and they would show too much tooth if they were extruded into occlusion.
Surgical correction of the vertical jaw discrepancy is required in these cases, if
they are to be treated at all.

As the teeth erupt into the intermaxillary space, they are guided towards one
another by the tongue, lips and cheeks. Thus dento-alveolar compensation will
often minimize any occlusal mismatch that would otherwise have arisen from
variations in apical base relationships. The compensation may be inadequate to
establish a normal occlusion where there are severe apical base discrepancies,
and may break down altogether when the soft tissue pattern is unfavourable. For
example, in the child with a Class II skeletal pattern and incompetent lips, a
Class II, division 1 relationship may be established that is more severe than the

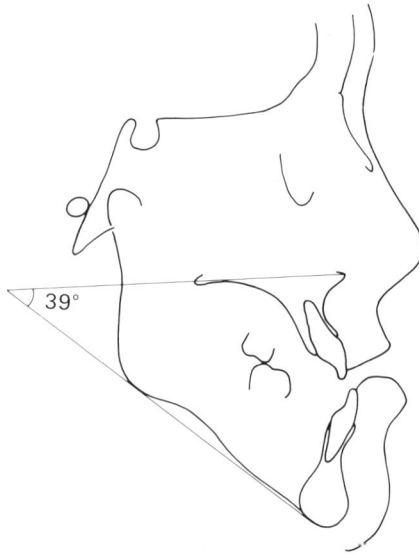

Fig. 4.11. A skeletal anterior open bite. The anterior intermaxillary space is too great to be bridged by growth of the teeth and alveolar processes.

dental base discrepancy because the lower lip fails to control the upper incisor position.

PREDICTION OF FACIAL GROWTH

In certain cases it would be useful to be able to predict the pattern of facial growth and the timing of the pubertal growth spurt. Jaw relationship can change appreciably during growth and, particularly for cases at the limits of appliance correction of their malocclusion, even minor changes in skeletal relationships may be important. The average tendency is for the mandible to become more prognathic than the maxilla, which is helpful in Class II cases but may make a Class III case untreatable, or may cause it to relapse. Currently available methods of growth prediction depend upon adding average increments of growth to the existing skeletal patterns.[34] As the major part of facial growth has already been completed by the age that orthodontic treatment is usually started, and because most individuals do not differ greatly from the average in their growth pattern, this procedure gives a reasonably reliable estimate of future changes due to growth in most cases. However, some cases differ appreciably from the average and it is in these individuals, for whom growth prediction would be most important, that it is least reliable.

Growth changes during the average course of orthodontic treatment are not usually great enough to interfere with the outcome of treatment, and provided that good, stable occlusal relationships are established, dento-alveolar adaptation will maintain the occlusion in spite of minor changes in jaw relationship. It is normally prudent to plan treatment for Class II cases on the basis of the existing jaw relationship, and any growth changes that occur will usually be favourable and enhance stability. Orthodontic treatment is directed towards attaining specific occlusal goals, and the clinician will automatically allow for any growth changes during treatment, often being unaware of them and taking credit for favourable changes. Class III cases at the limits of orthodontic correction should be evaluated conservatively: growth changes in jaw relationships are often unfavourable and if this would prejudice the result, it may be more prudent to defer intervention until growth is nearly complete.

REFERENCES

1. Noel J. F., Wright E. A. (1972) The growth of transplanted mouse vertebrae. *J. Embryol. Exp. Morphol.* **28**; 633–45.
2. Chalmers J. and Ray R. D. (1962) The growth of transplanted foetal bones in different immunological environments. *J. Bone Joint Surg.* **44B**; 149–64.
3. Crilly R. G. (1972) Longitudinal overgrowth of chicken radius. *J. Anat. (Lond.)* **112**; 11–18.
4. Enlow D. H. (1968) Wolff's law and the factor of architectonic circumstance. *Am. J. Orthodont.* **54**; 803–22.
5. Wright K. W. and Yettram A. L. (1979) Analytical investigation into possible mechanical causes of bone remodelling. *J. Biomech. Eng.* **1**; 41–9.
6. Bassett C. A. L. and Becker R. O. (1962) Generation of electric potentials by bone in response to mechanical stress. *Science (New York)* **137**; 1063–4.
7. Davidovich Z., Mathew M. D., Finkelson B. S. et al. (1980) Electric currents, bone remodelling and orthodontic tooth movement. *Am. J. Orthodont.* **77**; 14–32, 33–47.
8. Norton L. A., Hanley K. J. and Turkewicz J. (1984) Bioelectric perturbations of bone. *Angle Orthodont.* **54**; 73–87.
9. Crawford G. N. C. (1954) An experimental study of muscle growth in the rabbit. *J. Bone Joint Surg.* **36B**; 294–303.
10. Scammon R. E. (1930) The measurement of the body in childhood. In: Harris J. A., Jackson C. M., Paterson D. G. et al. (ed) *The Measurement of Man.* University of Minnesota Press.
11. Tanner J. M., Whitehouse R. H., Marubini E. et al. (1976) The adolescent growth spurt of boys and girls of the Harpendon growth study. *Ann. Hum. Biol.* **3**; 109–26.
12. Houston W. J. B. (1980) Relationships between skeletal maturity estimated from hand–wrist radiographs and the timing of the adolescent growth spurt. *Eur. J. Orthodont.* **2**; 81–93.
13. Liebgott B. (1978) Dental age: its relation to skeletal age and the time of peak circumpuberal growth in length of the mandible. *J. Canad. Dent. Assoc.* **44**; 223–7.
14. Hägg U. and Tarranger J. (1980) Menarche and voice change as indicators of the pubertal growth spurt. *Acta Odontol. Scand.* **38**; 179–86.
15. Smith D. W. and Töndury G. (1978) Origin of the calvaria and its sutures, *Am. J. Dis. Child.* **132**; 662–6.
16. Persson K. M., Roy W. A., Persing J. A. et al. (1979) Craniofacial growth following experimental craniosynostosis and cranioectomy in rabbits. *J. Neurosurg.* **50**; 187–97.
17. Koski K. (1968) Cranial growth centres: facts or fallacies? *Am. J. Orthodont.* **54**; 566–83.
18. Young R. N. (1959) The influence of cranial contents on postnatal growth of the skull in the rat. *Am. J. Anat.* **105**; 383–409.
19. Ryöppy S. (1965) Transplantation of epiphyseal cartilage and cranial suture. *Acta Orthop. Scand.* Suppl. 82.
20. Melsen B. (1974) The cranial base. *Acta Odontol. Scand.* Suppl. 62.
21. Hopkin G. B., Houston W. J. B. and James G. A. (1968) The cranial base as an aetiological factor in malocclusion. *Angle Orthodont.* **38**; 250–5.
22. Björk A. and Skieller V. (1977) Growth at the maxilla in three dimensions as revealed radiographically by the implant method. *Br. J. Orthodont.* **4**; 53–64.
23. Scott J. H. (1953) The cartilage of the nasal septum. *Br. Dent. J.* **95**; 37–43.
24. Wexler M. R. and Sarnat B. G. (1965) Rabbit snout growth after dislocation of nasal septum. *Acta Otolaryng.* **81**; 305–13.
25. Fränkel R. (1980) A functional approach to orofacial orthopaedics. *Br. J. Orthodont.* **7**; 41–51.

26. Freng A. (1979) Dentofacial development in long lasting nasal stenosis. *Scand. J. Dent. Res.* **87**; 260–7.
27. Elder J. R. and Tuenge R. H. (1974) Cephalometric and histologic changes produced by extra-oral high-pull traction to the maxilla in *Macaca mulatta. Am. J. Orthodont.* **66**; 599–617.
28. Nanda R. (1978) Protraction of maxilla in rhesus monkeys by controlled extra-oral forces. *Am. J. Orthodont.* **74**; 121–41.
29. Moss M. L. (1969) The differential roles of periosteal and capsular functional matrices in oro-facial growth. *Trans. Eur. Orthodont. Soc.* pp. 193–206.
30. Avis V. (1961) The significance of the angle of the mandible: an experimental and comparative study. *Am. J. Phys. Anthropol.* **19**; 55–61.
31. Moss M. L. and Rankow R. M. (1968) The role of the functional matrix in mandibular growth. *Angle Orthod.* **38**, 95–103.
32. Rowe N. L. (1983) Ankylosis of the temporomandibular joint. *J. R. Coll. Surg. Edinb.* **27**, 167–209.
33. McNamara J. A. (1980) Functional determinants of craniofacial size and shape. *Eur. J. Orthodont.* **2**; 131–59.
34. Björk A. and Skieller V. (1972) Facial development and tooth eruption. *Am. J. Orthodont.* **62**; 339–83.
35. Houston W. J. B. (1979) The current status of facial growth prediction: a review. *Br. J. Orthodont.* **6**; 11–17.

Chapter 5

Occlusal and Skeletal Classification

Occlusal and facial patterns vary widely and in many circumstances it is convenient to categorize them into a small number of groups. The objective of any system of classification is to gather together cases with similar features or with a common aetiology. Individuals within a class should ideally resemble one another more closely in the relevant features than individuals in other classes. However, as with many biological attributes, there is a spectrum of continuous variation and the division between classes is arbitrary. This makes the designation of borderline cases difficult. Methods of classifying malocclusions and facial patterns have been developed intuitively, and when modern statistical techniques are used to investigate the most efficient systems, these generally do not correspond with the time-honoured patterns which nevertheless persist. However, the importance of classification in everyday clinical practice should not be exaggerated: the classification of a malocclusion cannot constitute an adequate description of it, nor is it the basis for the prescription of treatment.

Different methods of classification may be needed for different purposes, and an appropriate method must be adopted for the task in hand. The requirements for clinical categorization differ from those of epidemiology. Other methods of indexing are required for investigation into the relationships between dental irregularity and problems such as periodontal disease. For example, Angle's classification, which is the most commonly used classification in clinical practice, is not suitable for these purposes.

OCCLUSAL CLASSIFICATIONS

Angle's Classification

The only internationally recognized classification of malocclusion is that of Angle,[1] one of the founders of modern orthodontics. Angle divided the whole range of malocclusions into three main groups according to the anteroposterior relationship of the arches. Vertical and transverse malrelationships are not taken into account.

In brief, a normal anteroposterior arch relationship is Class I (sometimes called neutrocclusion); a more distal than normal relationship of the lower arch to the upper is Class II (distocclusion); and a more mesial than normal relationship is Class III (mesiocclusion). A more detailed description of these classes of malocclusion is given in *Fig.* 5.1. Angle believed that the permanent molars developed in a constant relationship to the jaws and that their occlusion

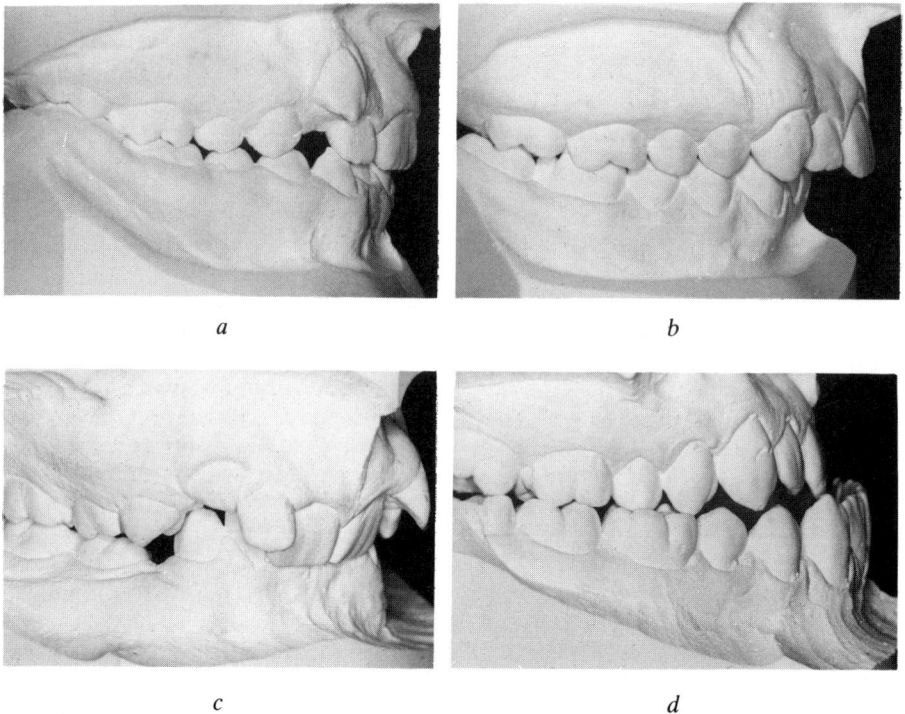

Fig 5.1. Angle's classes of malocclusion. *a*, Class I. A normal anteroposterior arch relationship. Angle stated that the mesiobuccal cusp of the upper first permanent molar should occlude with the anterior buccal groove of the lower first permanent molar. Note that this is not always the correct relationship (*see Fig.* 1.2). *b*, Class II, division 1. The lower arch lies at least one half cusp width distal to the correct relationship with the upper; and the upper incisors are of average inclination or are proclined so that the overjet is increased. *c*, Class II, division 2. The lower arch lies at least one half cusp width distal to the correct relationship with the upper; and the upper central incisors are retroclined. *d*, Class III. The lower arch lies at least one half cusp width mesial to the correct relationship with the upper.

could be used to classify jaw relationships. It is now recognized that this is not so and that skeletal and occlusal relationships must be assessed independently of one another.

There may be difficulties in using Angle's classification. He focused attention on the relationship of the first permanent molars and allowance is made where there has been drift of these teeth following early loss of deciduous molars, a judgement that may not be easy or reliable. Where first permanent molars are missing, the relationship of other teeth is used. In some cases where the upper first permanent molar is small, the correct relationship may be further back than described by Angle (*see Fig.* 1.2): the distobuccal cusp of the upper molar must occlude in the embrasure distal to the lower molar, otherwise it may not be possible to establish a correct premolar and canine relationship.[2] Because of these problems, it is important to take account of the general buccal segment occlusion, and in particular the canine relationships, before deciding on the classification.

Strictly interpreted, Angle's Class I includes anteroposterior buccal segment malrelationships of up to half a cusp width, and thus only quite severe discrepancies would be included in Class II and Class III. This requirement is generally relaxed, and milder arch malrelationships are included in Classes II and III.

Incisor Classification

Patients are generally more concerned with incisor rather than with buccal segment relationships, and their correction is a central concern of much orthodontic treatment. Accordingly, a classification of incisor relationships has been widely adopted. For general use, the incisor classification is simpler and more relevant than Angle's classification. Angle's terms are used, and in most cases the classifications are concordant.

The incisor classification is based upon the relationship between the lower incisor edges and the cingulum plateau of the upper central incisors (*Fig.* 5.2). Problems arise where the relationship differs between sides, but in these cases the classification should rest on the general features.

Definitions

Class I: The lower incisor edges occlude with or lie directly below the cingulum plateau of the upper central incisors (*Fig.* 5.2*a*).

Class II: The lower incisor edges lie posterior to the cingulum plateau of the upper central incisors. There are two divisions of Class II:

Division 1: the upper central incisors are of average inclination or are proclined. The overjet is thus increased (*Fig.* 5.2*b*).

Division 2: the upper central incisors are retroclined (*Fig.* 5.2*c*).

Class III: The lower incisor edges lie anterior to the cingulum plateau of the upper central incisors (*Fig.* 5.2*d*).

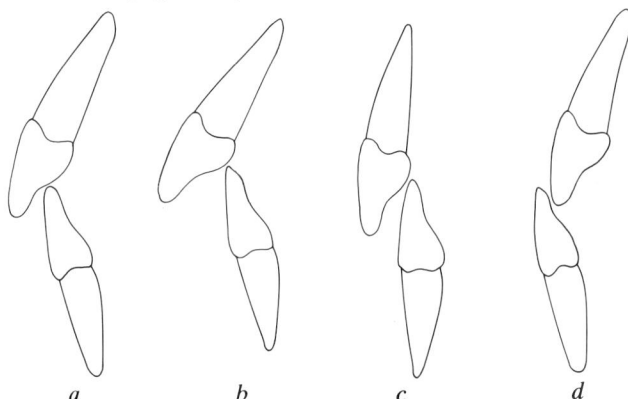

a   *b*   *c*   *d*

Fig. 5.2. Incisor classification. *a*, Class I. The lower incisor edges occlude with or lie below the cingulum plateau of the upper incisors. *b*, Class II, division 1. The lower incisor edges lie posterior to the cingulum plateau of the upper incisors, which are of average inclination or are proclined so that the overjet is increased. *c*, Class II, division 2. The lower incisor edges lie posterior to the cingulum plateau of the upper incisors; and the upper central incisors are retroclined so that the overjet is normal or only slightly increased. *d*, Class III. The lower incisor edges lie anterior to the cingulum plateau of the upper incisors.

Indices of Malocclusion

Neither Angle's nor the incisor classification provides a measure of the severity of a malocclusion. Thus different methods are required for estimating the prevalence of malocclusion in a population, for deciding on treatment priority where services are limited and for investigating the relationships between malocclusion and various aspects of dental health. Several indices of malocclusion have been proposed. None is entirely satisfactory and it is not likely that a single index will be suitable for all purposes. Before it is adopted, an index should be tested for validity (does it in fact measure what is required?) and reproducibility (do observers consistently obtain the same values for a series of test cases?).

The aim of using an index is to be able to rank occlusal disharmonies according to their severity. The index can then be used for epidemiological purposes and to establish priorities of treatment. There are many difficulties in devising a reliable index of malocclusion: for example a localized irregularity such as an instanding upper incisor may be a more serious problem than generalized mild crowding, which will almost inevitably attract a higher score.

Two of the best established indices of malocclusion are the Handicapping Malocclusion Assessment Record[3] and the Occlusal Index.[4] Both perform reasonably well for reproducibility and validity.[5]

The Handicapping Malocclusion Assessment Record (HMAR) allocates points for dental irregularities and arch malrelationships, which are multiplied by a weighting factor before the total score is assigned. This can be done from orthodontic models or at a clinical assessment. In the latter case, further points can be allotted for dentofacial deviations such as clefts of the lip and palate, facial asymmetry and functional disabilities. This assessment is quite rapid and does not require special instruments.

The Occlusal Index (OI) scores dental age, molar relations, overbite, overjet, posterior crossbite, posterior open bite, tooth displacement, midline relations and missing upper lateral incisors. A number of measurements are involved and the scoring is rather more complicated than for the HMAR, but it is a more reliable method of ranking malocclusion severity.

SKELETAL CLASSIFICATION

Angle believed that the first permanent molars had a definite developmental relationship to the jaws and so the skeletal pattern could be established from the molar occlusion. This is incorrect because the dental lamina which gives rise to the tooth germs does not develop in a constant relationship to the jaw. Although jaw relationship influences the arch relationship and the two will often correspond, they must be assessed separately. A detailed investigation of skeletal relationships can be undertaken only with the aid of a lateral skull radiograph (*see* Chapter 6), but a general evaluation sufficient for many clinical purposes can be obtained by clinical assessment.

The appearance of the nose and chin have a very important effect on the facial characteristics, but of more immediate concern to the orthodontist is the relationship of the dental bases, which are the parts of the jaws that can be occupied by the apices of the teeth. Little periosteal remodelling occurs at this level in response to tooth movement and so the anteroposterior dental base relationship (the skeletal pattern) imposes limitations on the possible tooth positions. Ideally the skeletal pattern would be assessed at apical level, but there are no suitable landmarks and so the depths of the concavities of the profiles of maxilla and mandible, named points A and B respectively, are used instead (*Fig.* 5.3). The soft tissue, or integumental, profile does not follow the skeletal profile exactly, but variations in the thickness of the lips are rarely sufficient to give a misleading impression of the skeletal pattern. Some clinicians prefer to retract

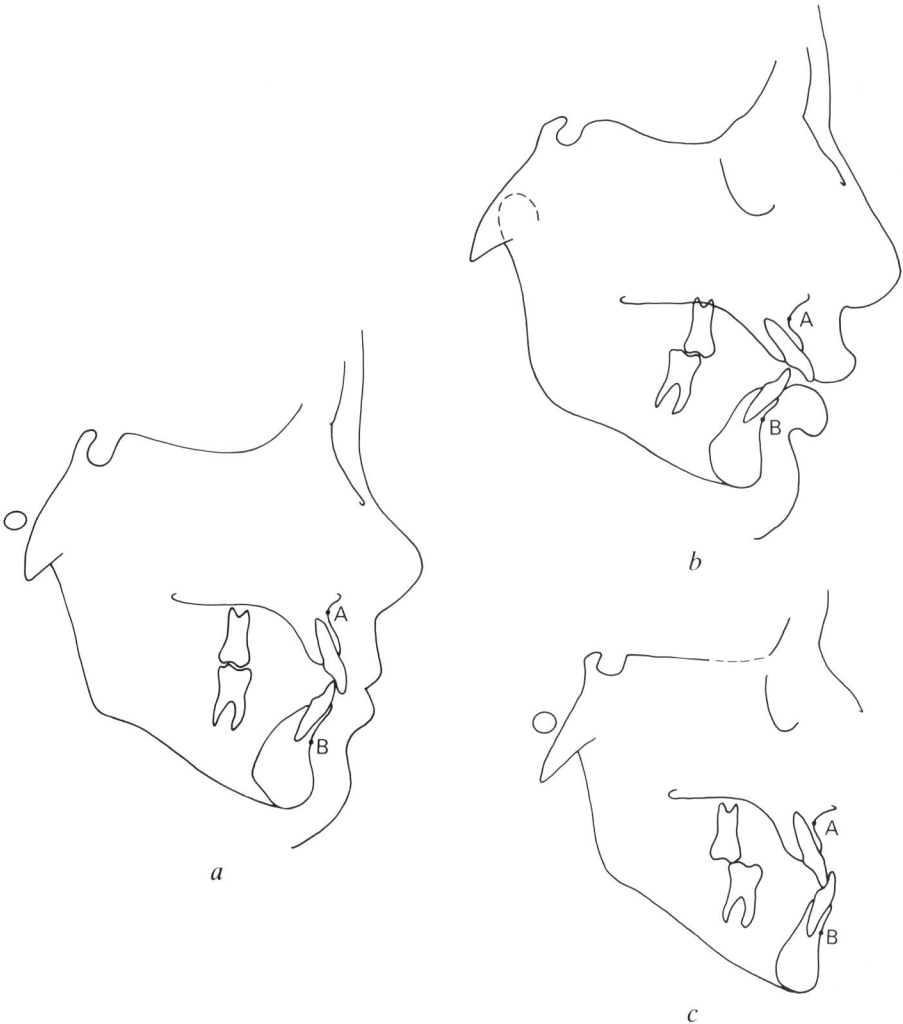

Fig. 5.3. Skeletal classification. *a*, Class I. The mandible is correctly related to the middle facial skeleton. The facial profile will generally be well balanced. *b*, Class II. The mandible is retruded relative to the middle facial skeleton. This may be the result of true mandibular retrusion, or maxillary protrusion, or a combination of both. *c*, Class III. The mandible is prominent in relation to the middle facial skeleton. As in Class II, the problem may lie in the maxilla, the mandible or both.

the lips and examine the skeletal relationship at about the level of the muco-gingival junction. When assessing the skeletal pattern, the patient should sit or stand unsupported with the head in the free postural position. It helps if the patient looks at an object at eye-level, ideally at the reflection of their own eyes in a wall-mounted mirror. The Frankfort plane should be more or less horizontal when the head is positioned correctly. The clinical assessment of the skeletal pattern is subjective and so the definitions are qualitative. With experience, the clinical assessment of the skeletal pattern should closely match its measurement from a lateral skull radiograph (*see* Chapter 6).

Definitions

Class I: The lower dental base is normally related to upper. Point B lies a few millimetres behind point A (*Fig. 5.3a*).

Class II: The lower dental base is retruded relative to upper (*Fig. 5.3b*).

Class III: The lower dental base is protruded relative to the upper (*Fig. 5.3c*).

REFERENCES

1. Angle E. H. (1898) Classification of malocclusion. *Dental Cosmos* **41**; 248–64.
2. Andrews L. F. (1972) The six keys to normal occlusion. *Am. J. Orthodont.* **62**; 296–309.
3. Salzmann J. A. (1967) Malocclusion severity assessment. *Am. J. Orthodont.* **53**; 109–19.
4. Summers C. J. (1971) The occlusal index: a system for identifying and scoring occlusal disorders. *Am. J. Orthodont.* **59**; 552–67.
5. Gray A. S. and Demirjian A. (1977) Indexing occlusions for dental public health programs. *Am. J. Orthodont.* **72**; 191–7.

Chapter 6

Cephalometric Analysis

Skull radiographs have been used for a variety of purposes from the early days of radiography, but it was only in 1931 that Broadbent[1] in the USA and Hofrath in Germany, independently of one another, developed a standardized system of cephalometric radiography that could be of use to the orthodontist. Subsequent research into facial growth and the results of orthodontic treatment had a major impact on orthodontic theory and practice. On the basis of early cross-sectional studies, where average values for cephalometric measurements at different ages were compared with one another, it was concluded that the pattern of facial growth was rather stable[2,3] and that orthodontic treatment had little or no effect upon it. However, this method of analysis obscures individual variability and the work of Björk[4] in particular has demonstrated the extent of this. The possible effects of orthodontic treatment upon facial growth are still a matter of controversy (*see* Chapter 4).

In clinical practice, cephalometric analysis is of value in assessing facial and dentoskeletal relationships as an aid to treatment planning. Evaluation of changes attributable to growth and treatment is important in monitoring treatment progress and standards. Broadbent[2] emphasized the three-dimensional nature of facial relationships and recommended that postero-anterior (PA) as well as lateral skull views should be obtained. Others have suggested that views of the skull base are of value for some measurements. However, cephalometric analysis has come to mean, almost exclusively, the measurement of lateral skull radiographs (*Fig.* 6.1). In part this is because the facial variations of greatest orthodontic importance are in the sagittal plane, and in part because other views are difficult to interpret and measure. In the PA view (*Fig.* 6.2), for example, few landmarks that are important in lateral skull radiographs can be identified and so the possibilities of three-dimensional analysis are very limited. Furthermore, even minor variations in head position can result in distortion so that the apparent asymmetry of the skeletal structures can be exaggerated or even reversed.

Cephalometric radiographs are taken under standardized conditions so that measurements can be compared between patients and for the same patient on different occasions. The head is held in a cephalostat so that the mid-sagittal plane is at a fixed distance from, and parallel to, the film (*Fig.* 6.3). The target of the X-ray tube is also at a fixed distance from the film, with the central ray directed through the ear rods of the cephalostat so that the enlargement at the mid-sagittal plane is constant (*Fig.* 6.4). Various recommendations have been made that the distances should be agreed internationally so that the enlargement

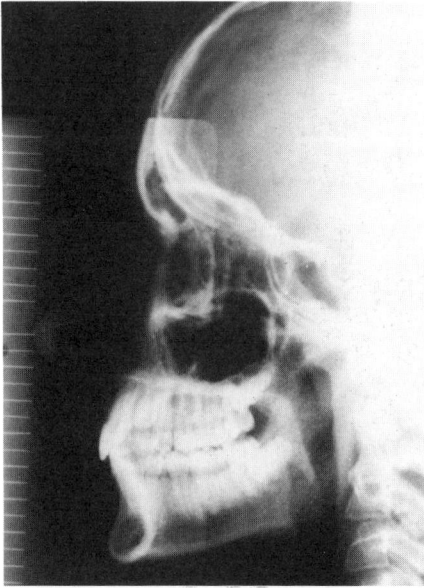

Fig .6.1. A lateral skull radiograph. Note the scale at the mid-sagittal plane which provides a permanent record of the enlargement of the radiograph.

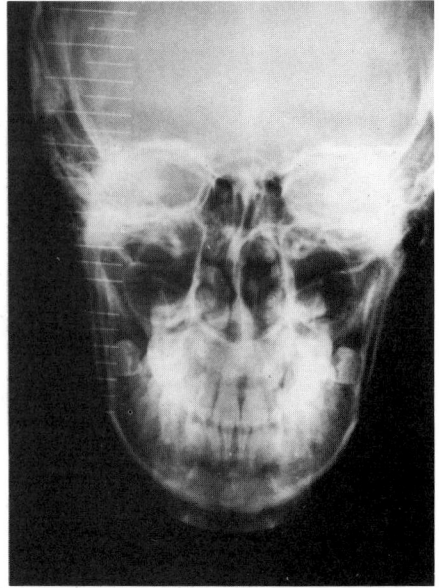

Fig. 6.2. Postero-anterior view of the patient shown in *Fig.* 6.1. Few landmarks common to both views can be identified reliably.

would be standardized, but unfortunately these have not been adhered to. In most installations, the magnification is in the order of 10 per cent and provided that this is known, linear enlargement can be compensated for. To this end it is good practice to suspend a metal scale of known length at the mid-sagittal plane of the head so that it appears in every film and provides a permanent record of the enlargement of that film (*Fig.* 6.1).

When the patient is positioned in the cephalostat, care should be taken to ensure that the ear rods are in fact in the ear canals and that the Frankfort plane is horizontal. The teeth should be in centric occlusion unless there is a mandibular displacement, in which case the mandible should be positioned in centric relation with the teeth in the initial contact relationship. If this is not done, a misleading impression of the skeletal relationships will be obtained. The patient should be posed with the lips in their habitual position.

ANATOMY VISUALIZED ON SKULL RADIOGRAPHS

The skull consists of three major components: the calvarium, the cranial base and the facial skeleton. The calvarium is of little relevance to orthodontic assessment and in the interests of radiation protection, the radiographic beam should be collimated to exclude unnecessary areas (*Fig.* 6.1). The radiographic anatomy of these views is shown in *Fig.* 6.5. Measurements are usually made on tracings (*see Fig.* 6.6) and the relevant aspects of the anatomy will be mentioned in the description of the tracing procedure.

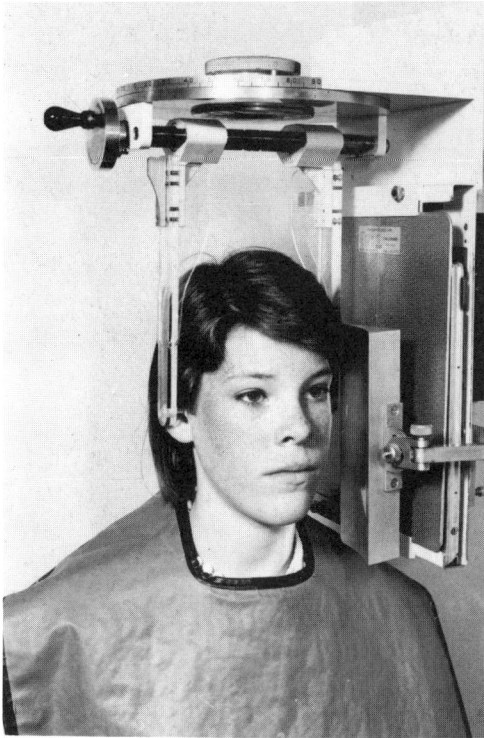

Fig. 6.3. The cephalostat maintains the patient's head in a definite relationship to the film.

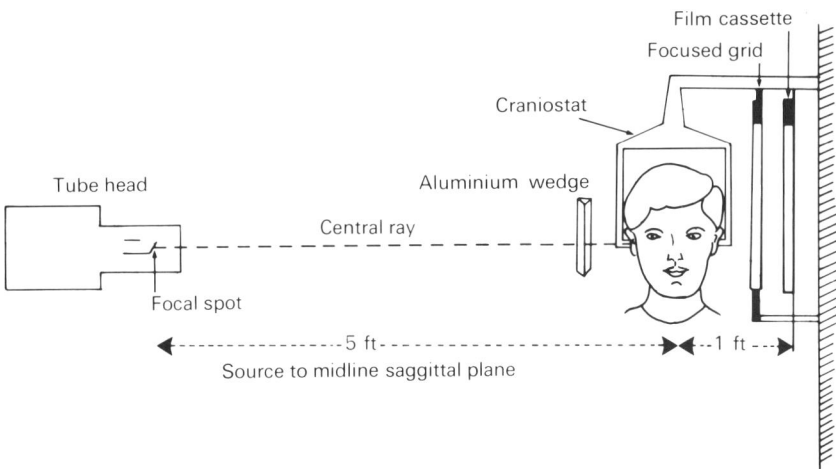

Fig. 6.4. The relationship of film, patient's head and tube in a cephalometric installation.

Tracing a Lateral Skull Radiograph

It is helpful when learning to identify the landmarks to obtain a radiograph of a dry skull. The absence of soft tissues improves the definition of the bony landmarks and it is instructive to compare the radiographic anatomy with the skull itself. Landmarks difficult to locate on the radiograph can be confirmed by fixing pieces of wire or lead shot to the skull before obtaining a further view.

The tracing should be made under suitable conditions, i.e., a darkened room, a well-illuminated viewing screen blanked off with card to leave a window just large enough for the radiograph, a good quality tracing sheet fixed to the radiograph with clear adhesive tape and a hard pencil (4H or 6H). The radiograph should be orientated with the Frankfort plane parallel to the bottom edge of the screen, because a number of landmark definitions depend on head orientation.

The Cranial Base (Fig. 6.5)

Identify sella turcica and trace its outline, including the anterior and posterior clinoid processes. Proceed forwards along the planum sphenoidale, across the spheno-ethmoidal synchondrosis and along the cribriform plate of the ethmoid.

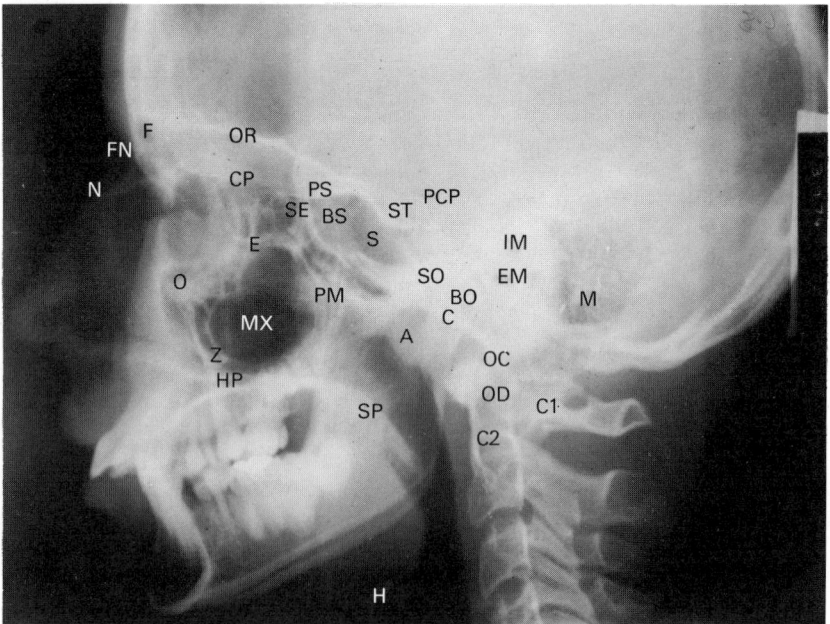

Fig. 6.5. Anatomical features on a lateral skull radiograph. Key: A=adenoids; BO=basiocciput; BS=basisphenoid; C=condyle; CP=cribriform plate of ethmoid; C1=atlas; C2=axis; E=ethmoid air cells; EM=external acoustic meatus; F=frontal sinus; FN=frontonasal suture; H=hyoid bone; HP=hard palate; IM=internal acoustic meatus; M=mastoid air cells; MX=maxillary sinus; N=nasal bone; O=orbital margin; OC=occipital condyle; OD=odontoid process of axis; OR=orbital roof; PCP=posterior clinoid process; PM=pterygoid maxillary fissure; PS=planum sphenoidale; S=sphenoid air sinus; SE=site of spheno-ethmoidal synchondrosis; SO=spheno-occipital synchondrosis; SP=soft palate; ST=sella turcica, the pituitary fossa; Z=zygomatic process of maxilla.

The latter can be difficult to identify and must not be confused with the roofs of the orbits: the cribriform plate is flat or concave superiorly. The wedge-shaped contour of the posterior cranial base is traced easily, except at its posterior limit where the occipital condyles overshadow the basiocciput at the anterior margin of foramen magnum: the basiocciput in the midline does not curve inferiorly and terminates directly above the tip of the odontoid process of the second cervical vertebra.

The anterior surfaces of the frontal and nasal bones should now be traced. The nasal bone is thin and in an overexposed radiograph the anterior surface may be difficult to locate and care must be taken to trace it correctly. The frontonasal suture should also be indicated because the landmark nasion lies at its anterior limit. The frontal and nasal bones are, of course, not part of the cranial base but nasion is taken to represent its anterior limit because there is no alternative reliably identifiable landmark. (For full discussion of cephalometric landmarks, *see* pp. 63–66.)

The Facial Skeleton (Fig. 6.5)

The outline of hard palate is traced without difficulty. The posterior nasal spine may be obscured by unerupted upper molar teeth, but it lies directly below the inferior limit of the pterygomaxillary fissure and so the landmark can be constructed by dropping a perpendicular from the fissure to a line parallel to the nasal floor along the middle of the hard palate. The anterior nasal spine is difficult to locate, unless a wedge filter has been used (*see Fig.* 6.4). It must not be confused with the alar cartilages of the nose which are superimposed upon it and project further forwards. The maxillary profile between anterior nasal spine and the alveolar crest can be very difficult to locate as the labial plate of bone is thin and the image of the soft tissues of the cheeks may be projected over it. The roots of the upper incisors give an approximate guide to its position.

The lateral and inferior borders of the orbit should be traced. Note their outline when viewed from the lateral aspect (*Fig.* 6.6). The inferior border can be particularly difficult to identify because of the complex pattern of bony trabeculae in this region, but the roof of the maxillary antrum, which lies just below it, helps in its location. The root of the zygomatic process of the maxilla may also be identifiable below the orbit.

The external auditory meatus is difficult to locate: the headholder of some cephalostats obscures it and if the central ray does not pass directly through both external auditory meati, the petrous parts of the temporal bones are superimposed upon them. The internal auditory meatus is often much clearer but should not be traced: it lies above and behind the external meatus. The glenoid fossa is level with the upper margin of the meatus and the mandibular condylar head, if it can be seen, gives a good indication of its height. Some authors recommend that the ear rods of the cephalostat should be traced instead of the auditory meatus. This is not acceptable because at best they are positioned in the cartilaginous ear canals and may lie at some distance from the bony meati.

The posterior and inferior borders of the mandible are clearly visible. Where the sides are not superimposed both should be traced and the 'average' position indicated by an interrupted line. The condylar heads can seldom reliably be identified on the lateral skull view, but if they are visible, their position can be

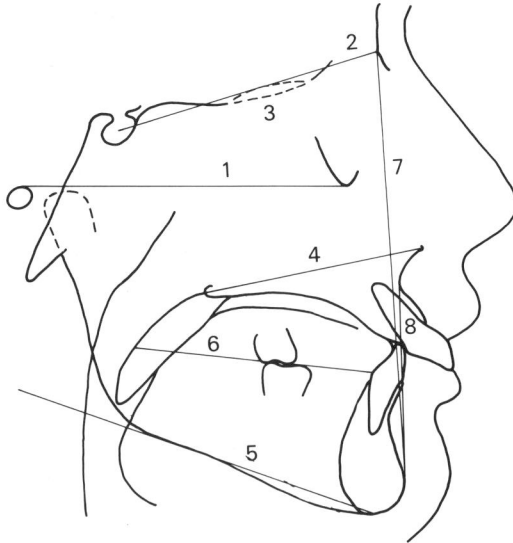

Fig. 6.6. Lines of reference. 1=Frankfort plane; 2=sella–nasion line; 3=De Coster's line; 4=maxillary plane; 5=mandibular plane; 6=functional occlusal plane; 7=facial plane; 8=A–pogonion line.

indicated on the tracing. However, this should not encourage the use of landmarks on the condylar heads. If measurements are to be made to the condylar head, a second lateral skull view should be taken with the mouth open, so that it is forward on the articular eminentia. This allows mandibular length to be measured but would seldom be of sufficient clinical importance to justify a second radiograph.

The exact outlines of the teeth can be difficult to identify with confidence due to their superimposition upon one another. The upper and lower central incisors and first permanent molars are traced. Because it is most clearly seen, the most prominent incisor is outlined, but in some cases this can give a misleading impression of the general position of the incisors and care should be taken in interpreting the results of a tracing where one incisor is particularly proclined or crowded labially. In these circumstances, the other central incisor should be traced as well. Many clinicians use a commercially produced stencil of tooth shapes to produce a clear outline of the tooth. Provided that the tooth to be traced is of average form and size, and provided that the stencil is located correctly so that the incisor edge and apex, and thus the long axis, are correctly shown, this is acceptable. However, there are considerable variations in incisor root length and crown–root angle and a misleading impression of tooth form and position can be given when a stencil is used.

Soft Tissues (Fig. 6.6)

The lips and facial integument, tongue, soft palate and nasopharynx may be traced to give an impression of their relation to the facial skeleton. However, unless the patient was carefully posed when the radiograph was taken, the positions of the lips in particular may be very misleading. If the lips are parted, no conclusions can be drawn about the mechanism of obtaining an anterior oral seal. A posterior oral seal is usually formed by contact between soft palate and tongue, but this may not appear patent on the radiograph if the patient was swallowing at the instant of exposure. The adenoids may be seen on the postero-superior wall of the nasopharynx but no firm conclusions should be drawn about the adequacy or otherwise of the airway, from their appearance: even if they are large, the airway may be sufficient if the nasopharynx is wide; and if they seem to be small or absent, the airway may still be inadequate elsewhere.[5]

CEPHALOMETRIC LANDMARKS (Fig. 6.7)

The definitions assume that the radiograph is orientated with the Frankfort plane horizontal. Many landmarks are bilateral but where the two sides are superimposed perfectly, only a single point is identifiable. Where the two sides are distinct, both should be traced and the midpoint taken as the landmark.

ANTERIOR NASAL SPINE (ANS)

The tip of the anterior nasal spine   This may be difficult to locate if a wedge filter has not been used to enhance profile detail. The spine must not be confused with the alar cartilages which may be visible superimposed upon it.

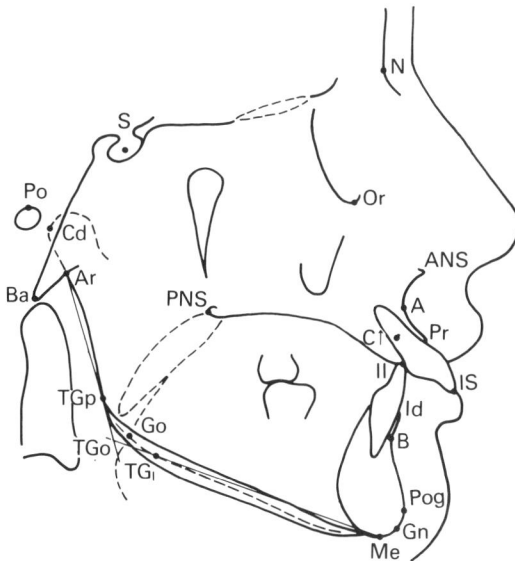

Fig. 6.7. Cephalometric landmarks. A=point A; ANS=anterior nasal spine; Ar=articulare; B=point B; Ba=basion; C↑=centroid of upper incisor; Cd=condylion; Gn=gnathion; Go=gonion; II=incision inferius; IS=incision superius; Id=infradentale; Me=menton; N=nasion; Or=orbitale; Po=porion; Pog=pogonion; PNS=posterior nasal spine; Pr=prosthion; S=sella; TG$_I$=inferior tangent point; TG$_P$=posterior tangent point; TG$_O$=constructed gonion.

ARTICULARE (Ar)

The intersection of the posterior border of the neck of the mandibular condyle and the lower margin of the posterior cranial base   This constructed point does not exist anatomically but is used to indicate the position of the mandibular joint relative to the cranial base. In some studies it has been used as an alternative to basion, which can be difficult to identify, in measurements of the cranial base. Others use it as an alternative to condylion in measuring mandibular length.

BASION (Ba)

The most posterior inferior point on the clivus (basiocciput)   It lies on the anterior margin of foramen magnum and may be difficult to locate because it is overshadowed by the occipital condyles. It represents the posterior limit of the midline cranial base.

CENTROID OF THE UPPER INCISOR ROOT (C↑)

The midpoint on the root axis of the most prominent upper incisor

CONDYLION (Cd)

The most superior posterior point on the head of the mandibular condyle   This point cannot be located reliably on a standard lateral skull radiograph because the shadow of petrous temporal obscures the condylar head. Articulare is often used as an alternative point.

GNATHION (Gn)

The most anterior inferior point on the mandibular symphysis in the midline   It may be located by inspection or may be constructed as the intersection of the margin of the symphysis with the bisector of the angle between the facial line (N–Pog) and the mandibular line (TG_IMe).

GONION (Go)

The most posterior inferior point on the angle of the mandible   It may be located by inspection or may be constructed using the bisector of the angle between the ramal line ($Ar–TG_p$) and the mandibular line (TG_IMe). The constructed point TG_o may be used instead.

INCISION INFERIUS (II)

The tip of the crown of the most prominent lower incisor In this text the point is also referred to as E↓, the lower incisor edge.

INCISION SUPERIUS (IS)

The tip of the crown of the most prominent upper incisor

INFRADENTALE (Id)

The intersection of the alveolar crest and the outline of the most prominent mandibular incisor

MENTON (Me)

The lowermost point of the mandibular symphysis in the midline Where the chin is grooved, the most inferior points are bilateral but the midline contour can be seen slightly above them.

NASION (N)

The most anterior point on the frontonasal suture Where the frontonasal suture cannot be identified, the deepest point of the profile between the frontal and nasal bones should be taken. This is often slightly below true nasion and for consistency of identification might be a better point to use routinely. In dense radiographs, the anterior border of the nasal bone is difficult to see and care should be taken not to locate nasion too far back.

ORBITALE (Or)

The most inferior anterior point on the margin of the orbit Strictly speaking, the left orbitale should be used for orientating the Frankfort plane but, unless there is a pointer to the lower border of the left orbit or a radio-opaque mark is attached to the skin before the radiograph is taken, it is not possible to tell left from right and so the sides should be averaged. Orbitale is a rather unreliable landmark.

POGONION (Pog)

The most anterior point on the bony chin

POINT A *(also known as subspinale)*

The most posterior point on the profile of the maxilla between the anterior nasal spine and the alveolar crest It is taken to represent the anterior limit of the maxillary apical base. It is difficult to locate reliably because the soft tissues of the cheeks may be superimposed upon it. Sometimes there is a ridge of bone passing inferiorly from the anterior nasal spine, which lies further forward than point A.

POINT B *(also known as supramentale)*

The most posterior point on the profile of the mandible between the chin point and the alveolar crest It represents the anterior limit of the mandibular apical base.

PORION (Po)

The uppermost outermost point on the bony external auditory meatus This can be difficult to locate but it is on the same level as the upper border of the condylar heads, which may act as a guide if they can be seen.

POSTERIOR NASAL SPINE (PNS)

The tip of the posterior nasal spine   This may be obscured by unerupted molars in which case the landmark is constructed as the intersection of the line parallel to the nasal floor along the middle of the hard palate and the line perpendicular to it through the lower limit of the pterygomaxillary fissure.

PROSTHION (Pr)

The intersection of the alveolar crest and the outline of the most prominent maxillary incisor

SELLA (S)

The midpoint of the sella turcica

TG_1

The inferior tangent point at the angle of the mandible   It is identified as the point of contact of the tangent to the angle of the mandible that passes through menton.

TG_p

The posterior tangent point at the angle of the mandible   It is identified as the point of contact of the tangent to the angle of the mandible that passes through articulare.

TG_o

The intersection of the lines TG_1 Me and Ar–TG_p   It is a constructed point that can be used as an alternative to gonion.

CEPHALOMETRIC MEASUREMENTS

While cephalometric radiographs can be measured directly with computer supported digitizers, most commonly the measurements are made on tracings. Both methods are subject to similar errors. Provided that due care is taken at each stage from positioning the patient to recording the measurement, errors should not be large. However, the validity and reproducibility of each measurement must be considered.

Validity

This is the extent to which the measurement represents the structure under consideration. If a measurement involves a landmark of questionable validity, it

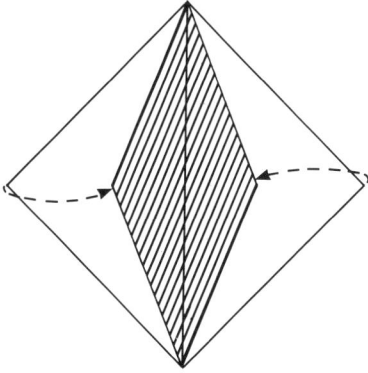

Fig. 6.8. Effects of perspective. When a rectangle is viewed obliquely, the edges are foreshortened and the angles are affected according to the laws of perspective.

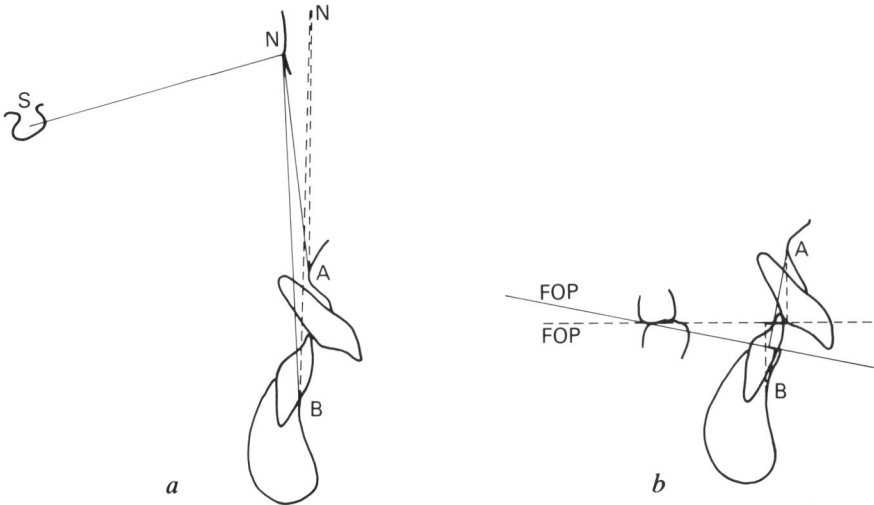

Fig. 6.9. Variations in a reference point or plane give misleading results. *a*, Anatomical variations in the position of nasion can affect the size of the angle ANB. *b*, Variation in the orientation of the functional occlusal plane affects the estimate of the skeletal pattern from projections to it.

must be treated with caution. This problem has been discussed with the definition of landmarks. Measurements where the defining landmarks are not all in a plane parallel to the film are distorted according to the laws of perspective: linear measurements are foreshortened and angles are distorted (*Fig.* 6.8). If the lateral displacement of the landmarks is known, true values can be obtained but this is rarely done because most landmarks are difficult to identify on a PA film and because it has become conventional cephalometric practice to use projections of measurements on to the film plane. Finally, where the relationship between pairs of points is measured as an angle subtended at a third point, or as the projected distance on to a line, variations in the position of the base point or line can give a misleading impression of the relationship of primary interest (*Fig.* 6.9).

Reproducibility

Reproducibility is the closeness of repeated measurements of the same structure. This depends on a number of factors, including the quality of the radiograph, the clarity of the landmark and of its definition, and the skill and care of the observer. Some measurements, such as the angle SNB, should be highly reproducible because the landmarks are clear, while others such as SNA, where A may be difficult to locate, are less reliable. It is instructive for the clinician to trace the same group of radiographs on two separate occasions and to compare the reproducibility with results published by others.

Norms

If a measurement is to be intelligible, its average value and range of variation must be known. Most linear and some angular measurements vary according to age, sex and race and so for these many different norm values are required. For this reason most clinical cephalometric analyses use angular values which differ little with age or sex and so a single series of norms can be used for each racial group. The values used in this text are Caucasian and are derived from a number of groups of individuals with normal occlusions. Comparative values for some other racial groups are given in *Table* 6.1. Ninety-five per cent of values lie within 2 standard deviations on either side of the mean (or average) and so measurements that fall beyond this range may be regarded as extreme.

Norms are of value in description, but they should not necessarily be taken as an indication of the need for treatment, nor as a treatment goal. Even in an individual with a good occlusion and a pleasing facial appearance, it is not uncommon to find several measurements at the limits of normal variation; and planning treatment to the average of a value, for example inclination of the lower incisors, is no guarantee of stability.

Cephalometric measurements must not be evaluated singly and in isolation. It may well be the case that an extreme value for one measurement is compensated by variation in different structures. Thus true cephalometric analysis is the exploration of a pattern: how have the different dentofacial components fitted

Table 6.1. Some cephalometric norms for different racial groups

| | Caucasian[1] | | Negro[2] | | Chinese[3] | |
	Mean	s.d.	Mean	s.d.	Mean	s.d.
SNA	81.4	3.6	88.2	4.4	83.8	3.5
SNB	77.7	3.4	83.9	4.4	79.9	3.8
ANB	3.7	2.4	4.3	2.5	3.9	2.0
LI/Mn	94.7	6.5	101.2	7.0	98.4	7.6
UI/LI	125.5	10.0	112.8	9.5	121.7	7.8

[1]Data derived from: Riolo M. L., Moyers R. E., McNamara J. A. et al. (1974) An atlas of craniofacial growth. Monograph No. 2., Center for Human Growth and Development, University of Michigan. (Sample: 12-year-old girls with no orthodontic treatment).

[2]Fonseca R. J. and Klein W. D. (1978) A cephalometric evaluation of American Negro women. *Am. J. Orthodont.* **73**; 152–60. (Sample: 40 adult women with Class I malocclusions).

[3]Chan G. K. (1972) A cephalometric appraisal of the Chinese. *Am. J. Orthodont.* **61**; 279–85. (Sample: 30 adult men with excellent occlusions.)

together to give the observed skeletal and occlusal relationships? Treatment is planned on the basis of alterations of some of the components (generally dentoskeletal relationships) in a way that will harmonize with the overall facial pattern as well as giving a result that is aesthetically and functionally acceptable and which will be stable.

CEPHALOMETRIC ANALYSIS

Many different cephalometric analyses have been proposed. A number of these are elaborate and the usefulness of some of the measurements is obscure. Practical cephalometric analysis should concentrate upon features that have an immediate bearing on the orthodontic problem and its treatment and the clinical relevance of each measurement should be clear. Cephalometric analysis may encompass: description of the dentofacial pattern; prediction of the changes that are expected to occur with growth; prescription of treatment objectives; and retrospective evaluation of growth and treatment changes.

It is desirable to avoid superfluity, but there is value in examining some relationships in two different ways because, for structural reasons, one measurement may be misleading. For example the use of the angle ANB to measure the skeletal pattern may be misleading because of anatomical variation in the position of nasion (*see Fig.* 6.9); and an independent measurement such as the angulation of the line AB to the occlusal plane gives a useful check.

When two independent measurements reinforce one another, they can be accepted with confidence, but when they do not, the reason for any discrepancy must be sought. The cephalometric findings should be integrated to give a coherent picture of the facial pattern of the individual. An integrated approach to cephalometric analysis will be illustrated by later examples, but first the individual measurements will be discussed.

Descriptive Analysis

Skeletal and dental relationships are generally measured by reference to a point or plane. Variations in the position or orientation of the reference structure can affect the measurement. It is important to recognize that such structural effects can give erroneous results, which can usually be discovered by looking at the general pattern of measurements or by making a separate assessment of the relationship in question, relative to a different reference structure.

Lines of Reference (Fig. 6.6)

THE TRUE HORIZONTAL

If the patient can be posed with the head in the natural postural position when the radiograph is taken, the true horizontal may be identified.[6] It is also possible to record this by attaching radio-opaque markers to the skin before taking the radiograph.[7] The problem lies in posing the patient reliably. The true horizontal would be particularly useful for the assessment of anteroposterior jaw relationships but, because positioning the patient correctly can be time-consuming, this is seldom done. Attempts have been made to orientate cephalometric radiographs by reference to the semicircular canals of the vestibular apparatus, but these cannot be located reliably and so this approach has little application to clinical assessment.

FRANKFORT PLANE

This plane, which passes through porion and orbitale, was defined at a conference of craniometrists held in Frankfort in 1884 as approximating the true horizontal when the head is held in the normal postural position. It was designed to allow a comparison of the skulls of different species, and races of man, and was subsequently adopted for use in cephalometric analysis. In fact, there is appreciable variation in the orientation of the Frankfort plane (up to 10° on either side of the true horizontal) and its identification on a lateral skull radiograph can be unreliable owing to difficulty in locating its reference landmarks. However, it is one of the few planes that can be identified clinically as well as radiographically and so it can be useful in relating clinical impressions to radiographic findings, and in orientating profile photographs to match lateral skull radiographs.

SELLA–NASION LINE

This line is taken to represent the anterior cranial base, which undergoes little change from growth or remodelling after about 6 years of age when the spheno-ethmoidal synchondrosis fuses. This stable area is therefore valuable as a baseline in the measurement and comparison of jaw relationships between individuals and within the one case at different ages. A further advantage of this line is that the landmarks (S and N) are comparatively easy to locate reliably. Unfortunately, nasion does not in fact lie on the anterior cranial base but at the

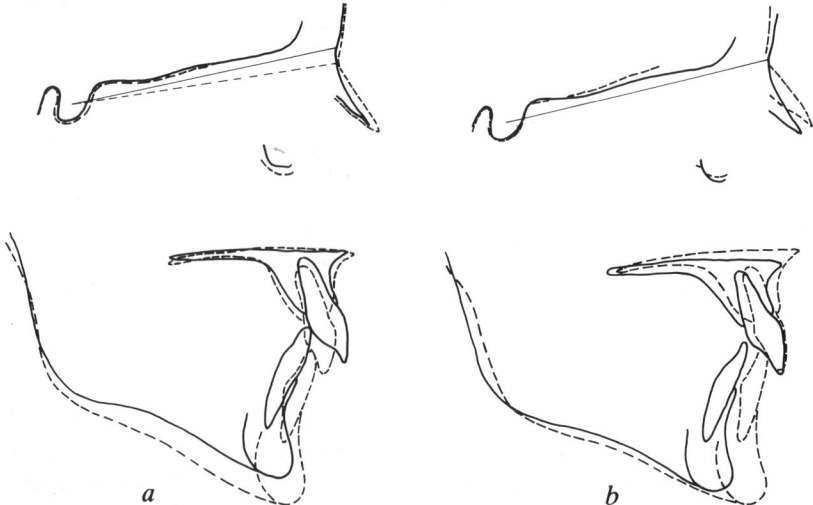

Fig. 6.10. Superimposition of serial radiographs. *a*, Superimposition on de Coster's line shows that nasion has drifted downwards with growth. *b*, Superimposition of the same tracings on the sella–nasion line gives a different and misleading impression of facial growth in this case.

outer limit of the frontonasal suture, which does remodel with growth. In most children, nasion drifts forwards along the original sella–nasion line, but it can drift vertically and this will give an incorrect impression of the way that the face has grown if serial radiographs are related to one another by means of this line (*Fig.* 6.10).

When jaw relationships are measured relative to the SN line, it is important to recognize that variations in its orientation, and in the position of nasion in particular, can give a false impression of the true relationships (*see Fig.* 6.9).

DE COSTER'S LINE (*see Fig.* 6.6)

This follows the floor of the anterior cranial base close to the midline from the anterior margin of the ethmoid bone to sella turcica. It passes along the cribriform plate of the ethmoid, and the planum sphenoidale, and includes the anterior wall and base of sella turcica. Little remodelling with growth takes place in the midline anterior cranial base after fusion of the spheno-ethmoidal synchondrosis[8] and so it is possible to use de Coster's line for the superimposition of serial radiographs taken after 7 years of age. Experience is required to do this reliably, and care has to be taken not to confuse the correct reference line with the roofs of the orbits or the crista galli, which may be more clearly visible on the radiograph. Minor remodelling changes do occur and so the comparison of serial radiographs taken more than 4 or 5 years apart must be undertaken with reservations.

MAXILLARY LINE (ANS–PNS)

The inclination of the upper incisors is commonly measured to this line. Where the anterior nasal spine curves upwards or downwards markedly, the maxillary line should be orientated parallel to the nasal floor (*see Fig.* 6.5), as is done when the posterior nasal spine cannot be seen.

MANDIBULAR LINE

The inclination of the lower incisors is measured to the mandibular line and its angulation to the maxillary line gives a measure of lower anterior face height. The mandibular line is defined in a number of different ways: the anterior landmark may be menton or gnathion and the posterior landmark may be TG_I or gonion. The measurements obtained will differ slightly according to the line used. The most convenient line, which is used in this book, passes through menton and TG_I.

OCCLUSAL LINE

As with the mandibular line, several different definitions are found. Many authors use the line passing midway between the tips of the mesiobuccal cusps of the upper and lower first permanent molars, and the lower incisor edges. This may give an unreliable assessment of the general line of the occlusion where there is a deep overbite.

The functional occlusal plane (FOP) is perhaps more useful for most purposes: it passes through the occlusion of the premolars or deciduous molars and the first permanent molars. The cuspal outlines of these teeth are often not clear and it may be difficult to locate the functional occlusal plane accurately, particularly in the mixed dentition when only the first permanent molars may meet in occlusion.

It is important to recognize that whatever occlusal line or plane is used, its orientation may change with growth or treatment and so it is not an entirely satisfactory reference from which to evaluate other relationships.

THE FACIAL LINE (N–POG)

This was used as a line of reference by Downs[9] to help to assess the facial profile. The angle of the facial line to the Frankfort horizontal (the facial angle) indicates whether the profile is prognathic, retrognathic or orthognathic (the lower face is protrusive, retrusive or upright, respectively).

THE LINE FROM POINT A TO POGONION (A–POG)

This line has been used in a number of cephalometric analyses to measure the anteroposterior position of the crowns of the incisor teeth. Raleigh Williams[10] stated that the best aesthetic results were obtained when the lower incisor edges lay on the A-Pog line; but it does not necessarily indicate a position of stability for these teeth.

Many other cephalometric lines and planes of reference have been proposed, but in general they have little application to modern cephalometric analysis.

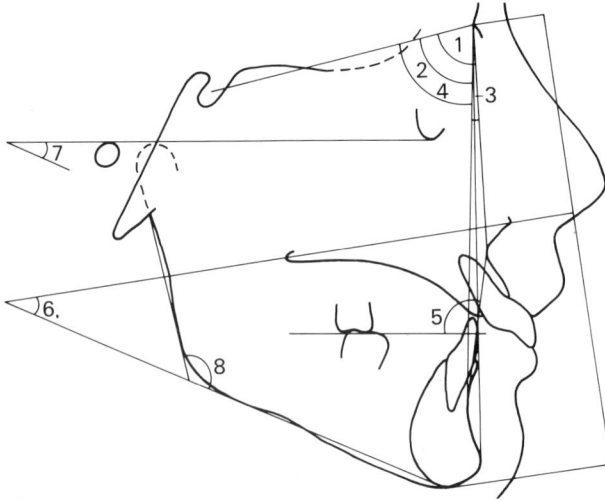

Fig. 6.11. Cephalometric measurements of skeletal relationships. 1=SNA; 2=SNB; 3=ANB; 4=SNPog; 5=A–B/FOP; 6=MM angle; 7=FM angle; 8=gonial angle.

Measurement of Skeletal Relationships (Fig. 6.11)

The values given for each measurement are the standard deviations from Caucasian norms (*see* p. 68).

ANGLE S–N–A (82±3°)

Prognathism of the maxillary apical base   The average value is 82° and a marked deviation from this usually indicates that either the position of nasion or the orientation of the S–N line is aberrant (*see Fig.* 6.9). Variation in the size of angle S–N–A is not usually important *per se* unless surgical change in the position of the maxilla is to be planned; but it should be taken into account when other measurements involving nasion, and in particular A–N–B, are interpreted.

ANGLE S–N–B $(79\pm3°)$
Prognathism of the mandibular apical base

ANGLE S–N–POG $(80\pm3°)$
Mandibular prognathism   It is interesting to compare the values of S–N–B and S–N–Pog. Where there is a well-developed chin but mandibular apical base retrusion, the facial appearance may be good but the apical base relationship is unfavourable, as is often the case in Class II, division 2 cases. Where S–N–Pog is smaller than S–N–B in Class II cases, the facial appearance is usually less good than the apical base relationship would suggest.

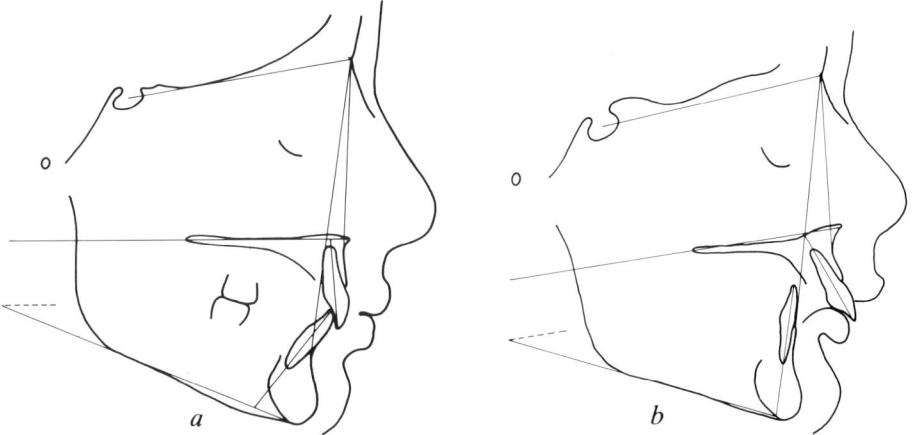

Fig. 6.12. *a*, Dento-alveolar compensation. There is a Class II skeletal pattern (ANB=6°) with the MM angle=22°. The skeletal pattern is largely compensated by the proclined lower incisors (LI/Mn=107°) and there is some compensation in the upper incisors (UI/Mx=94°). The skeletal malrelationship is fully compensated and the incisor relationship is Class I. *b*, Dento-alveolar exacerbation. The Class II skeletal pattern is moderately severe (ANB=10°) and the MM angle is 25°. The overjet is even larger than would be expected from the skeletal pattern because the upper incisors are proclined (UI/Mx=113°) and the lower incisors are retroclined (LI/Mn=82°).

ANGLE A–N–B (3±1°)

The anteroposterior apical base relationship (skeletal pattern)   Where the antero-posterior apical base relationship is favourable for a Class I occlusion, the A–N–B angle is usually in the range of 2–4°. However, apical base relationships beyond this range can be associated with a Class I occlusion if there is appropriate dento-alveolar compensation; and arch malrelationships occur even with favourable apical base relationships, where the inclinations of the teeth are unfavourable (*Fig.* 6.12). Following Angle's classification of arch malrela-

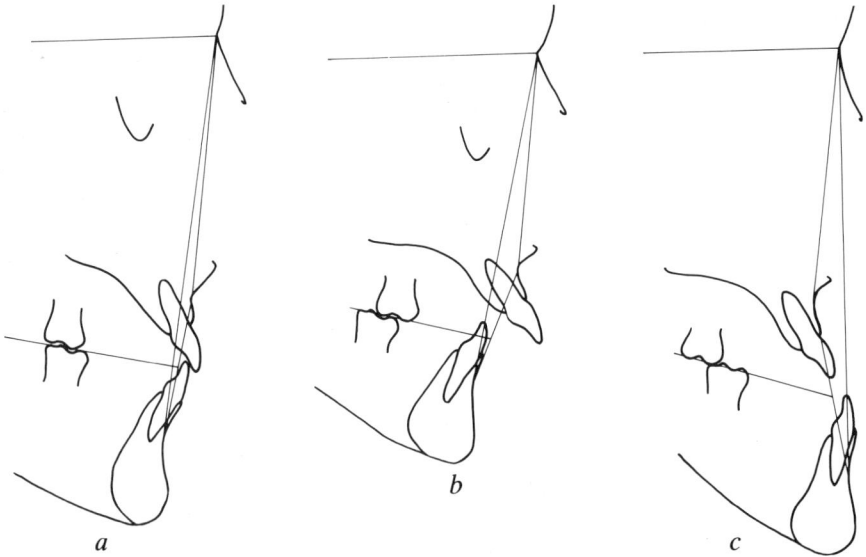

Fig. 6.13. Different skeletal patterns. *a*, Class I: ANB 2.5°, A–B/FOP 90°. *b*, Class II: ANB 6°, A–B/FOP 100°. *c*, Class III: ANB −7°, A–B/FOP 62°.

tionships, the skeletal pattern is described as being Class I where the A–N–B angle is in the range 2–4°, and where the angle is greater than +4° degrees or less than +2°, as Class II or Class III, respectively (*Fig.* 6.13). As has been emphasized previously, the occlusal and skeletal relationships do not always match and they must be assessed independently.

The value of A–N–B may be misleading where the position of nasion is unusual (*see Fig.* 6.9), and while a warning of this may be given by the value of S–N–A, this is not completely reliable.

ANGLE A–B/FOP (90±5°)

This measures the apical base relationship by reference to the functional occlusion plane. In a Class I skeletal pattern, the range is 85–95°. Clearly variation in the orientation of the occlusal plane will affect this angle and changes in its size must not be taken as evidence of change in the skeletal pattern in treated cases where the orientation of the occlusal plane may have been altered.

If the functional occlusal plane is to be used as a reference line, its angulation to the maxillary line should be checked: if this angle is within the range 6–14°, the orientation of the FOP is within 1 standard deviation of the mean and it may be used with reasonable confidence to evaluate the skeletal pattern.

Harvold[11] used the distance between perpendicular projection of the points *A* and *B* on to the FOP to indicate the skeletal pattern, and this was subsequently adopted at the University of Witwatersrand and became known as the 'Wits analysis'.[12] No figures for the range of normal variation were given and its construction is less convenient than the angle described above.

MAXILLARY–MANDIBULAR PLANES ANGLE (Mx–Mn or MM angle) (27±5°)

This angle provides a measure of the divergence of the intermaxillary space anteriorly. Variations are usually attributable to the slope of the mandibular plane. The anterior intermaxillary height is of interest because if it is appreciably increased or reduced, there is often an anterior open bite or a deep overbite respectively, and these being of skeletal origin can be difficult to correct. A high MM angle is often associated with a posterior pattern of mandibular growth rotation, and a low angle with an anterior growth rotation.

The size of the MM angle is, of course, largely determined by the ratio of anterior and posterior intermaxillary heights and so an independent estimate of the anterior intermaxillary height is desirable. This is provided by the ratio of lower and middle facial heights.

FACE/HEIGHT RATIO (Me–Mx/N–Me) (50–55 per cent)

This ratio is used to estimate anterior intermaxillary height but it can, of course, be affected by variations in midfacial height. When the MM angle and the face height ratio are inconsistent, they must be interpreted with caution and the reason for the discrepancy should be sought.

FRANKFORT–MANDIBULAR PLANES ANGLE (FM angle) (27±5°)

This angle is highly correlated with the MM angle and there is little point in measuring both. The FM angle is less reliable, due to problems in locating the landmarks that determine the Frankfort plane. It does, however, have the advantage that it can be measured clinically.

GONIAL ANGLE (Ar–TG_P/TG_IMe) (126±5°)

The slope of the posterior border of the mandibular ramus varies little and so this angle essentially measures the slope of the mandibular plane and is highly correlated with the MM angle. There is little value in measuring both.

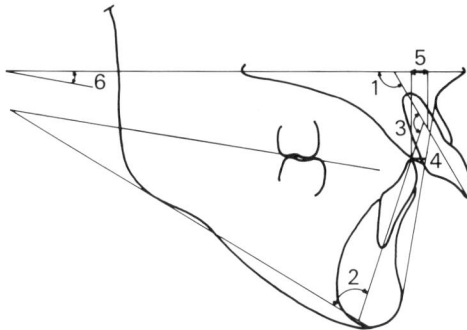

Fig. 6.14. Dentoskeletal relationships. 1=Upper incisor to maxillary planes angle (UI/Mx). 2=Lower incisor to mandibular planes angle (LI/Mn). 3=Interincisor angle (UI/LI). 4=Lower incisor edge to A–Pog distance (E ↓ –A–Pog). 5=Lower incisor edge to upper centroid projection (E ↓ C ↑). 6=Functional occlusal plane to maxillary planes angle (FOP/Mx).

Dentoskeletal Relationships (Fig. 6.14)

UPPER INCISOR TO MAXILLARY PLANE ANGLE (UI/Mx) (108±5°)

The orientation of the upper incisors is important functionally and aesthetically, and the existing inclination will determine the types of tooth movement that are required to correct any anomalies in the incisor relationships. For example, a case with a moderate Class II, division 1 incisor relationship is treated much more readily if the upper incisors are proclined than if they are retroclined. Further insight into the tooth movements required to correct incisor malrelationships is obtained from the edge–centroid relationships (*see below*).

Where there is an unusually large crown–root angle, this measurement may give an incorrect evaluation of the orientation of the incisor crowns, which is an important factor in appearance and occlusal relationships.

LOWER INCISOR TO MANDIBULAR PLANE ANGLE (LI/MN) (92±5°)

Although it is usually stated that this angle should ideally lie within the range indicated above, it cannot be evaluated adequately without taking account of other variables. The average and range of variation given above is appropriate only where the maxillary–mandibular planes angle and skeletal pattern are within normal limits.

The labiolingual position of the crowns of the lower incisors, and thus their inclination, is influenced by the balance between the lips and tongue and when the lower border of the mandible is inclined steeply relative to the maxillary plane, there tends to be compensatory retroclination of the lower incisors, and vice versa when the mandibular plane is more horizontal than average (*Fig.* 6.15). Thus there is an inverse relationship between the size of the MM angle and the expected inclination of the lower incisors to the mandibular plane, and for every degree that the MM angle exceeds 27°, the expected value of the lower incisor inclination (92°) should be reduced by 1°, and vice versa where the MM angle is less than 27°. In order to avoid adjusting the lower incisor angle in this way, some authorities measure the inclination of the lower incisors to the

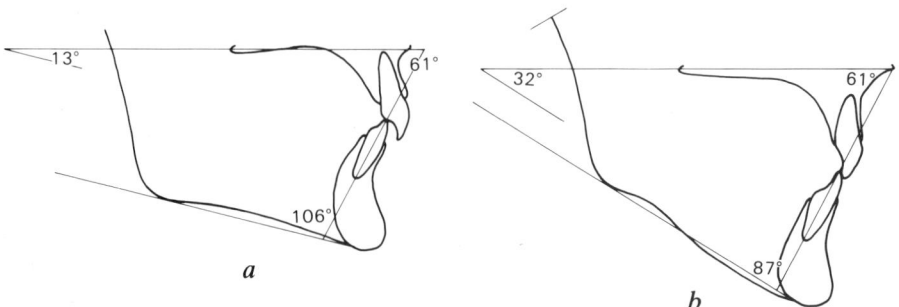

Fig. 6.15. The inverse relationship between the lower incisor angulation and the MM angle. *a*, The lower incisor angle is 106° (14° above the average) but the MM angle is 13° (14° below the average). The lower incisor angle is therefore considered to be 'normal' for this patient. *b*, The MM angle is 5° above the average (27°) and so the lower incisor angle, which is 5° below the average, is considered normal for this patient. Note that the lower incisor to maxillary plane angle is 61° in both cases, which is average for this population group.

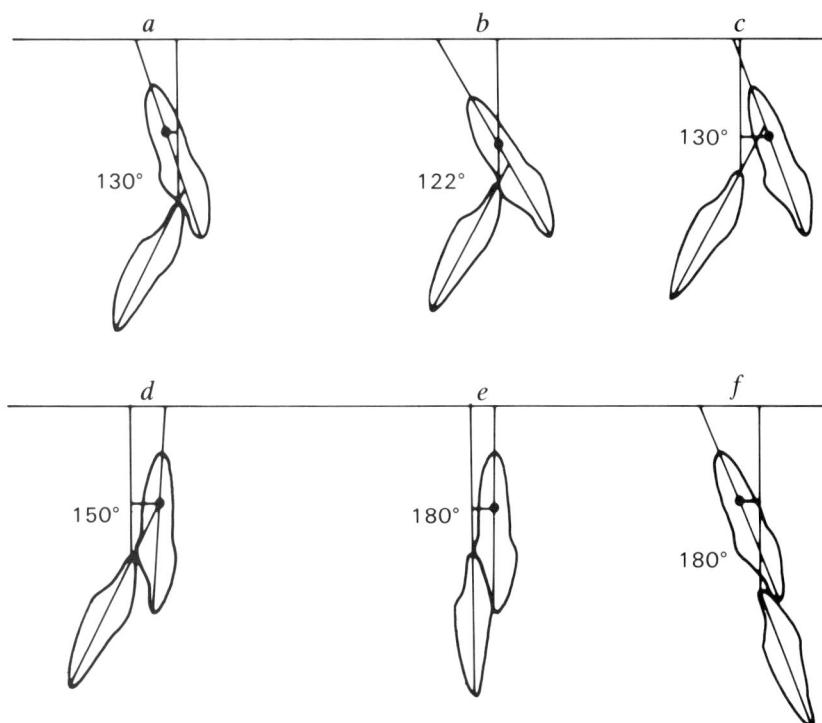

Fig. 6.16. Interincisor relationships and overbite. The interincisor angle is given on the diagrams. *a*, In a Class I incisor relationship with an average inclination of upper incisors, the lower incisor edge lies in advance of the upper incisor centroid and so the overbite is within normal limits. *b*, In this Class II incisor relationship, the upper incisors are proclined and so the interincisor angle is reduced. E ↓ is directly below C ↑ and so provided that the tooth is tipped back around the centroid, the overbite reduction should be stable. For greater security of overbite reduction, C ↑ should be moved 1–2 mm palatally. *c*, A Class II, division 1 incisor relationship where E ↓ lies well behind C ↑ . Simple tipping of the upper incisor will merely produce a Class II, division 2 incisor relationship, with a deep overbite. Stable overbite reduction depends upon a change in the E ↓ and C ↑ relationships. *d*, A Class II, division 2 incisor relationship. Overbite reduction will be stable only if the E ↓ and C ↑ relationship can be changed. *e, f*, In both these cases, the interincisor angle is very wide (180°). In (*e*), there is a Class II, division 2 incisor relationship with an adverse E ↓ C ↑ relationship. When the E ↓ lies in advance of C ↑ (*f*) then the overbite will not be deep, in spite of the wide interincisor angle.

maxillary or to the Frankfort plane, which does not vary with the slope of the mandibular plane.

Where there is a Class II or Class III skeletal pattern and the soft tissue pattern is favourable, dento-alveolar compensation is often found, and so the lower incisors may be proclined or retroclined respectively. This is of course a favourable feature and so the lower incisor angulation should not be interpreted without reference to the skeletal pattern. Formulae for the expected degree of dento-alveolar compensation according to the skeletal pattern have been suggested, but it is more instructive to assess this by taking account of the relationships of the lower incisor edge to the A–Pog line and to the upper incisor centroid as described below.

INTERINCISOR ANGLE (UI/LI) (133±10°)

The interincisor angle is associated with the depth of overbite when there is incisor contact: if the interincisor angle is wide, then even if incisor contact is achieved during the eruption of the teeth or as a result of orthodontic treatment, they will tend to erupt past one another (*Fig.* 6.16) and the wider the interincisor angle, the deeper the overbite. However, the importance of a wide interincisor angle is greater in cases with a Class II rather than a Class III skeletal pattern (*Fig.* 6.16). In fact, it is the anteroposterior relationship of the incisor apices, rather than the apical bases, that is important, but this is not usually assessed in cephalometric analysis. A better and more direct assessment is given by the lower edge/upper centroid relationship, as described below.

LOWER INCISOR EDGE TO A–POG DISTANCE (E ↓ A–POG) (0–2 MM)

It is found that in well-balanced faces with good occlusions, the lower incisor edge lies on or close to the A–Pog line; and in treated cases with a skeletal malrelationship, the most satisfactory occlusal and aesthetic relationships are generally obtained when the lower incisors are in this position. In many cases with a favourable soft tissue pattern this is also the position of lower incisor stability which the teeth will have adopted naturally. However, this is not always the case, and the A–Pog line should not be used to predict the position of lower incisor stability: it takes no account of soft tissue balance and its orientation is greatly influenced by the prominence of the chin. The A–Pog line does provide a measure of the extent of dento-alveolar compensation for skeletal malrelationships and it can be useful to monitor the changes in the position of the lower incisor crowns that have occurred during treatment.

LOWER INCISOR EDGE TO UPPER INCISOR CENTROID DISTANCE (E ↓ C ↑) (0–2 MM)

This is measured as the distance between the perpendicular projections of the lower incisor edge and the centroid of the upper incisor root (*Fig.* 6.16) on to the maxillary plane.[13] This relationship is closely associated with overbite depth in that the further behind the centroid the lower edge lies, the deeper the overbite is liable to be, except of course if it is incomplete. The edge–centroid relationship allows for the influence on the incisor relationship of both the skeletal pattern and the lower dento-alveolar compensation. In planning treatment it focuses attention on the tooth movements that will be required to obtain a satisfactory incisor relationship, and in particular a stable overbite.

FUNCTIONAL OCCLUSAL PLANE TO MAXILLARY PLANE ANGLE (FOP/MX) (10±4°)

This measurement is correlated with the divergence of the intermaxillary space (MM angle). If it is beyond the normal range, the FOP must be used with caution as a plane of reference (e.g. in the A–B/FOP angle) because the result may give a misleading impression of the relationship that it is intended to measure.

Soft Tissue Analysis

Changes in tooth position have a small but variable effect on lip positions[14] and one should be aware of this in planning treatment. For example, when upper incisors are retracted, the upper lip will drop back, more at the vermilion border than at the base, and the lip will tend to flatten. The form and position of the lower lip can alter markedly when a large overjet is corrected and it lies in front of the upper incisors rather than behind them. When a bimaxillary proclination is reduced, the lip protrusion is also affected, particularly in patients who previously had difficulties in obtaining a lip seal.

Lip position always changes less than tooth position and the relationship varies appreciably in different individuals. The dentist should be aware of the relationship of the teeth to the rest of the face and to the soft tissues in particular.

However, people rarely see themselves in profile and are seldom viewed by others, except orthodontists, in this way; and so some of the features that are evaluated may have little impact on the patient in everyday life.

There are a number of problems with soft tissue analysis. If cephalometric radiographs rather than profile photographs are used, the soft tissues may not be visualized readily unless a wedge filter has been used (*see Fig.* 6.4) and the patient may not have been posed correctly with the lips in their habitual posture. A major difficulty is that soft tissue assessment is purely aesthetic, and opinions differ as to what is acceptable; to one a slight fullness of the lower face may be pleasing, while to another this is considered unattractive.

The orthodontist's ability to produce changes in the soft tissue profile is strictly limited. Stability of treatment is imperative, and if it is acknowledged that facial growth cannot be controlled at will, the possible positions of the incisors are constrained by the skeletal relationships, by soft tissue balance and by growth. Thus it is facile to base treatment planning on changes in soft tissue profile. Naturally the possible effects on lip form of any proposed changes in incisor position should be evaluated when treatment is planned; and if alternative approaches to treatment are feasible, this is a factor to consider in choosing between them. It should be remembered that published cases illustrating the importance of soft tissue planning are selected specially for that purpose and may not be typical results of the approach to treatment planning that is being advocated. In many cases the major contribution to an improvement in integumental profile is growth and facial maturation. Soft tissue analysis has a more important role in planning surgical correction of skeletal malrelationships where there may be a wider choice of procedures and their effects on the integumental profile are greater than with tooth movement by orthodontic appliances.

Many reference lines have been proposed for analysis of the integumental profile, and some of these are shown in *Fig.* 6.17. They are an aid to description of facial appearance and of soft tissue change associated with growth and treatment. As explained above, they are of limited value in planning treatment, although manoeuvres that would cause deterioration in lip form should be avoided if possible.

Lines of Reference (Fig. 6.17)

UPPER LIP TANGENT[15]

This is a line perpendicular to the Frankfort plane and tangential to the vermilion border of the upper lip.

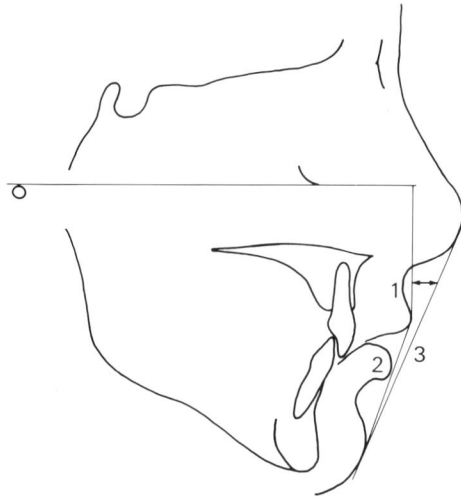

Fig. 6.17. Soft tissue profile analysis. 1, the upper lip tangent is perpendicular to the Frankfort plane. The depth of the concavity of the upper lip should lie 1–4 mm behind this. In this case the upper lip curl is 3 mm. 2, The H (or harmony) line of Holdaway is drawn tangential to the upper lip and chin. The vermilion border of the lower lip should lie within 1 mm of the H line. 3, The E (or aesthetic) line of Ricketts. The vermilion borders of both lips should lie close to this line. Note that during the later stages of facial growth, growth of the nose in particular carries the E line forwards so that the relation of the lips to it may well change after the completion of orthodontic treatment,

H LINE

The Harmony line of Holdaway[15]   This is the tangent to the soft tissue chin and to the vermilion border of the upper lip.

AESTHETIC LINE[16]

This is the tangent to the tip of the nose and chin.

Fig. 6.18. A 12-year-old boy with a Class II, division 1 malocclusion. SNA and SNB are both within normal limits although slightly below average. The ANB angle is within the range of a Class I skeletal pattern. This is supported by the A–B/FOP angle at 90°. The orientation of the FOP to the maxillary plane is within normal limits.

The face height ratio and the MM angle are both a little reduced but again within normal limits. Thus the skeletal relationships do not impose limitations on the correction of the malocclusion.

The lower incisors are quite proclined at 102° to the mandibular plane: even allowing for the slightly low MM angle, the adjusted value is 98°. However, the lower incisor edge is only slightly in advance of the A–Pog line, indicating that they are quite well placed within the face and should allow a satisfactory position of the upper incisor edges following their retraction.

The upper incisors are proclined and, as is to be expected from the inclination of upper and lower incisors, the interincisor angle is reduced. The lower incisor edge lies 2 mm in advance of the upper root centroid which indicates that tipping the upper incisors about a fulcrum close to the centroid should produce a satisfactory incisor relationship. There is liable to be a slight residual overjet due to the proclination of the lower incisors, but this should not present problems of aesthetics or stability.

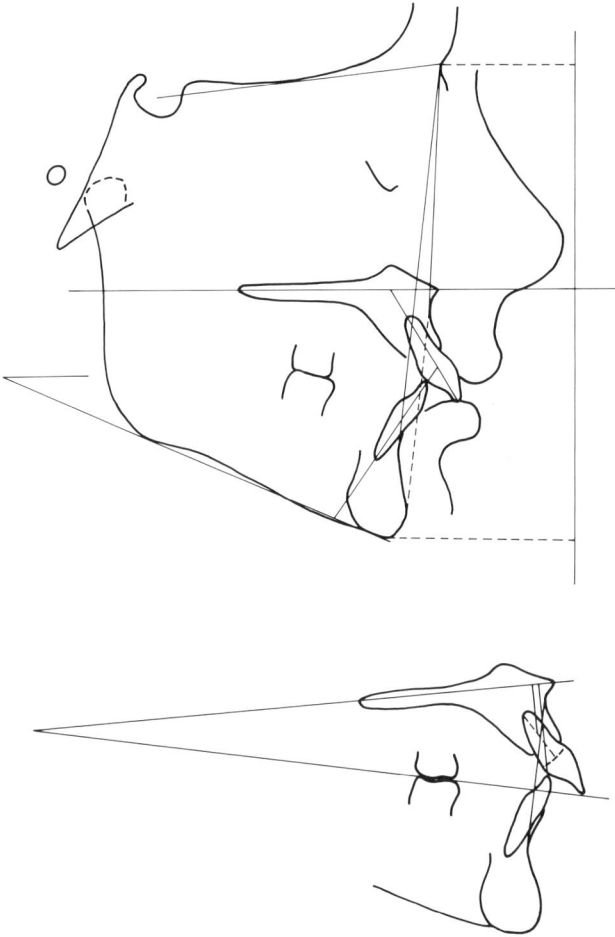

Measurement	Mean ± normal range	This case
SNA	82±3°	81°
SNB	79±3°	77°
ANB	3±1°	4°
A–B∕FOP	90±5°	90°
MM<	27±5°	23°
Face-height ratio	50–55%	49%
FOP∕Mx	10±4°	12°
UI∕Mx	108±5°	121°
LI∕Mn	92±5°	102°
UI∕LI	133±10°	114°
EI–APog	0–2 mm	+1·5 mm
EI C I	0–2 mm	+2 mm

Measurements

UPPER LIP CURL

The upper lip profile should be concave, the depth of the concavity lying 1–4 mm behind the upper lip tangent. This is a more useful measurement than the nasolabial angle, which can be misleading if the base of the nose slopes markedly.[15]

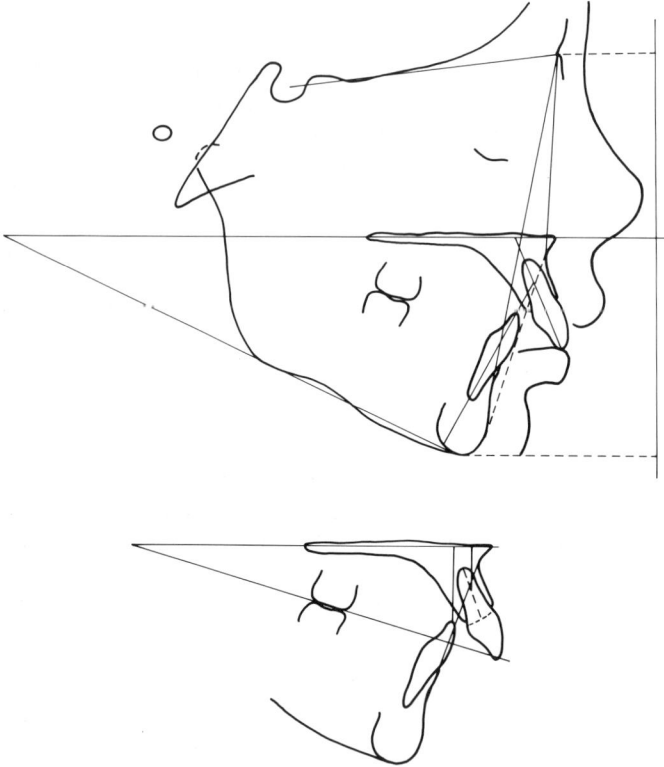

Measurement	Mean ± normal range	This case
SNA	82±3°	79°
SNB	79±3°	72°
ANB	3±1°	7°
A–B/FOP	90±5°	94°
MM<	27±5°	25°
Face-height ratio	50–55%	54%
FOP/Mx	10±4°	16°
Ul/Mx	108±5°	113°
Ll/Mn	92±5°	93°
Ul/Ll	133±10°	128°
El–APog	0–2 mm	−2 mm
El Cl	0–2 mm	−5 mm

LOWER LIP POUT

The vermilion border of the lower lip should be close to the H line, and preferably within 1 mm of it[15]

LIPS TO AESTHETIC LINE

The vermilion border of both lips should ideally lie close to the aesthetic line.[16]

Practical Cephalometric Analysis

The evaluation of single cephalometric film is concerned with description, prescription and prediction. Description involves comparison of the individual's values with cephalometric norms in order to build up a coherent picture of skeletal and dentoskeletal relationships. Inferences may then be made about the aetiology of the malocclusion; for example, what is the contribution of skeletal relationships and how much dento-alveolar compensation has taken place?

Prescription involves the planning of possible changes in incisor positions, together with an appraisal of their practicability and stability. This has to be done in conjunction with the clinical findings on the soft tissue pattern etc. Once the changes in incisor position and relationship have been decided, other tooth movements can be planned from the models and clinical findings. Prediction of the alterations that can be expected as a result of growth, and of the changes in tooth position that will be stable, is a necessary part of the treatment planning.

All prediction involves a margin of uncertainty. As discussed in Chapter 8, the best guide to stability of the labial segments is the existing position of the lower incisors. Many attempts have been made to discover some reliable basis for individualized prediction, but without success. The best that can be done is to

---

Fig. 6.19. An 11-year-old girl with a Class II, division 1 malocclusion. SNA and SNB are both reduced in value, SNB being particularly low; and the ANB angle is increased at 7°. As the angle SNA is reduced, the ANB angle may slightly underestimate the severity of the Class II skeletal pattern. The A–B/FOP angle is only slightly increased at 94° but this too underestimates the severity of the Class II skeletal pattern, because the FOP is rather steeply inclined. The skeletal pattern is definitely Class II and is more severe than the cephalometric measurements indicate, a conclusion reinforced by the clinical assessment. Lower face height appears to be close to average according to the MM angle and face height ratio.

The lower incisors are of average inclination but their edges lie a little behind the A–Pog line. Thus there is no lower incisor compensation for the Class II skeletal pattern. The upper incisors are a little proclined but the lower incisor edge–upper root centroid relationship is very unfavourable at −5 mm. This will have to be corrected either by advancement of the lower incisor edges or palatal movement of the upper incisor roots, or a combination of both. Bodily retraction of the upper incisors to reduce ...e overjet completely would be technically difficult and would set the upper incisors rather far back in the face. There is probably not enough palatal bone at apical level to retract the incisors fully. The patient does not suck a digit and the overbite is incomplete so ιh⁻ lower incisors have not been restrained by either of these factors. It is possible that when a lip seal is obtained anterior to the upper incisors, the lower labial segment might be stable if advanced a little, but this is questionable. As this is an 11-year-old girl, the face is still growing and it is reasonable to hope that the skeletal pattern will improve. If facial growth were adverse, orthodontic treatment would be very difficult. If this were an adult patient, serious consideration would have to be given to surgery to correct the skeletal pattern, in conjunction with orthodontic treatment.

assume that the individual will experience average growth changes. Fortunately the facial pattern remains fairly stable with growth and appreciable changes in jaw relationship are unusual, at least during a course of orthodontic treatment of average duration. However, it is important to be aware of the general trends of growth and to recognize whether these are liable to be helpful or otherwise (Chapter 4). For example, growth in facial height and forward growth of the mandible relative to the maxilla are helpful in Class II cases but adverse in Class III.

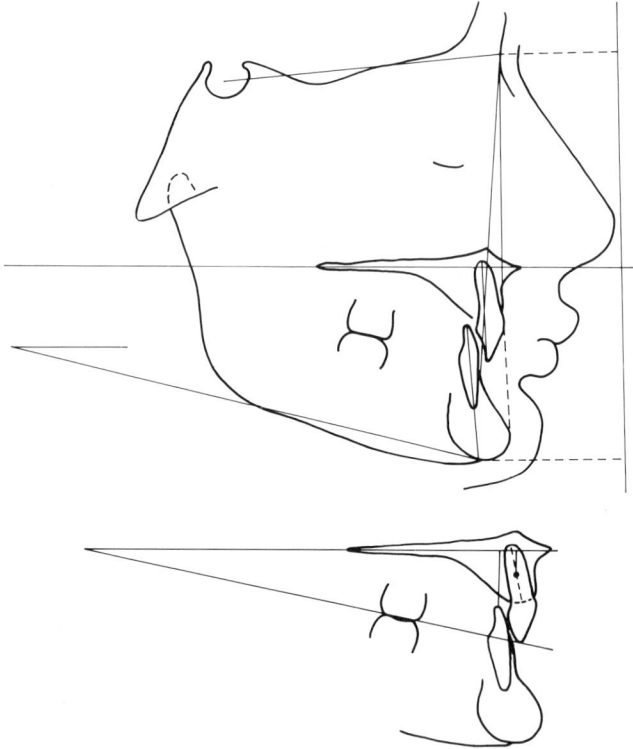

Measurement	Mean ± normal range	This case
SNA	82±3°	85°
SNB	79±3°	81°
ANB	3±1°	4°
A–B/FOP	90±5°	91°
MM<	27±5°	13°
Face-height ratio	50–55%	47%
FOP/Mx	10±4°	12°
UI/Mx	108±5°	93°
LI/Mn	92±5°	71°
UI/LI	133±10°	184°
EĪ–APog	0–2 mm	–10 mm
EĪCĪ	0–2 mm	–4·5 mm

Practical cephalometric analysis is best described by applying it to a number of cases (*Figs.* 6.18–6.21). Many cephalometric analyses have been described, but most have fallen into disuse. Downs'[9] and Steiner's[17] analyses are illustrated in *Figs.* 6.22 and 6.23. Simplistic analyses where one or two variables are considered to hold the key to the facial pattern are suspect; and analyses where measurements are used which have little obvious biological or clinical relevance are to be avoided.

EVALUATION OF GROWTH AND TREATMENT CHANGES

When growth and treatment changes are to be examined, a comparison of the cephalometric measurements from the two radiographs gives a general impression of the changes that have occurred, but a detailed investigation requires direct superimposition of the tracings (*Fig.* 6.24). A valid superimposition can be undertaken only by using reference structures that have not changed during the interval in question, and these are few in number. In order to obtain a realistic impression of the changes of interest, an appropriate region of superimposition must be used. In order to examine the overall changes in facial pattern, superimposition on the anterior cranial base is useful (*Fig.* 6.24*a*). For a clear impression of changes in the intermaxillary space and in upper incisor position, superimposition on maxillary structures is required; while superimposition on mandibular structures will reveal details of the changes in position of the lower teeth (*Fig.* 6.24*b*).

Fig. 6.20. An 11-year-old girl with a Class II, division 2 malocclusion. SNA and SNB are above average and so the ANB angle may be biased towards Class II. However, it is still within the range of normal at 4°. This is supported by the A–B/FOP angle of 91° which is probably reliable because the inclination of the FOP to the maxillary plane is within normal limits. Thus the skeletal pattern is Class I. It is apparent from inspection that the chin is well developed and this could be confirmed by measuring the S–N–Pog angle.

The MM angle is very low and lower face height is slightly small relative to total face height, a common finding in Class II, division 2 cases. The lower incisors are very retroclined, particularly when the low MM angle is taken into account. Their expected inclination would be 106° (14° above average) but they are only at 71° to the mandibular plane. Thus the lower incisor edge lies far behind the A–Pog line. Given the well developed chin, it is not surprising that the lower incisors are behind the A–Pog line, but they are severely retruded. This is a very unfavourable position for the lower incisor edge, as is confirmed by the lower edge upper root centroid projection of −4.5 mm. This together with the retroclination of the upper incisors and the large interincisor angle, explains the very deep overbite.

Treatment planning is difficult. It would not be possible to correct the incisor relationship by retraction and apical torque of the upper incisors: there is not sufficient bone palatal to the upper incisor apices. In addition, the incisors would be far too retruded within the face. It is possible that the lower incisor retroclination can be explained to some extent by unfavourable dento-alveolar adaptation during favourable mandibular growth: the lower incisors are trapped behind the upper incisors and even if the skeletal relationship had improved with growth after they had erupted, this would not be reflected by an improvement in the incisor relationship. If this had happened, some lower incisor advancement would be stable following a change in the upper incisor position, but this is difficult to quantitate. In addition, it is reasonable to expect favourable changes during further growth. Orthodontic correction of this incisor relationship is feasible only if the lower incisor edges can be advanced by several millimetres to a stable position.

Superimposition on Cranial Base Structures

Superimposition on the S–N line with registration at sella usually gives quite a reliable picture of overall facial growth, but if nasion has drifted upwards or downwards with growth, a rotational artefact will be introduced, which will produce the greatest errors at the mandibular symphysis as this is furthest

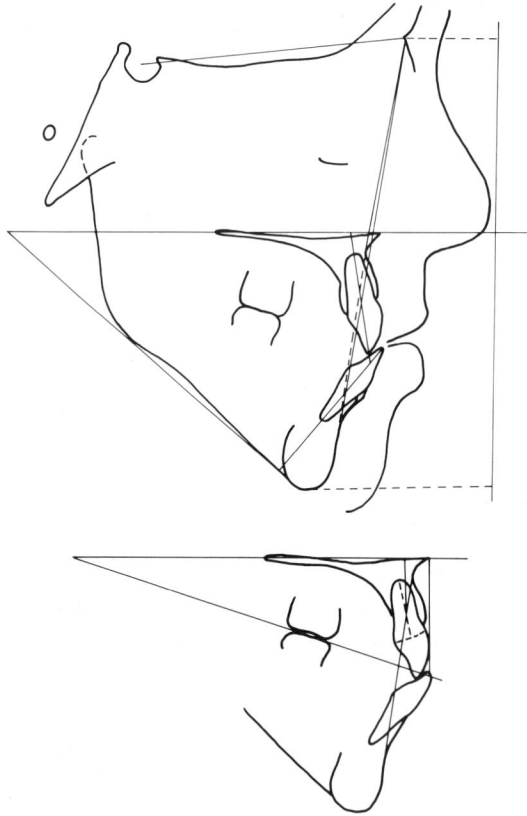

Measurement	Mean ± normal range	This case
SNA	82±3°	74°
SNB	79±3°	75°
ANB	3±1°	−1°
A–B/FOP	90±5°	81°
MM<	27±5°	41°
Face-height ratio	50–55%	57%
FOP/Mx	10±4°	18°
UI/Mx	108±5°	99°
LI/Mn	92±5°	90°
UI/LI	133±10°	131°
EI–APog	0–2 mm	−8 mm
EICI	0–2 mm	+6·5 mm

from the centre of rotation at sella[18] (*see Fig.* 6.10). Superimposition on de Coster's line is more reliable, provided it is done with expertise.

Various methods of relating the radiographic images by superimposition have been attempted, but tracing is simplest and is of sufficient accuracy for routine use. It is important that the tracing is done with great care, taking the precautions mentioned on p. 60. The cortical plate of the basisphenoid in particular is quite thick, and so its periosteal surface should be traced. A good knowledge of skull anatomy is necessary and it is quite common to see tracings superimposed upon the roofs of the orbits, which do undergo periosteal remodelling. The most accurate superimposition is obtained by tracing the first radiograph and superimposing that tracing on the second film, registering the appropriate cranial base structures.[19]

Although superimposition on cranial base structures is potentially accurate, large errors can arise if it is not done expertly, and this can give a misleading impression of the changes that have, in fact, occurred.

Superimposition on Maxillary Structures

Unfortunately, the maxilla is subject to extensive periosteal remodelling and there are no really satisfactory stable sites for superimposition. The maxillary plane is often used but the hard palate descends by apposition of bone on the oral surface and resorption on the nasal surface. This does not always take place uniformly along the length of the palate and so some rotational artefacts may be introduced by the use of the maxillary plane. However, at least where radiographs are taken within a few years of one another, these rotational effects are quite small and should not introduce serious errors.

The other problem is the anteroposterior registration of the superimposition. Errors here will give an erroneous impression of the tooth movements that have been achieved, and of the changes in the apical base relationship (*Fig.* 6.25).

Fig. 6.21. A Class III malocclusion in a 9-year-old boy. There is no mandibular displacement on closure. There is a definite Class III skeletal pattern with an ANB angle of $-1°$. However, both SNA and SNB are below average and this probably means that the severity of the Class III skeletal pattern is underestimated by the ANB angle. The A–B/FOP angle is considerably reduced at 81° and although to some extent this may reflect the steep cant of the FOP (18° to the maxillary plane), it still indicates a definite Class III skeletal pattern. The MM angle is very high and the lower face height is a larger than average proportion of total face height. This is not a favourable feature because it may mean that, with growth, the overbite will reduce and perhaps be lost altogether, which could prejudice the stability of any incisor correction.

The lower incisors are at 90° to Mn, but taking account of the MM angle, the expected value is 78° (92−14°) and so the lower incisors are very proclined. The upper incisors are a little retroclined and so there has been no dento-alveolar compensation for the Class III skeletal pattern. Retroclination of the lower incisors and proclination of the upper incisors could correct the reverse overjet without producing an unacceptable inclination of these teeth and, provided the overbite was maintained, this could be stable. However, the long term stability depends on growth. A 9-year-old boy expects appreciable further growth. Vertical growth will tend to reduce the overbite and anterior growth will tend to exacerbate the Class III skeletal pattern, both factors that may lead to relapse in the incisor relationship. Even if the incisor correction were to remain stable, the aesthetic acceptability of the skeletal pattern would have to be assessed clinically. Treatment planning is difficult and this case lies at the limits of orthodontic treatability.

Commonly the contour of the palate at the base of the alveolar process is used, but, although this is not affected by tooth movements, it is a site of periosteal remodelling with growth and is not entirely satisfactory. Björk,[20] on the basis of studies where metallic implants were inserted as markers in the jaws of children, found that the anterior surface of the zygomatic process of the maxilla is the one site in the maxilla that undergoes little periosteal remodelling

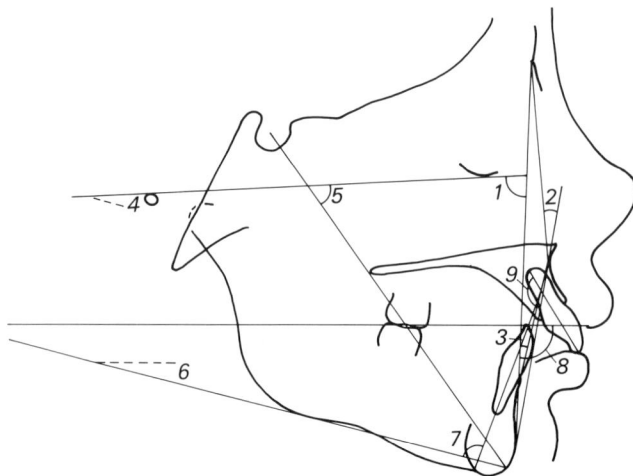

| | | Downs norm | | |
		Mean	Range	This case
1.	Facial angle	88°	82–95	84
2.	Angle of convexity	0°	–8·5–10	15
3.	AB/facial plane	–5°	–9–0	11
4.	FM angle	22°	17–28	17
5.	Y axis	60°	53–66	57
6.	Cant of occlusal plane	9°	1–14	14
7.	1 to mandibular plane	91°	81–97	96
8.	1 to occlusal plane	105°	93·5–110	111
9.	Interincisor angle	135°	130–150	128
10.	1 to A-Pog	3 mm	1-5	10

Fig. 6.22. Downs' analysis of case in *Fig.* 6.19. The interpretation of the measurements is as follows. The facial angle towards the lower end of the normal range indicates a retrognathic lower face. The large angle of convexity (AB to facial plane angles) reflects the Class II skeletal pattern. The FM angle is low, indicating a reduced lower facial height but it is surprising that the cant of the occlusal plane is at the upper end of the norm range: with a low FM angle it could have been expected to be low as well. The lower incisors are proclined, as shown by their angulation to the mandibular and occlusal planes, reflecting mild dento-alveolar compensation for the Class II skeletal pattern. The upper incisor edge is far in advance of the A–Pog line but the interincisor angle is low, indicating that the overjet should not be reduced by tipping the upper incisor teeth palatally, because they would become too retroclined.

Note that this analysis leads to slightly different conclusions about this case than the recommended procedure (*see* Fig. 6.19), which gives a more useful insight into the cephalometric relationships.

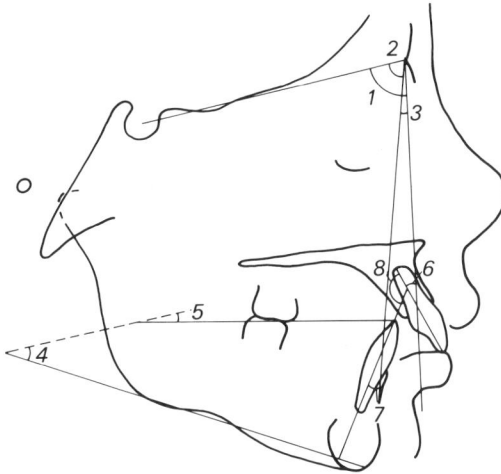

Measurement	Steiner norm	This case
1. SNA	82°	79
2. SNB	80°	72
3. ANB	2°	7
4. Go–Gn/S–N	32°	31
5. Occlusal plane/S–N	14°	12
6. 1̄ to NA	22°	27
	4 mm	6·5
7. 1̄ to NB	25°	18
	4 mm	3
8. Interincisor angle	131°	128

Fig. 6.23. Steiner's analysis of case in *Fig.* 6.19. The low values of angles SNA and SNB reflect a retrognathic lower face and ANB shows that the skeletal pattern is Class II. The orientation of the mandibular plane (Go–Gn) and of the occlusal plane to SN are about normal. The upper incisors are slightly more proclined and a little more ahead of NA than the norm. The lower incisors are a little retroclined and fractionally retruded to NB. The interincisor angle is slightly low.

Steiner's analysis does not give as detailed a picture of dentoskeletal variables as is desirable. Measurement of the incisor position relative to the lines NA and NB is not sufficiently informative about their positions.

with growth. This structure is not always easily seen on a lateral skull radiograph, and it is much too short to provide a satisfactory base for superimposition. However, it can be used for anteroposterior registration of superimposition on the maxillary plane (*see Fig.* 6.24*b*). This is a registration requiring great care.

Superimposition on Mandibular Structures

Björk[21] found that the mandible undergoes rather complex remodelling changes which may be associated with anterior or posterior growth rotations. However, he described a number of stable structures: the contour of the mandibular canal and the inner contour of the cortex of the mandibular symphysis being the most useful of these. This superimposition (*see Fig.* 6.24*c*) can be used to evaluate the

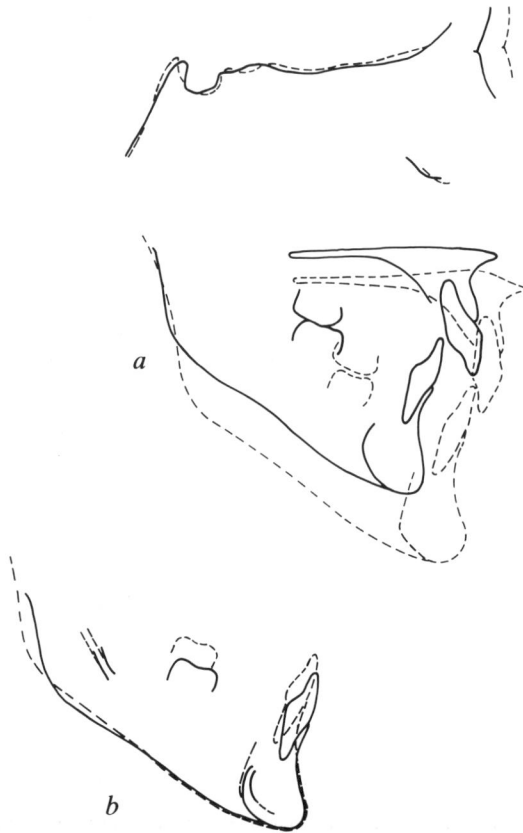

Fig. 6.24. *a*, Superimposition on stable structures gives a general impression of the overall changes in facial pattern that have occurred with growth. Here, nasion has grown forwards. The maxillary complex and palate have descended relative to the anterior cranial base, in part as a result of sutural growth, and in part as a result of periosteal drift. It is not possible to distinguish these contributions from this superimposition. The mandible has descended about twice as far as the maxillary complex and in this patient has grown forwards to a similar extent. *b*, Superimposition on stable structures in the mandible, in particular the inner cortex of the lingual and inferior border of the mandibular symphysis and the cortical outline of the mandibular canal. This reveals the periosteal remodelling that has occurred at the lower and posterior border of the mandible; and the amounts and directions of movement of the mandibular dentition.

Superimposition on maxillary structures is not very reliable and may be misleading (*see Fig.* 6.25). The palate has descended during growth as a result of periosteal remodelling and this superimposition does not reveal the full extent of eruption of the maxillary dentition.

remodelling in the mandible that has occurred with growth, and the changes in lower incisor position.

CONCLUSION

Cephalometric radiography is valuable in examining dental and skeletal relationships in difficult cases. However, it should be used only to supplement the

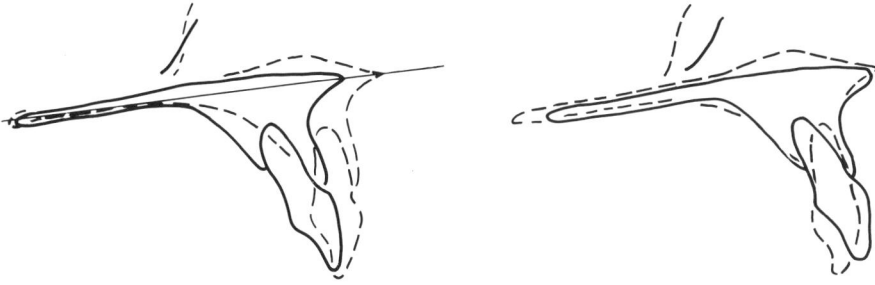

Fig. 6.25. Incorrect anteroposterior registration of the maxillary superimposition gives a totally erroneous impression of the nature of any orthodontic tooth movement. Apposition of bone takes place both at ANS and at PNS. Registration at ANS gives a misleading impression of the amount of palatal movement of the upper incisors that has been achieved by treatment. Registration at PNS gives a misleading impression of labial movement of the upper incisor apices. These problems are compounded by the inferior drift of the palate which obscures the descent of the dentition that may have occurred during growth and treatment. Unless metallic implants have been placed in the maxilla prior to taking the first radiograph, it is not possible to be confident about the reliability of this superimposition where appreciable growth has taken place between registrations.

clinical examination and not as a substitute for a clinically based diagnosis and treatment plan.

REFERENCES

1. Broadbent B. H. (1931) A new X-ray technique and its application to orthodontics. *Angle Orthodont.* **1**; 45–66.
2. Broadbent B. H. (1937) The face of the normal child: Bolton standards and technique. *Angle Orthodont.* **7**; 183–233.
3. Brodie A. G. (1941) Growth patterns of the human head from the third month to the eighth year of life. *Am. J. Anat.* **68**; 209–62.
4. Björk A. and Palling M. (1955) Adolescent age changes in sagittal jaw relation, alveolar prognathy and incisal inclination. *Acta Odontol. Scand.* **12**; 201–32.
5. Montgomery W. M., Vig P. S., Staab E. V. et al. (1979) Tomography: A three-dimensional study of the nasal airway. *Am. J. Orthodont.* **76**; 363–75.
6. Solow B. and Tallgren A. (1971) Natural head positioning in standing subjects. *Acta Odontol. Scand.* **29**; 591–607.
7. Showfety K. J., Vig P. S. and Matteson S. R. (1983) A simple method for taking natural head position cephalograms. *Am. J. Orthodont.* **83**; 495–500.
8. Melsen B. (1974) The cranial base. *Acta Odontol. Scand.* Suppl. 62.
9. Downs W. B. (1984) Variations in facial relationships; their significance in treatment and prognosis. *Am. J. Orthodont.* **34**; 812–40.
10. Williams R. (1969) The diagnostic line. *Am. J. Orthodont.* **55**; 458–76.
11. Harvold E. (1963) Some biologic aspects of orthodontic treatment in the transitional dentition. *Am. J. Orthodont.* **49**; 1–14.
12. Jacobson A. (1975) The 'Wits' appraisal of jaw disharmony. *Am. J. Orthodont.* **67**; 125–33.
13. Houston W. J. B. (1986) The incisor edge-centroid relationship as a factor influencing overbite. *Eur. J. Orthodont.* In the press.
14. Wisth P. (1974) Soft tissue response to incisor retraction in boys. *Br. J. Orthodont.* **1**; 199–204.
15. Holdaway R. A. (1983) A soft tissue cephalometric analysis and its use in orthodontic treatment planning, Part 1. *Am. J. Orthodont.* **84**; 1–28.
16. Ricketts R. M. (1957) Planning treatment on the basis of facial pattern and an estimate of its growth. *Angle Orthodont.* **27**; 14–37.

17. Steiner C. C. (1953) Cephalometrics for you and me. *Am. J. Orthodont.* **39**; 729–55.
18. Baumrind S., Miller D. and Molthen R. (1976) The reliability of head film measurements. *Am. J. Orthodont.* **70**; 617–44.
19. Ekström C. (1982) Facial growth rate and its relation to somatic maturation in healthy children. *Swedish Dent. J.* Suppl. 11, pp. 1–99.
20. Björk A. and Skieller V. (1979) Growth of the maxilla in three dimensions as revealed radiographically by the implant method. *Br. J. Orthodont.* **4**; 53–64.
21. Björk A. and Skeiller V. (1972) Facial development and tooth eruption. *Am. J. Orthodont.* **62**; 339–83.

Chapter 7

Case Assessment

A thorough and logical assessment of every case is essential. Failure to follow a consistent procedure can result in important features being overlooked. Provided that all relevant aspects are covered, the exact sequence of examination is a matter of individual preference. The approach outlined here is structured so that by the time the occlusion is examined in detail, the background information about the skeletal relationships, soft tissue pattern and dental status have been acquired, and this can be important in interpreting the occlusal findings. Clearly there is an interaction between the occlusion and lip activity, and the evaluation of the soft tissue pattern is not carried out in ignorance of the general features of the occlusion, which will be apparent from reference models, or from notes made on a previous occasion. However, it is desirable to assess lip pattern and activity before dental status is checked comprehensively because after the intra-oral examination the patient is less likely to behave in a relaxed and normal fashion. Indeed, much useful information about lip form and activity can be gained by observing the patient prior to the clinical investigation.

Before a thorough clinical examination is concluded, certain orthodontic records, usually study models and radiographs, are required. These will be discussed first.

ORTHODONTIC RECORDS

Reference Models

Study models are helpful in assessing details of the occlusion and, of course, they provide an essential basis for measuring treatment progress. Orthodontic study models should reproduce all the erupted teeth, the palate and the full depth of the buccal sulcus. Good impressions are most readily obtained in trays with deep flanges. It may be helpful to build up the tray margins with soft wax. Careful trimming of the models is important because visual judgement of symmetry and arch form is influenced by the framing provided by the sides of models. The bases are trimmed parallel to the occlusal plane, leaving enough thickness to give a balanced form to the models. The heels must be flush with one another so that when they are placed on a flat surface the correct arch relationship is registered (*Fig.* 7.1). The sides are trimmed symmetrically and equidistant from the median palatal raphé. Although the correct occlusal relationship of the arches should have been recorded with a wax wafer, it is necessary to check at the next visit of the patient that the models are correctly related to one another.

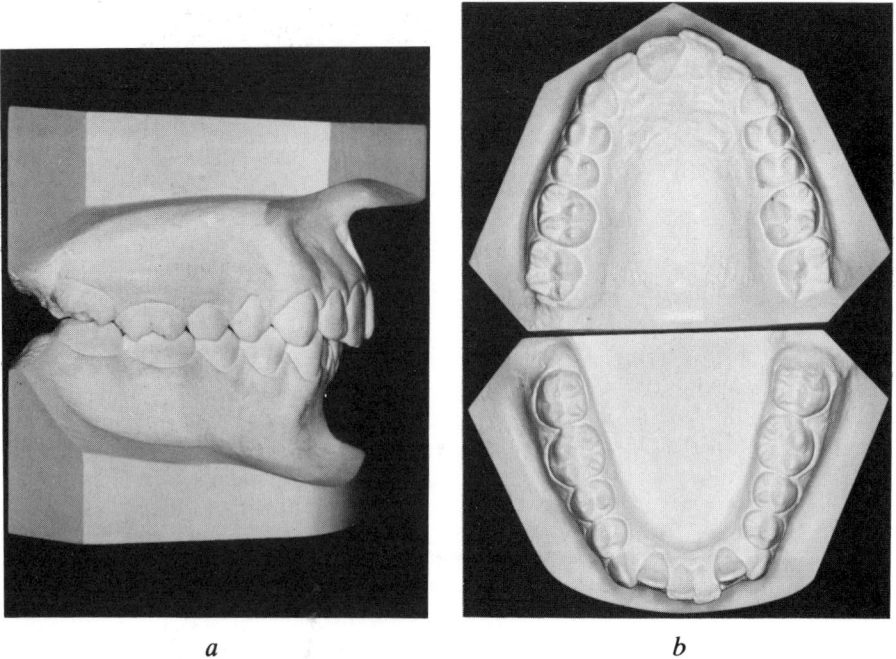

a   *b*

Fig. 7.1. Orthodontic models, correctly trimmed.

Model Analysis

While a visual assessment gives an impression of the space conditions in the arch, in some cases a more accurate estimate is required. Rather than arch size and tooth size *per se*, it is the amount of crowding and spacing that is of interest. Measurement can be helpful in marginal cases in deciding whether or not extractions will be required in the lower arch. A more reliable indication of upper arch space requirements is given by relating the upper and lower canine teeth and calculating how much space will be required to permit a Class I relationship. Allowance has to be made for any retraction of the lower canines to relieve lower labial segment crowding. Provided that the sizes of the upper and lower incisors match (*see below*), and the lower incisors are regular, a Class I canine relationship provides sufficient space to align the upper incisors with a normal overbite and overjet (*see Fig. 7.5a*).

Arch Size

In general it is the space conditions anterior to the first permanent molars that have to be assessed. Measuring the length of the arch segments (*Fig.* 7.2) will slightly underestimate the space available. A more precise measurement can be obtained by forming a length of soft wire to the general curve of the arch on which the approximal contact areas of the teeth should lie (*Fig.* 7.3a). The length of the straightened wire gives the arch length.

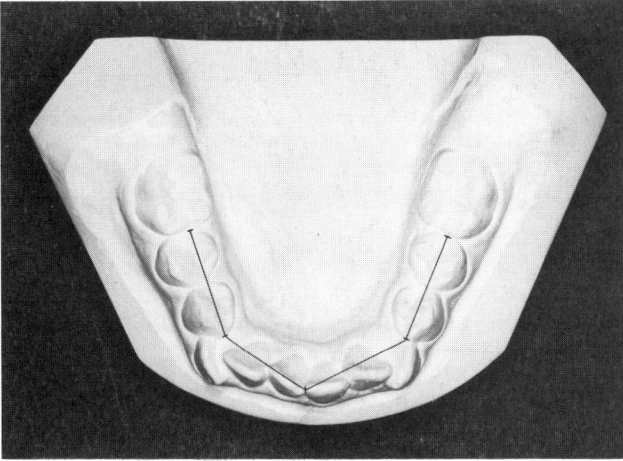

Fig. 7.2. Arch perimeter can be estimated from the sum of the segment lengths.

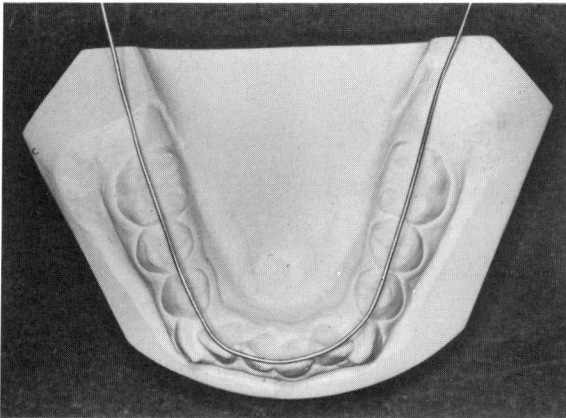

a

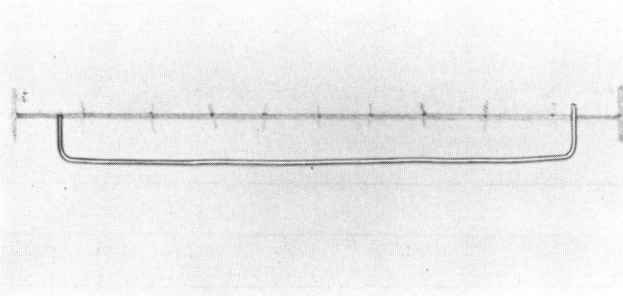

b

Fig. 7.3. Arch perimeter measured with a brass wire. *a*, The wire is formed to the arch. *b*, The mesiodistal tooth widths are marked on a card and compared with the arch perimeter measurement.

Tooth Size

The mesiodistal widths of erupted teeth are measured with dividers or callipers. If the tooth widths are recorded by punching them through a card (*Fig.* 7.3*b*), errors in reading the measurements are avoided.

The size of an unerupted tooth can be estimated from its antimere if this has erupted. Measurements taken from radiographs are not very reliable, even if enlargement is compensated for by a correction factor calculated from the image size of adjacent erupted teeth (*Fig.* 7.4). Average tooth widths can be used (*see* p. 13) but there is appreciable variability in size, particularly of lower second premolars. Moyers[1] published tables for estimating unerupted tooth sizes from the widths of the lower incisors with which they are correlated. This may be more accurate than the use of average tooth sizes but there is still an error associated with the estimate.

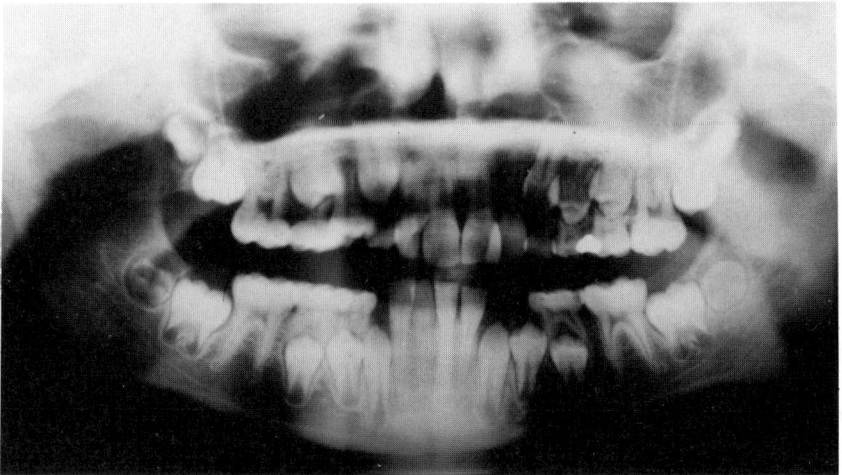

Fig. 7.4. Estimating unerupted tooth sizes from radiographs: enlargement factor=

$$\frac{\text{width of } \overline{\text{E}|} \text{ measured directly}}{\text{width of } \overline{\text{E}|}\uparrow \text{ measured on radiograph}} \quad \frac{10.1\,\text{mm}}{15.5\,\text{mm}} = 0.65.$$

width of $\overline{5|}$=measurement on radiograph×enlargement factor=11.0 mm×0.65=7.15 mm.
Note. Depending on their exact relationship to the film, the radiographic enlargement of the teeth will vary and so this is not a really reliable procedure.

Tooth Size Discrepancies

The upper incisor teeth are quite variable in size. If they are large in relation to the lowers and there is a Class I canine relationship with no lower arch spacing, then the upper incisors will be crowded or there will be an increase in overjet (*Fig.* 7.5). The converse applies when the upper incisors are small relative to the lowers (*Fig.* 7.5*c*). It is important to recognize this problem before treatment is started and to plan accordingly. Often the discrepancy in size is due to upper laterals that are small. Collectively, the widths of the upper incisors should equal the total width of the lower incisors plus one lower canine.

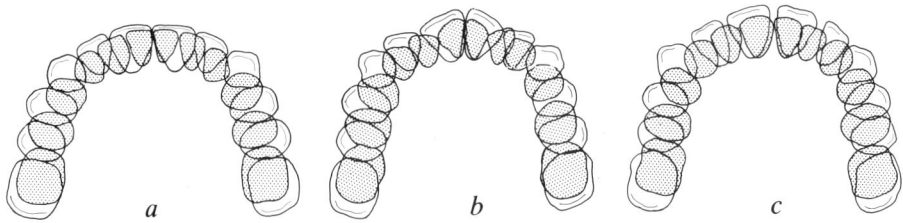

Fig. 7.5. The canine relationship is a key factor in determining whether or not the upper incisor teeth can be well aligned and in a Class I relationship to the lower arch. *a*, The lower labial segment is well aligned, and the upper canine occludes correctly in the embrasure between the lower canine and first premolar. Thus it is possible to fit the upper incisors around the lower incisors in good alignment and with a normal overjet. *b*, The lower labial segment is crowded and so there is insufficient room to align the upper incisors even although there is a correct canine relationship. The upper labial segment will either be crowded (as here) or there will be an increase in overjet. *c*, A discrepancy in the size of the upper and lower teeth will alter their balance. Here the upper incisors are relatively small and so they are spaced around the well-aligned lower incisors.

Space Discrepancy

Measurements obtained from the models give an indication of space discrepancy. This information is most useful in the lower arch in mildly crowded cases where a decision has to be made whether or not to extract teeth. Sometimes it is possible to align the lower teeth provided that the leeway space is not lost by forward movement of the first permanent molars, and a space maintainer may be fitted on exfoliation of second deciduous molars. At the other extreme where crowding is severe and extractions would provide just enough space, it is essential not to allow any forward movement of the permanent molars.

Space analysis in the upper arch is less useful than in the lower. Extractions in the upper arch are determined by the need to obtain a buccal segment relationship with the lower arch which will allow alignment of the upper incisors in a normal relationship with the lowers. This will be influenced by whether or not extractions are required in the lower (*see* Chapter 8).

Trial Set-up

Occasionally it is useful to reposition the teeth on the model to simulate their corrected positions and to evaluate whether a proposed treatment plan will give enough space. The value of this exercise is limited by the fact that plaster teeth are easily damaged on removing them from the model.

The technique of model preparation is described with the manufacture of positioners in Chapter 18. It is of very limited use for diagnostic purposes. Computer graphic techniques can also be used for this purpose, the size and positions of the teeth being recorded numerically by a digitizer. Although the procedure is impressive, it is doubtful whether it really aids treatment planning.

Radiographs

In order to confirm the presence and condition of all teeth, radiographs must be available at the clinical examination. A minimum requirement is a pan-oral or equivalent view and an intra-oral view of the upper labial segment. For the practitioner who does not possess the apparatus for obtaining a pan-oral type of film, lateral oblique jaw views obtained with a dental radiographic unit will suffice (*Fig.* 7.6). An intra-oral view of the upper labial segment is always needed because supernumerary teeth, which are not rare in this region, may not be visible on a panoramic view if they lie out of the plane of the arch. Cephalometric radiographs may be helpful in evaluating the more complex case, and their use is discussed in Chapter 6.

All possible precautions to minimize irradiation of the patient must be adopted. Filtration and collimation of the beam, the use of fast films and screening of the patient with a lead–rubber apron are all important. Where alternative views are possible, those involving less radiation to the patient should always be selected, and the number of films taken must be kept to the minimum required for adequate clinical evaluation.

A cursory review of radiographs may not reveal important information and it is essential that each film is examined carefully and in an orderly manner.

1   Identify and count the teeth, comparing the findings with the study models. By the age of 5 years, all permanent teeth except for third molars and possibly second premolars should be visible. Occasionally in boys second premolars may develop as late as 9 years; thus it can be difficult in a younger boy where there is not radiographic evidence of a second premolar to decide whether or not to extract the second deciduous molar in order to encourage space closure. Third molars are usually first visible on radiographs between 8 and 12 years of age but cases have been reported where they have not been evident until 15 years of age.

2   Examine the tooth crowns (*Fig.* 7.7). Although the views obtained may not be ideal for demonstrating defects in tooth structure, there may be clues that need to be followed up with supplementary radiographs. Caries, suspect areas below restorations, calcification of a pulp chamber, *dens in dente* involving the upper incisors and evidence of hypoplasia of the enamel of unerupted premolars

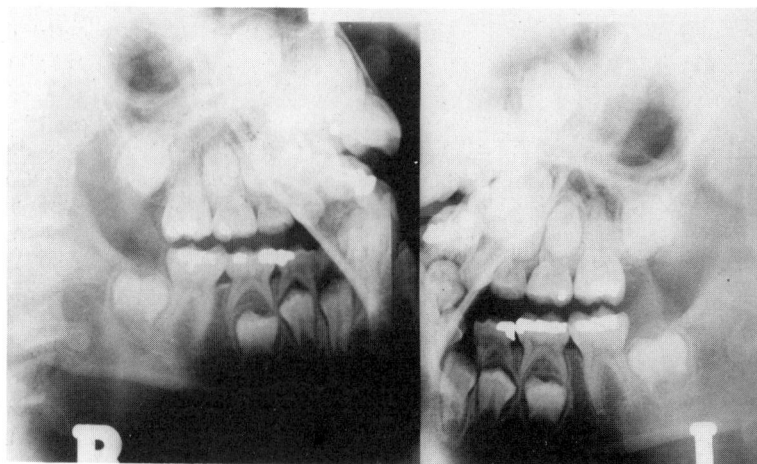

Fig. 7.6. Lateral oblique jaw views (bimolar views) can be taken with a dental X-ray set and should give an adequate view as far forward as the first premolars.

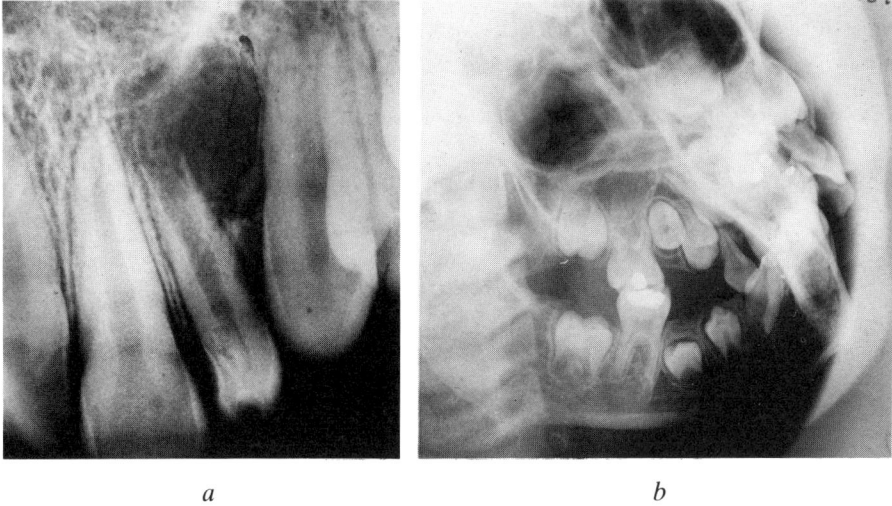

Fig. 7.7. Crown anomalies visualized on radiographs. *a*, *Dens-in-dente*. *b*, Hypoplasia of an unerupted lower first premolar.

are all features that may not be apparent clinically and yet need to be taken account of in planning treatment.

3   Examine the roots (*Fig.* 7.8). Dilaceration of roots may limit the possible correction of crown positions. Retarded root formation or failure of apical closure may indicate that the vitality of the tooth is in doubt and requires further investigation. Even in the absence of a history of trauma, fracture of upper incisor roots may be discovered and clearly influences the treatment plan: it may be best not to undertake orthodontic treatment or the decision may have to be made to extract the tooth, to remove the apical fragment and root-fill the tooth, or even occasionally, in the case of a hairline fracture, to root-treat the tooth and fit a metal post as an internal splint.

Root resorption is not uncommon, particularly in the upper incisor region. Sometimes there may be an obvious cause such as trauma or previous orthodontic treatment. More often there is no explanation and the resorption is termed idiopathic. Some individuals are susceptible to root resorption and several teeth may be affected. Teeth that have previously undergone root resorption seem to be particularly liable to suffer further resorption with orthodontic tooth movement, and even intact teeth in patients exhibiting idiopathic root resorption elsewhere may be at risk. It should also be remembered that teeth with short roots tip more than expected because the centre of rotation is closer to the crown. Clearly in patients exhibiting serious root resorption appliance treatment should be undertaken with reluctance. If treatment is commenced, extensive movement of the root apex should be avoided and the patient should be made aware of the dangers of further root loss.

Apical or lateral root resorption may be caused by the crypt of an adjacent unerupted tooth (*Fig.* 7.9). This is sometimes seen on an upper lateral incisor where the permanent canine is impacted against it.

4   Supporting bone. Areas of radiolucency or sclerosis may indicate some pathological process. Most common are periapical radiolucencies indicating that

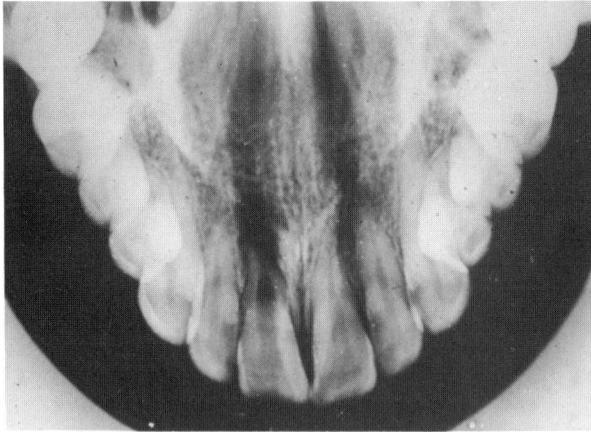

a

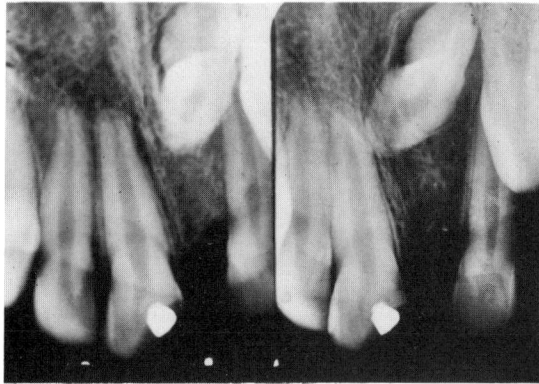

b

Fig. 7.8. Root anomalies visualized on radiographs. *a*, Open apex indicating cessation of root formation. *b*, Dilacerated root.

the tooth is not vital. The crypts around teeth whose eruption has been delayed should be examined for cyst formation.

PREVIOUS DENTAL AND MEDICAL HISTORY

Previous dental history is of relevance in that irregular attendance and general dental neglect indicate a lack of interest that may prejudice cooperation with subsequent orthodontic treatment.

A medical history should be taken for all patients. Many orthodontic patients require extractions and it is important to be aware of conditions such as bleeding disorders or congenital heart disease that could influence patient management.

Of direct orthodontic relevance are epilepsy, bleeding disorders and heart lesions where transient bacteriaemia could be dangerous. The epileptic patient controlled with phenytoin sodium or one of its derivatives is particularly

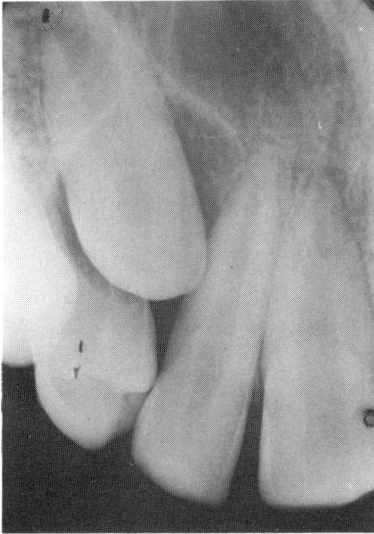

Fig. 7.9. Root resorption of an upper first premolar associated with impaction of an upper canine tooth.

susceptible to gingival hyperplasia and this is aggravated by poor oral hygiene. Oral hygiene control is often more difficult when appliances are worn and so there is the risk of precipitating gingival hyperplasia. In the event of an epileptic fit, there is the danger that the tongue, cheeks and lips could be lacerated by the appliance.

While bleeding disorders and heart lesions are not by themselves contraindications to orthodontic treatment, particular care needs to be taken not to carry out other procedures, such as extractions, that could be hazardous to the patient without due precautions.

CLINICAL ASSESSMENT

The Soft Tissue

The teeth lie in a zone of balance between the lips, cheeks and tongue. It is the habitual posture of these organs rather than transient activity that is important in determining tooth position.

Tongue position cannot be observed directly and any attempts to do so could interfere with what is to be investigated. Even tongue size cannot be measured reliably and it is only gross variations from the normal that are worthy of record. Some variations in tongue position and activity can be inferred from the occlusion of the teeth and from the position and activity of the lips. For example, if there is an incomplete overbite or anterior open bite, it is probable that the tongue comes forwards into the gap to help form an anterior oral seal; and if the lower lip lies behind the upper incisors, the seal will usually be formed by contact between lip, tongue and palatal mucosa. These variations in tongue position and activity are generally adaptations to provide an anterior oral seal and will readapt to corrected tooth positions provided that the patient is then able to maintain a lip seal. The rare primary tongue thrust will not adapt to corrected

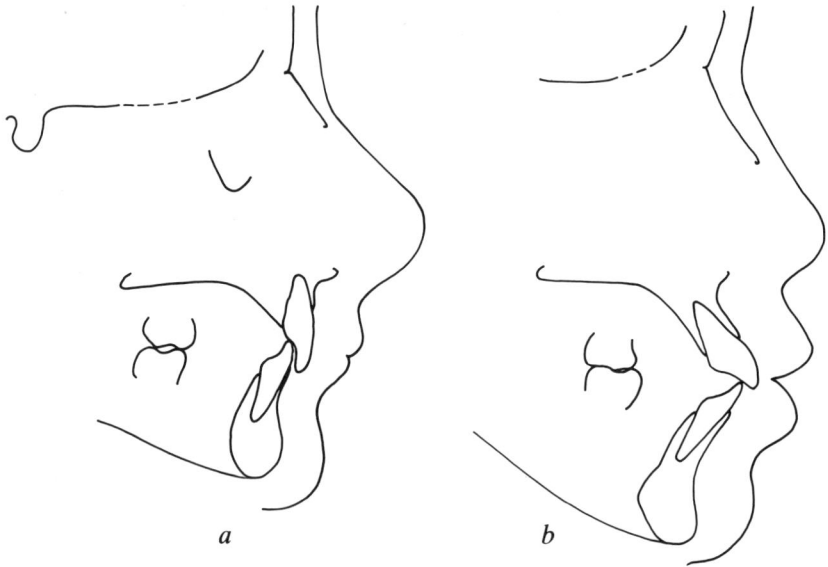

Fig. 7.10. Variations in soft tissue profile. *a*, Thin and vertical lips associated with bimaxillary retroclination. *b*, Full and everted lips associated with bimaxillary proclination.

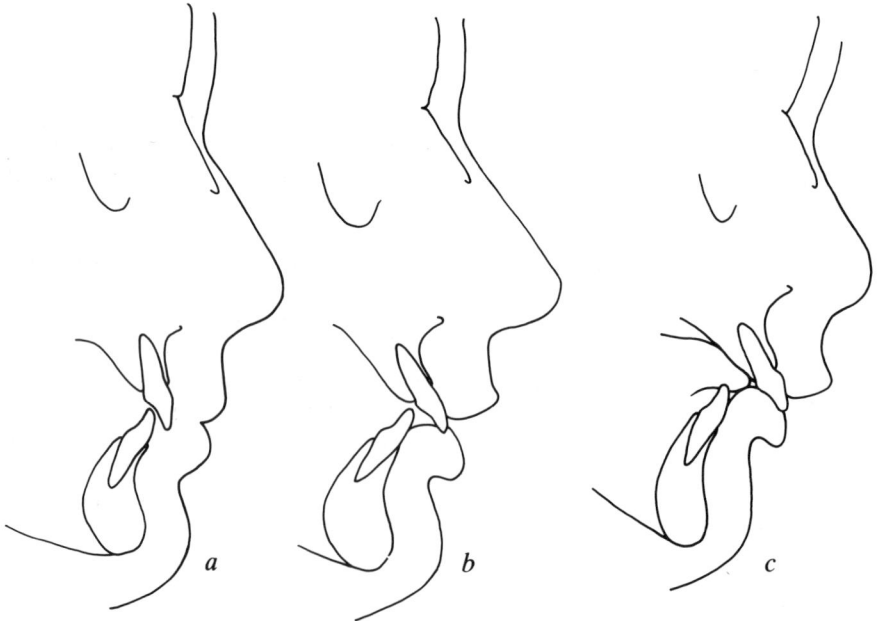

Fig. 7.11. Relationships between the lower lips and upper incisors. *a*, Ideally there is an habitual lip seal and the lower lip covers the incisal third of the upper incisor crown. *b*, Where the lower lip lies below or behind the upper incisor teeth they will usually be proclined. Their position is in part influenced by the form and level of the upper lip. *c*, Where the overjet is increased, an anterior oral seal is usually formed by contact between the lower lip or tongue and the alveolar mucosa palatal to the upper incisors.

tooth positions and so imposes limitations on treatment. These anomalies are discussed at greater length in Chapter 3.

The general form of the lips should be noted: are they everted or retracted? Full and everted lips are usually associated with a bimaxillary proclination, while more retracted lips often cause a bimaxillary retroclination of the incisor teeth (*Fig. 7.10*).

The manner of obtaining an anterior oral seal is of importance. Many individuals have lips parted at rest (incompetent lips) but habitually hold them together with minimal circumoral contraction. Provided that there is a habitual lip seal with the lip line above the upper incisor edges, the lower lip will control the upper incisor position (*Fig. 7.11a*). A very high lip line is often associated with retroclined upper incisors while a lip line below the upper incisor edges means that their inclination is controlled by the upper lip and they may be proclined (*Fig. 7.11b*). If the lips are habitually parted and an anterior oral seal is formed between lower lip, tongue and palatal mucosa, the overjet is usually increased (*Fig. 7.11c*). In these cases it is important to try to assess whether the patient will be capable of achieving a lip seal when the tooth positions are changed.

The position and activity of the soft tissues will vary, particularly in the child who is aware of being observed, and so it is important to try to evaluate them unobtrusively. With experience it is possible to do so while talking to the parent or patient before commencing the formal clinical examination.

Skeletal Relationships

Facial form should be assessed in all three dimensions. Transversely some facial asymmetry is normal but any unusual degree of imbalance should be noted. More important from an orthodontic viewpoint is whether the midpoint of the chin coincides with that of the rest of the face. A divergence can reflect a true asymmetry of the mandible, for example due to unilateral condylar hyperplasia or hypoplasia; or it can be due to a lateral mandibular displacement resulting from premature contacts of the teeth.

Anteroposterior jaw relationships are assessed from the profile with the patient sitting unsupported with the head in the normal postural position. While variations in lip thickness may disguise the skeletal relationships, it is usually possible to obtain a reliable impression of the underlying jaw relationship. Vertically the anterior lower facial height is assessed from the Frankfort–mandibular planes angle, or by comparing the height of lower and middle facial thirds. An excessively large or small lower facial height may be associated with a corresponding variation in the depth of overbite.

Mandibular Path of Closure

Both at rest and with the teeth in maximum occlusion the mandible should be in positions of centric relation with both condyles in retruded, unstrained positions in the glenoid fossae. The path of closure from rest to occlusion should be a hinge movement. Premature contacts of the teeth may result in a displacement of the mandible, anteriorly or laterally. Anterior displacements are commonly

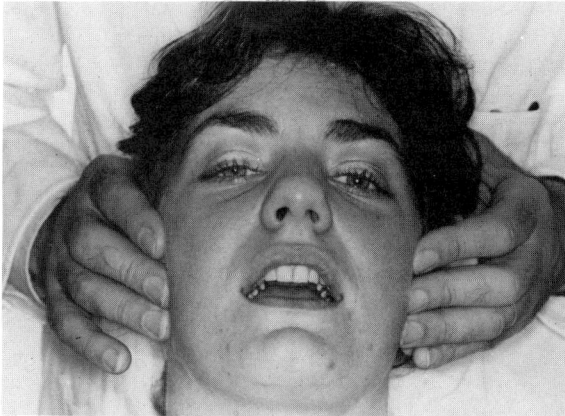

Fig. 7.12. When examining mandibular movements and path of closure, the patient should be viewed from above and behind. Gentle palpation allows condylar movements to be monitored.

found where incisors are instanding and lateral displacements are often caused by unilateral crossbites. The path of closure should be assessed with particular attention when such malocclusions are present, and care should be taken that closure starts from a position of centric relation because such patients often position their mandibles in a way that disguises the displacement. It is often helpful to observe the patient from above and behind and to palpate lightly just anterior to the ears in order to monitor the movement of the condylar heads (*Fig.* 7.12).

Mandibular displacements, where the occlusal position of the mandible is not one of centric relation, must be distinguished from mandibular deviations where the path of closure starts from a postured position of the mandible.

Intra-oral Examination

First identify and count the teeth, with the aid of radiographs for unerupted teeth as appropriate. The general condition of the mouth is then evaluated, with further assessment of teeth of poor prognosis. Oral cleanliness, gingival and periodontal conditions are then recorded.

Orthodontic treatment should be withheld from the patient with a poor standard of oral care, at least until plaque control is mastered. A gingival bleeding index is a useful control that is quickly undertaken and readily understood by the patient.

Particular attention should be paid to gingival or periodontal problems that may be associated with the malocclusion: for example, gingival recession around a labially crowded lower incisor.

Individual tooth malpositions are recorded. There is little value in detailing every minor irregularity but certain malpositions are particularly important: for example, the inclinations of the canine and incisor teeth may dictate the complexity of treatment and even which teeth need to be extracted.

Finally, buccal and labial segment relationships are examined. For labial segments, overjet, overbite and midline relationships, and for the buccal segments, any anomalies in anteroposterior, transverse and vertical relationships of the teeth are noted. This allows classification of the malocclusion (*see* Chapter 5). For the purposes of clinical description, the incisor classification together with a note of any buccal segment discrepancies is usually most informative. If Angle's classification is to be used, any drift of the first permanent molar teeth must be allowed for.

THE SUMMARY OF FINDINGS

The case assessment must follow a standardized procedure but many of the findings will not be of direct relevance to the treatment of that patient. It is therefore important to be able to recognize the relevant features and their inter-relationships, and to summarize them in a coherent manner. A summary should include:

1   Details about the patient:
     name, sex and age
     attitude to the malocclusion and to treatment
     relevant medical history
2   General features of the malocclusion and dentition:
     classification of the malocclusion
     crowding or spacing
     general standard of dental care
     teeth present and their condition
3   Skeletal relationships
4   Path of mandibular closure
5   Soft tissue features

The prominence given to a particular heading will depend on the features of the individual case.

REFERENCE

1. Moyers R. E. (1973) *Handbook of Orthodontics*, 3rd ed. Chicago, Year Book.

Chapter 8
Planning Treatment and Extractions

OBJECTIVES OF ORTHODONTIC TREATMENT

Orthodontic treatment can be justified only where it is reasonable to expect that it will produce a worthwhile and lasting improvement in dental appearance and/or in the health of the masticatory system. Thus the aims of orthodontic treatment are to produce an occlusion that is stable, functionally adequate and aesthetically satisfactory.

Stability is a primary requirement and imposes limitations on the scope of acceptable changes in tooth positions. For example, proclination of lower incisors to correct a Class II incisor relationship, or expansion of the arches to relieve crowding might superficially seem to be attractive; but in general will not be stable and so should not be undertaken except in special circumstances that are discussed in Chapters 10–13 on the different malocclusions.

Whatever the reason for orthodontic treatment, it is important that the result is functionally acceptable. Premature contacts, non-working side contacts in lateral excursion and other causes of occlusal dysfunction should not remain after orthodontic treatment. Incompetent orthodontic treatment may create these occlusal anomalies and leave the patient worse off than before. With simple removable appliance treatment, it may not be possible to correct all potentially traumatic tooth relationships, but provided that no new malfunctions are introduced and the expectation of future functional problems is remote, this may have to be accepted. However, where fixed appliance treatment is undertaken, care should be taken to correct functional malrelationships, even if these were not the primary justification for the orthodontic treatment. It is not acceptable to deal with post-treatment occlusal functional irregularities in the mixed and early permanent dentition stages by grinding the permanent teeth. Subsequent minor occlusal changes associated with continuing facial growth may well mean that the occlusal reshaping which has been undertaken prejudices the future functional status of the occlusion and of any later occlusal adjustment that might be required.

Aesthetic considerations apply principally to the alignment and relationship of the labial segments. Particularly where there are severe incisor rotations or the overbite and overjet are greatly increased, correction may be difficult. Although the patient's main concern may be the appearance of the teeth, the requirements of function and stability must not be sacrificed to this. Where these three requirements are not mutually compatible, priority should usually be given to function and stability. Only in exceptional circumstances should permanent artificial retention of an unstable occlusal result be planned as the culmination of orthodontic treatment.

Permanent retention is acceptable in malocclusions associated with clefts of the lip and palate and other cases where a denture or bridgework that would be required to replace missing teeth, can be used as an orthodontic retainer. In an adult a deep, traumatic overbite that cannot readily be treated in any other way, or drifting of teeth following periodontal disease and bone loss, may reasonably be stabilized with a permanent retainer. However, the problems of long term appliances should not be underestimated. If plaque control is not of a high order, there will be a deterioration in oral health; and if the retainer is abandoned by the patient, rapid relapse of the corrected tooth positions can be expected.

PRINCIPLES OF TREATMENT PLANNING

The Lower Arch

In general it is good practice to consider the lower arch first. In most cases the size and form of the lower arch has to be accepted because the zone of soft tissue balance is narrow and changes in arch form are very liable to relapse. Lower arch treatment should be based soundly upon the initial labiolingual position of the incisor teeth. In these circumstances, an important decision is whether to accept the lower arch as it is or whether to extract teeth to relieve crowding.

Choice of Extraction of Teeth in the Lower Arch

Incisors and canines The temptation to relieve lower labial segment crowding by extraction of an incisor or canine should be resisted except in a few well-defined circumstances. Following loss of a lower canine the contact relationship between the lateral incisor and first premolar is rarely satisfactory because of the shape of the crowns (*Fig.* 8.1). In general a lower canine should be extracted only when it is in an ectopic position.

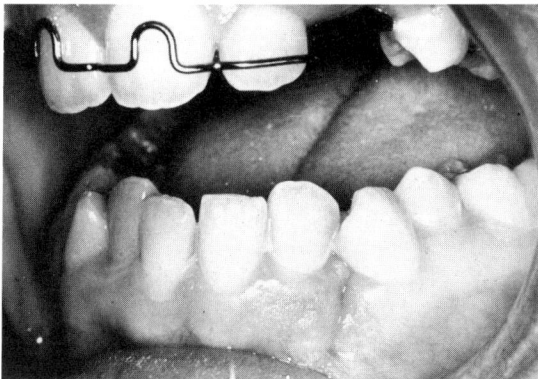

Fig. 8.1. The contact relationship between a lower lateral incisor and first premolar is rarely satisfactory because of the morphology of the teeth.

Loss of a lower incisor is often followed by a gradual decrease in lower intercanine width, with development of crowding in the remaining lower incisors. To some extent upper intercanine width is buttressed by the lower arch and so secondary reduction in upper intercanine width and upper incisor crowding may follow, particularly in the child whose face is still growing.

The circumstances in which a lower incisor may be extracted are where:

(a) a lower incisor is of poor prognosis because of trauma, caries or gingival recession;

(b) the lower labial segment is fanned with distal inclination of the canines and it would technically be very difficult to correct this by extractions further back in the arch (the most upright incisor should usually be selected for extraction so that the other teeth can be tipped into the correct positions);

(c) previous orthodontic treatment involving extraction of upper premolars has left a well-aligned upper arch and a good buccal segment intercuspation but unacceptable crowding of the lower incisors (*Fig. 8.2*) (in these cases, the lower incisors may be large relative to the uppers);

(d) a mild Class III incisor relationship with an acceptable upper arch, and lower incisor crowding: this is still usually better treated by extraction of lower first premolars.

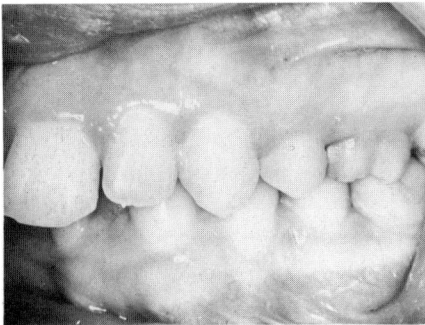
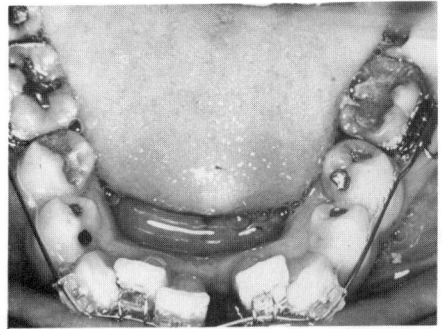

a   b

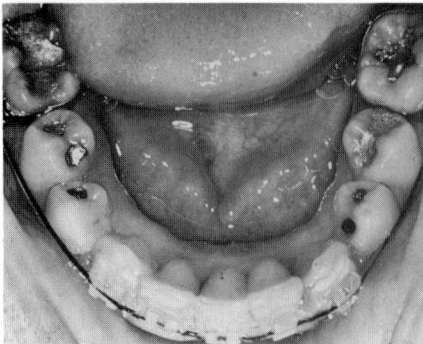
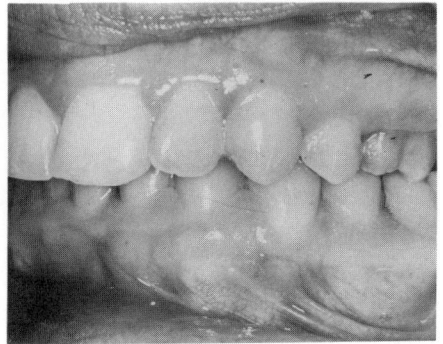

c   d

Fig. 8.2. This adult patient had been treated by extraction of upper first premolars but the lower incisor crowding had subsequently become worse. Treatment involved the extraction of a lower incisor and use of a fixed appliance. The upper incisor spacing was closed with a removable appliance. Note that the overjet is still increased at the end of treatment.

In all these circumstances, treatment should, if possible, be delayed until the patient has stopped growing, and generally fixed appliance treatment will be required to align the lower teeth. Arranging four upper incisors around three lowers is often difficult and may necessitate the extraction of an upper premolar so that one canine can be positioned to occlude between the lower premolars. This in turn can mean that the upper centre line is displaced.

These difficult cases should, whenever possible, be referred to an orthodontic specialist because of the complexities of planning treatment, the technical difficulties and the uncertainty about long term stability.

Premolars First premolars are the teeth of choice for extraction to relieve lower labial segment crowding which is moderate to severe. Where the canines are mesially inclined, spontaneous improvement in lower incisor alignment will usually follow (*Fig.* 8.3). Space closure occurs most rapidly during the first 6 months and will continue gradually for a number of years provided the occlusion allows this. In the growing child, with sufficient crowding, an acceptable contact will usually be established between the canine and second premolar. Often there is some tipping of the canine and second premolar towards one another but, unless food packing occurs, there is no evidence that this is detrimental to periodontal health.

Active alignment and space closure with a fixed appliance will usually be required (*a*) where lower canines are not mesially inclined; (*b*) where space requirements are minor; and (*c*) in adults. If an appliance is to be fitted, it is best not to delay this for too long after the extractions, because alveolar process

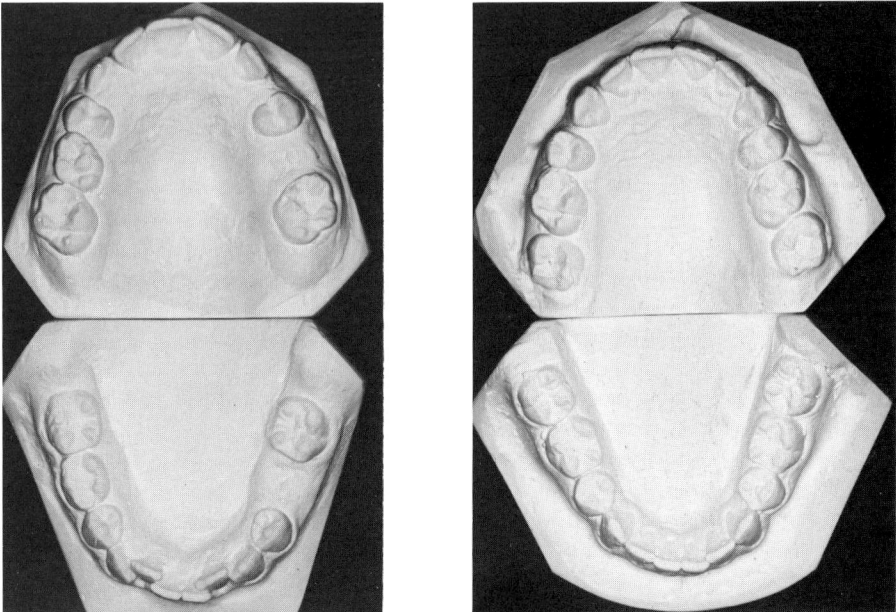

Fig. 8.3. Where lower first premolars are extracted at the optimal time in a child and there is moderate crowding with favourably inclined teeth, alignment of incisors and closure of the extraction space may occur spontaneously to a satisfactory extent.

resorption at the extraction site may delay tooth movement and there may be a permanent constriction of alveolar process at the extraction site (*Fig.* 8.4).

Second premolars should be extracted when they are excluded completely from the arch. This may happen following early loss of the second deciduous molars and the premolar will usually erupt lingually. Where there is more than 2–3 mm of residual space at the second premolar site, spontaneous space closure following its extraction is usually rather unsatisfactory, with mesial tipping of the first permanent molar and disruption of the occlusion. Spontaneous alignment of the lower incisors is much less satisfactory than where first premolars have been removed.

On the other hand, with mild lower incisor crowding which is to be treated with fixed appliances, second premolars can be a good choice for extraction as space closure can be completed by controlled forward movement of the lower molars, without the danger of unwanted retraction of the labial segment which can occur in such cases where first premolars have been extracted. The presence of the first premolar anterior to the extraction site alters the anchorage balance in a way that favours closure from behind.

Molars First permanent molars are seldom teeth of choice for extraction for orthodontic reasons because even when they are removed at the optimal time, the contact relationship between the second premolar and the second permanent molar is rarely ideal (*Fig.* 8.5) and can be poor (*Fig.* 8.6). The guidelines for management of cases where at least one first permanent molar is of poor prognosis are discussed in Chapter 9. Lower second permanent molars may be extracted to relieve impaction of the second premolar or of the third molar. Where the second premolar is slightly short of space due to forward drift of the first permanent molar, extraction of the second molar will allow the distal movement of the first molar (*Fig.* 8.7). This may occur spontaneously if a vertically impacted premolar forces its way in, or an appliance may have to be used. Little, if any, relief of incisor crowding is to be expected and it is not generally practical to retract entire lower buccal segments, because of the difficulties of applying extra-oral traction to the lower arch.

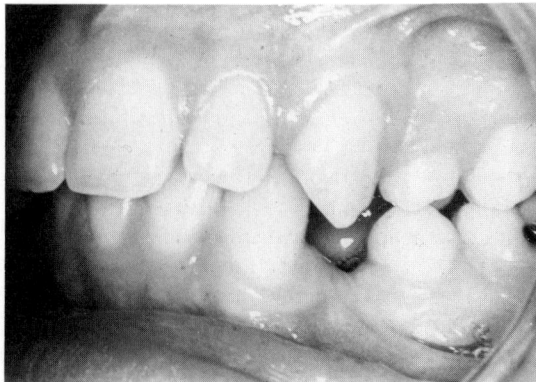

Fig. 8.4. Where space closure has not rapidly followed extraction, alveolar bone resorption produces a constricted alveolar process, and space closure, even with a fixed appliance, is liable to be slow and more difficult.

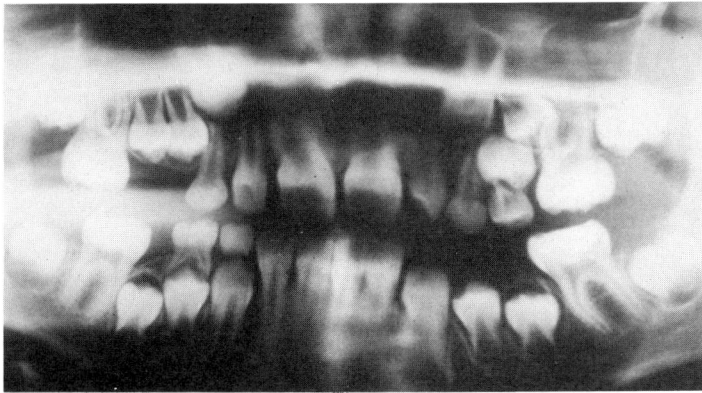

a

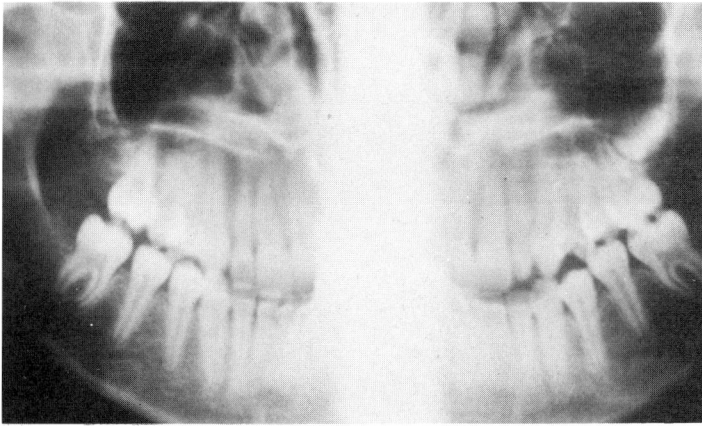

b

Fig. 8.5. A good result following early extraction of first permanent molars.

While the removal of a lower second permanent molar will usually allow the third molar to erupt, it will rarely come into an ideal position (*Fig.* 8.7). Thus, if the only problem is impaction of the third molar, it is preferable to remove this tooth. Where crowding further forward in the arch will be relieved by the loss of the second permanent molar, or where it is in a poor condition, then its extraction may be justified provided that the third molar is in a favourable position. The buccolingual and mesiodistal inclinations must be checked. The cuspal pattern on the radiograph will indicate whether there is an unfavourable lingual inclination of the tooth (*Fig.* 8.8). If the tooth is inclined mesially at more than 30° to the long axis of the second molar, the prospects of satisfactory eruption are again poor and extraction of the third molar is advisable. Spacing between the developing third molar and the second molar is a further unfavourable sign. Even when the position of the third molar seems to be ideal, surprising changes in its inclination may occur following extraction of the second molar (*Fig.* 8.7) and it may be necessary to institute local fixed appliance treatment after it erupts.

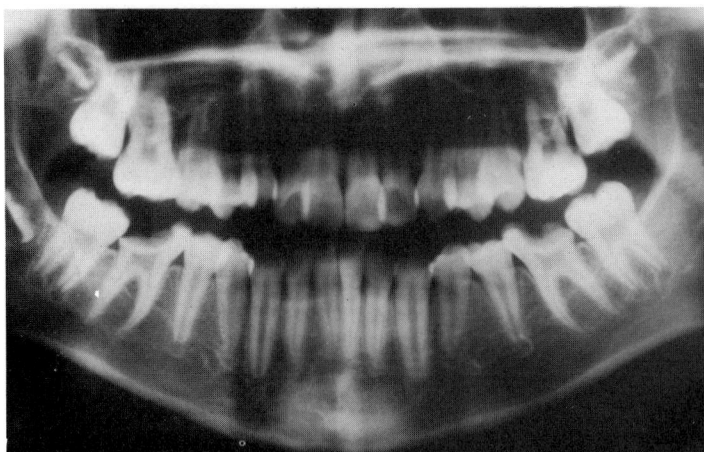

a

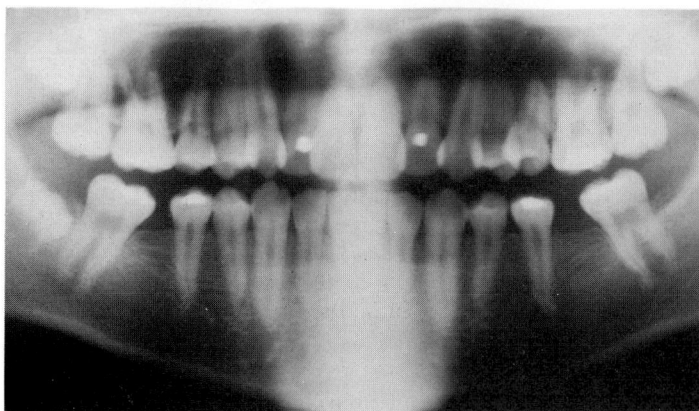

b

Fig. 8.6. A poor result following late extraction of lower first permanent molars.

When in spite of the problems mentioned it is decided to extract the second molar, timing is important. If premolar crowding is to be relieved, the second molar should be extracted before the premolar becomes deflected lingually, which generally means as soon after eruption of the second molar as is convenient. If the extraction is delayed until after the third molar roots are more than one-third formed, the prospects for its satisfactory eruption are reduced.

Third molars are commonly impacted and have to be removed. This can happen even when other teeth have been extracted. Impacted third molars have been implicated in the late crowding of lower incisor teeth, although the evidence is not clear-cut (*see* Chapter 3). If they are left until pericoronitis develops, not only may the patient be inconvenienced, but permanent bone loss and pocket formation may occur distal to the second molar. The conventional timing of extraction of a third molar is when two-thirds of its root has formed

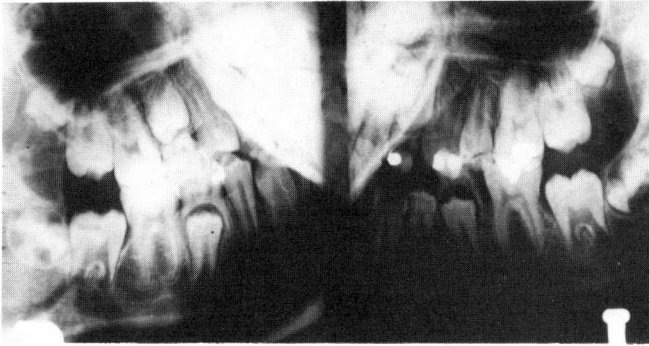

a

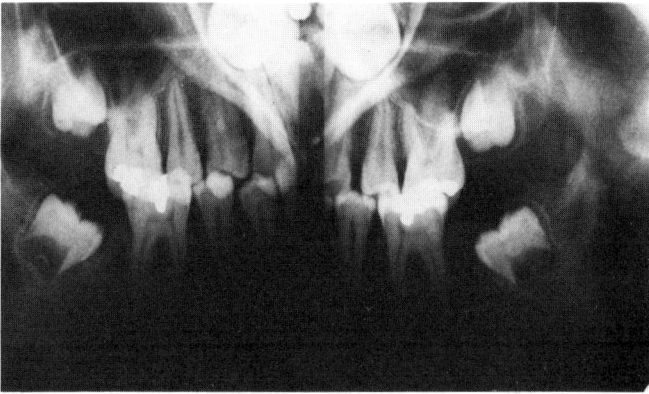

b

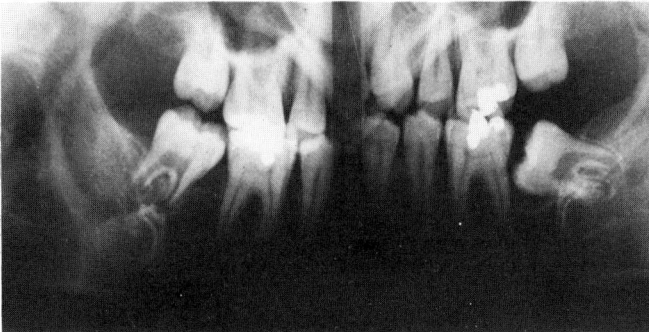

c

Fig. 8.7. In this case it was considered that the slight lower buccal segment crowding could best be relieved by extraction of the second molars, which were removed at the optimal time. The premolar alignment improved, but although both lower third molars had appeared to be favourably positioned at the outset, one became impacted. The position of the other is fairly typical of the result following second molar loss.

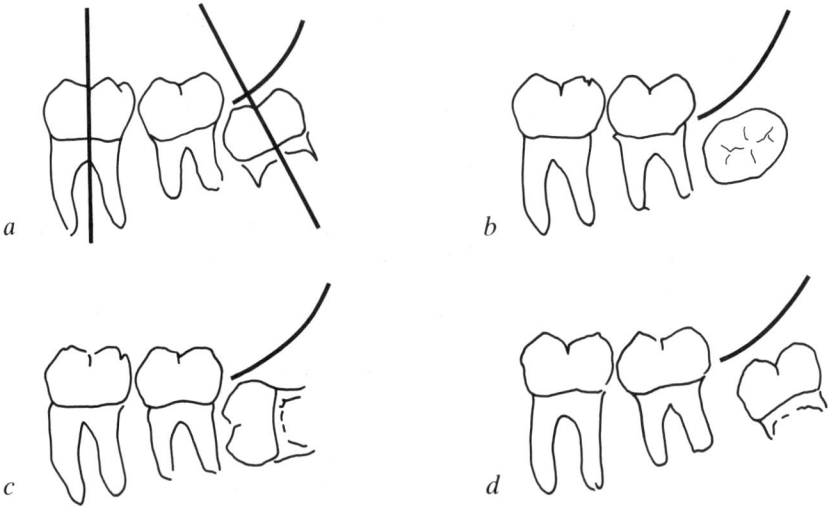

Fig. 8.8. Different developmental positions of lower third molars. *a*, This would be considered favourable for satisfactory eruption following second molar removal. A transversely positioned third molar (*b*) and a horizontally impacted tooth (*c*) should be removed surgically before root formation is complete. Where the third molar is spaced from the second molar (*d*), the prognosis for its satisfactory eruption following loss of the second molar is not good.

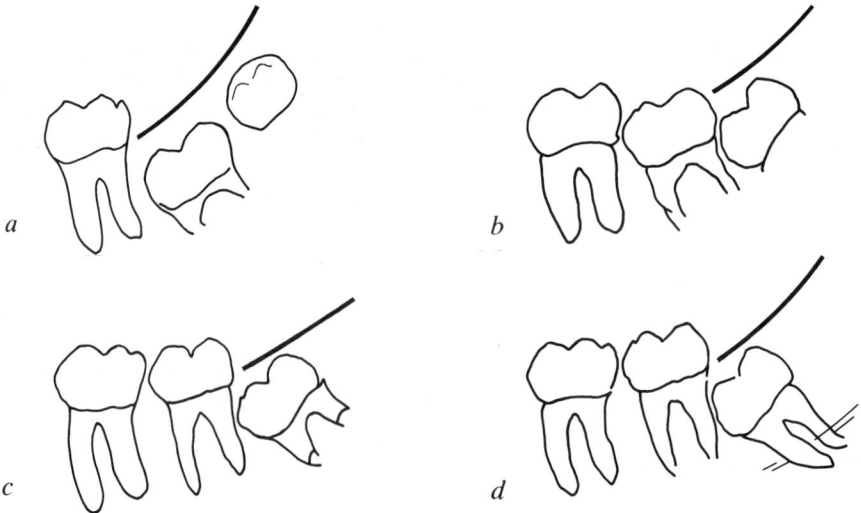

Fig. 8.9. Stages of development at which lower third molars may be removed surgically. *a*, The crypt is visible radiographically and the cusps are calcifying. Enucleation is possible but not recommended. *b*, The crown is complete. If it is obvious that the third molar will have to be removed surgically at some time, this can be done by lateral trepanation at this stage. *c*, The conventional time of removal of impacted third molars is when two-thirds of the roots are formed. *d*, If removal is delayed until the roots are complete, there is a danger of pericoronitis resulting in pocket formation distal to the second molar; the surgical removal is more complicated; and there is the danger of damage to the neuro-vascular bundle.

(*Fig.* 8.9*c*). Later than this, there is the danger of root dilaceration which may make removal more difficult and may risk damage to the mandibular nerve if the roots are close to the canal (*Fig.* 8.9*d*). Earlier removal by a conventional approach is technically difficult because the tooth is almost spherical and rotates when attempts are made to elevate it.

It has been argued that if there is the risk that pressure from third molars may accentuate mesial drift of buccal segments and aggravate incisor crowding, they should be removed before root formation commences. Enucleation at a very early stage, when only the cusps had calcified (*Fig.* 8.9*a*) was suggested by Bowdler Henry.[1] This has fallen into disfavour because it commits the child to surgery at an early age before it is possible to assess whether other extractions for orthodontic reasons would avoid the need, and even before third molar impaction can be predicted with confidence. Subsequently, Bowdler Henry[2] pioneered the technique of lateral trepanation, in which the completed crown of the tooth is removed by lateral approach (*Fig.* 8.9*b*). When undertaken by an oral surgeon experienced in this technique, it is safe and relatively atraumatic, but it is not simple and has not been adopted widely. It is indicated only when it is quite certain that third molars will have to be removed at some stage and there are positive indications for early removal, for example a low impaction against the second molar where any root development could involve the mandibular canal. There is no evidence at the present time that removal at this, rather than at a more conventional time, prevents crowding of the lower incisors.

The Upper Arch

The upper arch should be built up around the lower. The aim in most cases will be to align the upper teeth with a normal overbite and overjet of the incisors. Provided that the lower labial segment is well aligned and matches the upper incisors in size (*see* p. 97), this should be possible if the upper canines occlude in the correct relationship with the lowers. In planning treatment, it is easy to estimate how much space will be required to permit this relation of the canines, allowing for any distal movement of the lower canine teeth that is required to relieve lower incisor crowding. If crowding in the lower labial segment is to be accepted, or if the upper incisors are large relative to the lowers, then either corresponding upper incisor crowding or an increase in overjet will have to be accepted. The exception would be where a stable position of the upper canines can be attained that is further back than the normal relationship to the lowers. Conversely, if the lower incisors are spaced or the upper incisors are small, or if they are retroclined (*see Fig.* 12.5), it is not necessary to retract the upper canines as far as Class I.

Choice of Extraction of Teeth in the Upper Arch

Extraction of upper teeth may be required to relieve crowding or reduce an overjet. As a general rule, in Class I and Class II cases, if lower buccal teeth are to be removed, teeth at least as far forward should be removed from the upper arch. Thus, if lower first premolars are to be removed, it will usually be appropriate to extract upper first premolars, but if lower second or third molars are to be extracted, there is a greater freedom of choice in the upper arch. The removal of lower second premolars should be accompanied by extraction of upper first or second premolars, the latter choice usually giving a situation that is easier to manage, at least with fixed appliances. These are guidelines only and should not be adhered to rigidly. Clearly they do not apply when a lower incisor or canine is extracted. In Class III cases, the reverse applies and it will usually be appropriate to remove teeth from the lower arch at least as far forwards as from the upper.

Incisors and canines   If an upper central incisor has been lost or irretrievably damaged, the space may be used to relieve crowding elsewhere and the lateral incisor on the side of loss can be crowned to simulate a central incisor (*Fig. 8.10*). It may not be possible to obtain an ideal result as the neck of the tooth is rather narrow, but this is usually preferable to extracting another tooth to relieve crowding and fitting a prosthetic replacement for the lost incisor.

Where lateral incisors are peg shaped or badly displaced and there is crowding in the labial segment, their extraction may allow alignment of the teeth with a reasonable appearance, provided that the canines are recontoured, just as can be done where lateral incisors are developmentally absent (*see* Chapter 9). This can offer a simple solution to the case where the upper lateral incisors are palatally displaced and the canines are erupting labial to them and are vertical or inclined distally (*Fig. 8.11*). The more conventional solution of extracting first premolars and using a fixed appliance to align the teeth may give an aesthetic result that is only marginally better in spite of the long and difficult course of treatment. Lateral incisors should not be removed where the canines would look unsightly adjacent to the central incisors because of their colour or form.

The permanent canines are important teeth, and where possible should be retained. However, the upper permanent canines are not uncommonly ectopically positioned and their alignment with orthodontic appliances can be difficult or even impossible. Sometimes transplantation of the canine is feasible (*see* Chapter 19), but if the situation is not favourable, the solution may be to extract the canine itself. Provided that the first premolar has erupted or can be moved

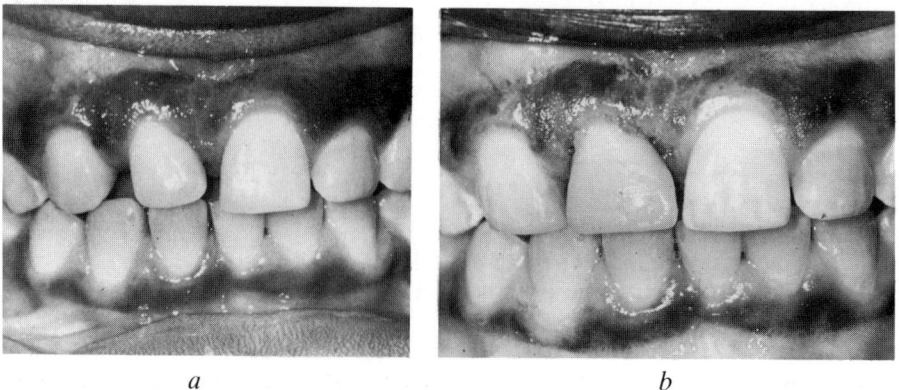

| *a* | *b* |

Fig. 8.10. *a*, Following loss of a central incisor, the remaining teeth were aligned and the lateral incisor moved into the centre of the residual space. *b*, A temporary composite restoration suffices until a jacket crown can be made. Note that before the permanent crown is made the gingival level should be adjusted for a good aesthetic result.

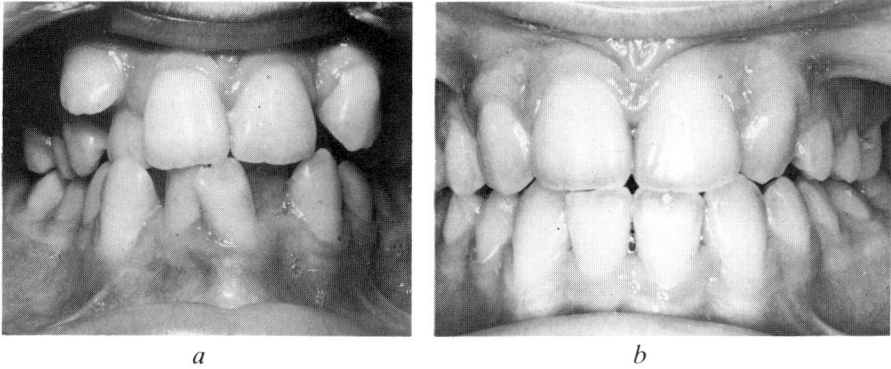

Fig. 8.11. Very occasionally, the extraction of a poorly positioned upper lateral incisor provides a simple solution to an orthodontic problem. Note that in this patient, there were originally only three lower incisors and the lower central incisor was removed because of its poor position and lack of labial plate of bone.

adjacent to the lateral incisor so that its palatal cusp does not show and does not interfere with lateral excursions of the mandible, the result may be very good (*Fig.* 8.12). Certainly, it is a mistake to remove a well-positioned first premolar and then achieve only partial alignment of the permanent canine.

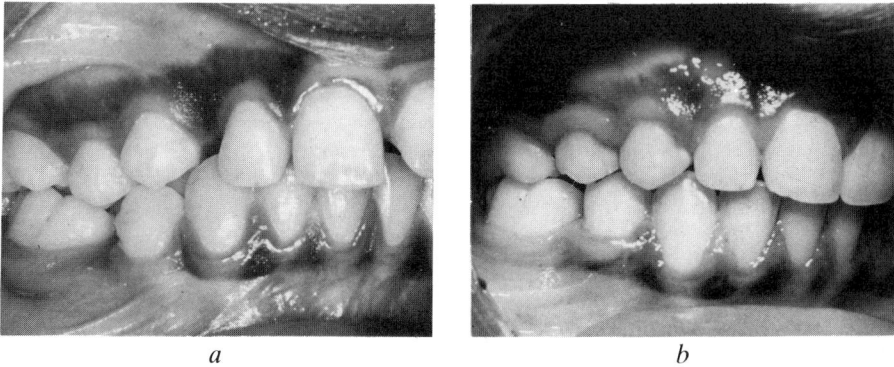

Fig. 8.12. The extraction of a poorly positioned upper canine and closure of any residual space can give a good result.

Premolars First premolars are the teeth most commonly extracted to relieve appreciable upper labial segment crowding or to allow reduction of a moderate or large overjet. Where upper canines have to be retracted by more than 3–4 mm, good results can be obtained following loss of first premolars, more readily than by any other extractions. This also applies in Class I and Class II cases where space requirements are less but where it is necessary to extract lower first premolars to relieve lower arch crowding. The optimal timing of extraction of these teeth in crowded cases is as the upper canine teeth start to emerge (*Fig.* 8.13). Maximum spontaneous alignment and dropping back of the canines will follow. If the premolars are extracted earlier, it is difficult to be confident that the canines are mesially inclined, and unplanned space loss may occur. Delayed

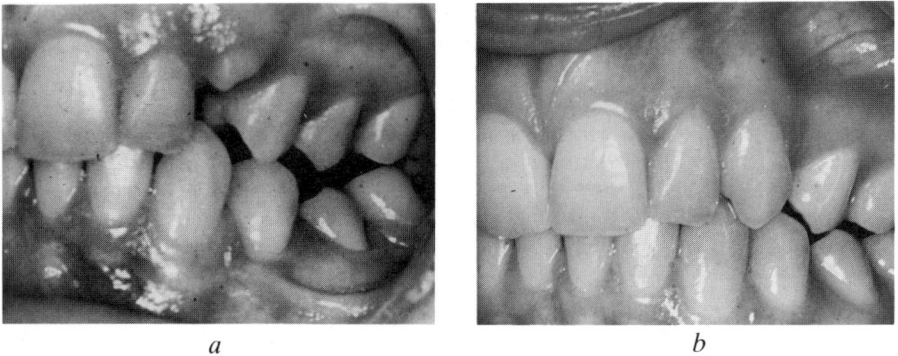

Fig. 8.13. Removal of an upper first premolar at the optimal time allows satisfactory spontaneous alignment of a buccally crowded canine. In this case the canine was more upright than is ideal.

extraction of the premolar may well mean that the canine erupts along a forward path so that the position of the apex is less favourable and spontaneous improvement and the ultimate position of the tooth may be prejudiced. On average, it takes 9 months from the emergence of the canine until it reaches the occlusal level. If space requirements are critical, a space-maintaining appliance should be fitted. If this is not done, the situation should be reviewed at 3-monthly intervals.

When upper second premolars are excluded completely from the arch due to forward drift of the first permanent molars following breakdown or early loss of deciduous molars, it will usually be best to extract them when they erupt palatally. The removal of upper second premolars to provide space for canine retraction with removable appliances is often rather unsatisfactory because the first premolar tilts and the first permanent molar rotates around its palatal root. Generally, where removable appliances are to be used, it is better to extract first premolars if an appreciable amount of space is required, or to retract buccal segments if space requirements are small. However, where fixed appliances are to be used and less than half a unit of space is required, excellent results can be obtained following loss of second premolars. Adequate space is provided for correction of the incisor problem and closure of residual space can be obtained without the risk of excessive retraction of the labial segments, which can sometimes happen when first premolars are extracted in mildly crowded cases.

Molars   Although the consequences of loss of upper first permanent molars in the upper arch are less serious than in the lower, these teeth should rarely be chosen for extraction unless one or more has a poor long-term prognosis. Guidelines for the management of cases where the extraction of first permanent molars is enforced are given in Chapter 9. In mildly crowded cases where less than 3–4 mm of space is required for the labial segments, good results can be obtained following retraction of the buccal segments. This is difficult when upper second permanent molars are erupting or have erupted, and is facilitated by their extraction. The retraction of first permanent molars to make space for crowded second premolars is also simpler when the second molars have been removed. Provided that the upper third molars are of good size and are favourably positioned, they will usually erupt satisfactorily following the loss of the upper second permanent molars. The extraction of upper second permanent molars is contraindicated when the upper third molars are absent and where lower arch crowding is to be treated by the extraction of premolars. A successful combination can be the loss of lower third molars and upper second molars. This can leave the lower second molars unopposed but they will not overerupt provided that the upper first molars are moved back into the correct occlusal relationship with them. In due course, the upper third molars will erupt into occlusion.

Upper third molars are frequently short of space where no other upper extractions have been undertaken. They rarely give rise to problems but will usually erupt buccally and distally inclined, when they can be extracted. There is generally little advantage in removing them prior to their eruption and their proximity to the maxillary antrum can make this hazardous.

Planned Extraction of Deciduous Teeth

In some circumstances the timely extraction of deciduous teeth can simplify later treatment: this is known as 'guidance of eruption'. Clearly the extraction of deciduous teeth can, at best, only relieve crowding temporarily and there is the danger of space loss due to forward drift of the first permanent molar teeth. Extraction of a deciduous tooth is, of course, indicated where it is deflecting or interfering with the eruption of its permanent successor.

Crowding of the permanent incisors can sometimes be relieved by extraction of deciduous canines, at the expense of space for the permanent canines. An important indication for this is where upper lateral incisors are trapped in a palatal position. The removal of the upper deciduous canines just before or as the permanent lateral incisors are emerging can allow them to escape labially. This is advantageous because if they are allowed to erupt fully in a palatal position, it will usually be found that their apices are palatally positioned and a fixed appliance may be required to move them labially. In the lower arch, a labially crowded incisor may have a very thin mucoperiosteal covering with little or no bony labial plate. Rapid gingival recession may occur due to poor plaque control, toothbrushing trauma or even without any obvious explanation. The extraction of lower deciduous canines allows the crowded incisors to align with improved prospects for their periodontal health. The removal of deciduous canines to relieve incisor crowding in either arch almost always means that the first premolars in that arch have to be extracted at a later date to provide space for the permanent canines. The ideal timing for the premolar extractions is just as the permanent canines are emerging through the alveolar mucosa.

Serial Extractions

This approach, of the planned extraction of certain deciduous teeth followed by the removal of first premolars, in order to encourage spontaneous correction of incisor irregularities, was given the name 'serial extraction' by Kjellgren,[3] although the technique is much older and was described by Bunon in 1745. Kjellgren recommended three stages:

1   All deciduous canines are extracted just as the upper permanent lateral incisors are emerging, at about 8½–9½ years of age in a child with average dental development. The objective of this stage, as described above, is to promote incisor alignment. In suitable cases, this is usually successful.

2   All first deciduous molars are extracted 1 year later, ideally when the first premolar roots are about half formed. The objective of this stage is to encourage the eruption of the first premolars in advance of the canines. In fact, upper first premolars usually erupt before the permanent canines, without any stimulus from the extraction of their deciduous predecessors. The lower permanent canine may still erupt before the first premolar and, if the first deciduous molar has been extracted, the premolar will become impacted between the canine and second deciduous molar. It may then be necessary to remove the second deciduous molar to allow the first premolar to erupt, with the risk of mesial drift of the first permanent molar unless a space maintainer is fitted. It is obvious that the extraction of the first deciduous molar is of doubtful benefit and it may result in loss of space from forward drift of the buccal segment. This stage is not recommended.

3   The first premolars are extracted as the permanent canines are emerging, to provide space for them to erupt into the line of the arch. Before extracting these teeth it is essential to re-evaluate the case and in particular to assess the conditions and positions of the other permanent teeth. It is particularly important to check that the upper canines are favourably placed: they should be mesially inclined and should be palpable buccally. The first premolars must not be extracted too early because the inclinations of the canines cannot be assessed reliably before they are about to emerge. Moreover, undue space loss may follow too early an extraction. If on re-evaluation it is decided that the extraction of first premolars is not the most appropriate course of action, then treatment must be re-planned. The full serial extraction procedure subjects the child to the extraction of 12 teeth and has little to commend it. However, in some cases, the timely removal of some or all of the deciduous canines can simplify later treatment; and whenever first premolars are to be extracted for orthodontic reasons, the timing can be important. If there is sufficient space in the line of the arch, extractions are often best deferred until the canines have reached the occlusal level. However, if the canines are crowded, subsequent treatment may be simplified if they are allowed to erupt into the line of the arch following the removal of first premolars as described above.

Serial extraction procedure as described by Kjellgren has little place in modern orthodontics. It was developed at a time when orthodontic appliances were crude and when treatment was not widely available. However, the concept of guidance of eruption to simplify orthodontic appliance treatment is still important and can be used to advantage in some cases.

REFERENCES

1. Bowdler H. C. (1938) Prophylactic odontectomy of the developing mandibular third molar. *Am. J. Orthodont. Oral Surg.* **24**; 72–84.
2. Bowdler H. C. (1969) Excision of the developing mandibular third molar by lateral trepanation. *Br. Dent. J.* **127**; 111–8.
3. Kjellgren B. (1948) Serial extraction as a corrective procedure in dental orthopaedic therapy. *Acta Odontol. Scand.* **8**; 17–43.

Chapter 9

Local Dental Irregularities
In collaboration with D. Poswillo

A number of well-defined factors operate locally on the dental arches to affect the developing dentition.[1] Their effects vary according to whether there is a 'normal' underlying development pattern or whether a degree of malocclusion already exists. In some cases treatment may take the form of a brief interceptive procedure. In other cases it may be part of a more complex plan of treatment.

The following are the main factors to be considered:

1 Abnormalities in the size, number and form of teeth.
2 Premature loss of deciduous teeth due to caries.
3 Loss of permanent teeth due to caries.
4 Prolonged retention of deciduous teeth.
5 Sucking habits.
6 Trauma: fractures and direct displacement of permanent teeth.
7 Large persistent labial fraenum.
8 Abnormal development in the position of tooth germs.

ABNORMALITIES IN SIZE, NUMBER AND FORM OF TEETH
Small Teeth and Missing Teeth

Small or missing teeth cause spacing in arches which are of normal or above average size. In rare cases of true hypodontia, or 'oligodontia', many teeth are missing and those present may be small and abnormal in shape (*Fig.* 9.1). The prevalence of missing teeth varies from 1.5 to 3 per cent according to the sample. Patients presenting for orthodontic treatment cannot be taken as a true cross-section of the population, but one sample showed that 4.3 per cent had one or more teeth missing.

Missing Upper Lateral Incisors

These teeth may be absent unilaterally or bilaterally. If one is absent the other may be of normal size but is often small and conical in shape (*Fig.* 9.2).

The local problem varies according to arch size and relationship. In a crowded arch or when the deciduous canine is retained, the permanent canine may erupt into contact with the central incisor. If the canine is not too pointed, a reasonable aesthetic result may be obtained by reducing its tip (*Fig.* 9.3). Where necessary, the crown can be recontoured using an acid etch composite technique.

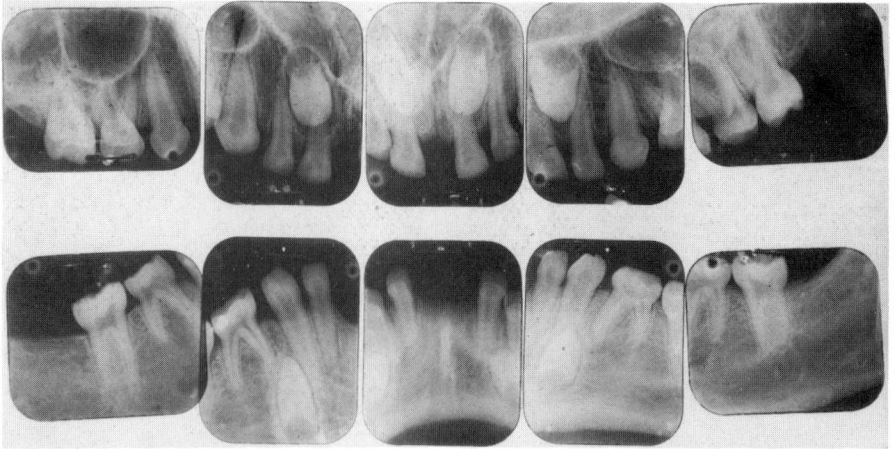

Fig. 9.1. Radiograph of a case of hypodontia showing many teeth missing. The only permanent teeth present are two small upper incisors and two lower caniniform teeth.

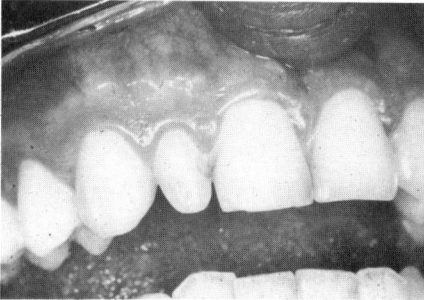

Fig. 9.2. Missing upper left lateral incisor with the contra-lateral tooth small and conical.

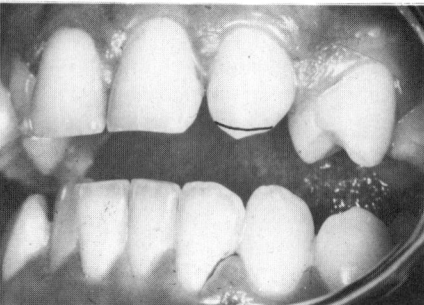

Fig. 9.3. Missing upper left lateral incisor with canine erupted next to central incisor. The canine can be stoned to give a better appearance, as indicated by the line.

In the average to large arch, spacing can be dealt with in several ways. Where it is minimal it may be acceptable to the patient. Where it is not acceptable to the patient (*Fig*. 9.4), sufficient space for a denture or a bridge may be obtained by retracting the canine and approximating the central incisors to concentrate the spacing at the site of the missing tooth. A removable appliance with finger springs will usually be satisfactory. In cases with an increased overjet, the space may be closed by retraction of the central incisors.

a   *b*

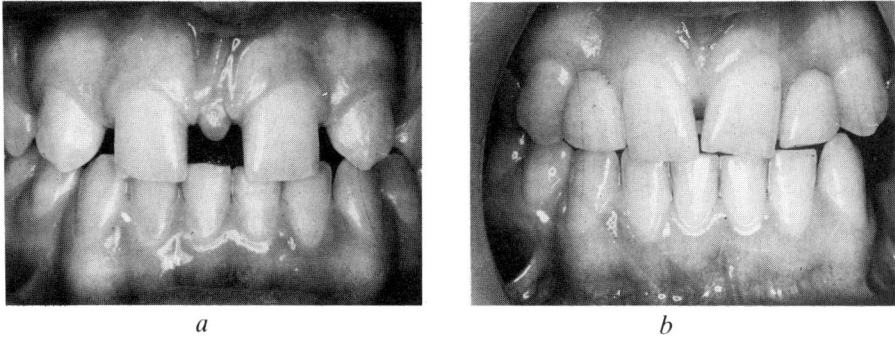

Fig. 9.4. Missing upper lateral incisors. Distal movement of the upper canines and mesial movement of the upper centrals has created space for a denture carrying upper laterals.

Commonly, the space for the upper lateral incisor is too large to be accepted but too small to accommodate a reasonably sized pontic. In such instances there are a number of possible options:

1   Create adequate space for a lateral incisor pontic by distal movement of upper buccal segments, following the extraction of upper second or third molars if posterior crowding is present, or by extraction of a premolar in order to create adequate space for a lateral incisor pontic, after canine retraction.

2   Closure of the anterior spacing by forward movement of posterior teeth. Fixed appliances and prolonged retention are required.

It should be remembered that opening up space will have to be followed by a lifetime's wear of a prosthetic device with all its attendant problems. Acceptance of a canine next to the central incisor is to be preferred in many cases.

Where there is a Class III incisor relationship and missing upper lateral incisors, advancement of the upper labial segment tends to open up the spaces further so that a pontic may be necessary.

Missing Premolars

The fact that lower second premolars, and less frequently upper second premolars, may be missing makes it essential to take routine radiographs before contemplating the extraction of any permanent teeth for relief of crowding (*Fig.* 9.5). In many cases where there is potential crowding, absence of lower premolars means that the extraction of permanent teeth can be confined to the upper arch. The lower second deciduous molars are then removed as part of the treatment of lower arch crowding. It should be pointed out, however, that space closure may require a fixed appliance. It is worth remembering that some premolars develop late and they should not be assumed to be missing until 9 years of age. When the lower premolars are missing and the arch is of ample size, second deciduous molars that are not resorbing may be left in situ until 30–40 years of age unless they show signs of submergence or are of poor quality. Retention of such teeth does mean that at a later stage there will be more than enough space to fit a pontic.

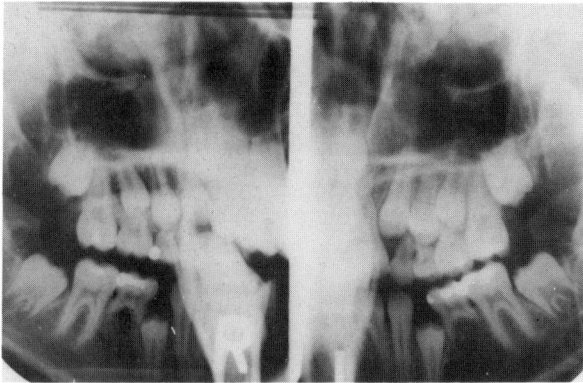

Fig. 9.5. Standard lateral oblique radiograph showing missing lower second premolars.

Missing Lower Third Molars

Absence of these teeth has little adverse effect on the developing occlusion and may be of some benefit, as impactions are common and there may be less chance of later deterioration in incisor alignment. Second permanent molars should not be extracted for orthodontic reasons before the presence of third molars has been confirmed. Third molar development is very variable and may start as early as 7 years or as late as 14 years of age.

Missing Lower Central Incisors

Although this is not a common occurrence, when one or more lower incisors are missing their replacement is a difficult technical procedure. Where the arch is of adequate size and the space is unlikely to close, deciduous teeth should be left in situ for as long as possible. Where the lower arch is crowded the space may close quite readily, although controlled movement with a fixed appliance may be needed. Absence of teeth in the lower labial segment may have an adverse secondary effect on the upper labial segment, particularly when the overbite is deep.

Teeth of Abnormal Form

Dens in Dente (*Fig.* 9.6)

Where the lateral incisors are small and conical it is important to check with a radiograph to see whether there is some abnormality. The radiograph may reveal an appearance described as *dens in dente* (tooth within a tooth), produced by a coronal invagination. The deep cingulum pit leads into a cavity with a deficient enamel lining, which allows bacteria to gain ingress to the pulp. The pulp may become infected soon after the tooth emerges into the mouth. If the cingulum pit can be sealed promptly this process may be prevented, but in other cases the tooth may have to be extracted due to the difficulties of adequate root treatment following abscess formation or because of the general deformity of the crown.

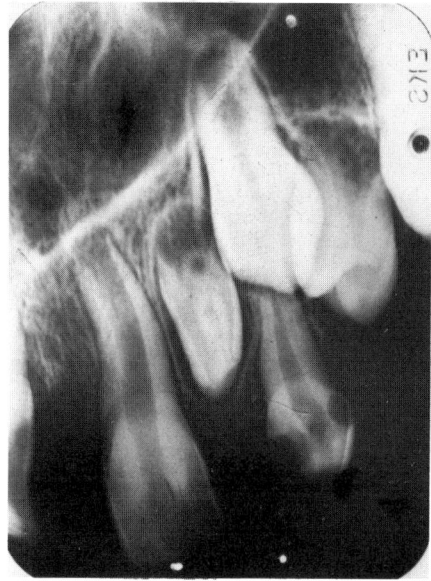

Fig. 9.6. *Dens-in-dente* involving upper left lateral incisor. The pulp may become infected after eruption of the tooth.

Dilaceration

This term describes an abnormal angulation between the crown and root of a tooth or within the root (*Fig*. 9.7). The site of deformation depends on the timing of the disturbance during the tooth's development. It is usually due to a blow to a deciduous tooth, driving it up into the alveolar process. Sometimes the deciduous tooth re-erupts, but the forming permanent incisor is damaged because of its developmental position close and palatal to the root of its predecessor. Little can be done to prevent this type of trauma as young children are liable to falls and other accidents. Occasionally dilaceration occurs without any history of trauma.

A dilacerated upper incisor may fail to erupt or may remain high in the labial sulcus (*Fig*. 9.8). In most instances it has to be removed surgically. Only rarely where there is minimal malformation can a dilacerated tooth be brought into the arch.

Other Malformations

Other abnormalities of tooth form may cause a local problem. Compound or complex odontomes sometimes replace teeth of the normal series. A complex odontome is a diffuse mass of dental tissue which is totally disorganized. Compound odontomes may be a series of denticles. These odontomes have to be removed.

Rarely, one or more teeth in the labial segments are 'connate': two crowns appear to be fused into one (*Fig*. 9.9). Such teeth are rarely acceptable aesthetically and are better extracted and replaced by a denture or bridge. Partially geminated teeth give similar problems.

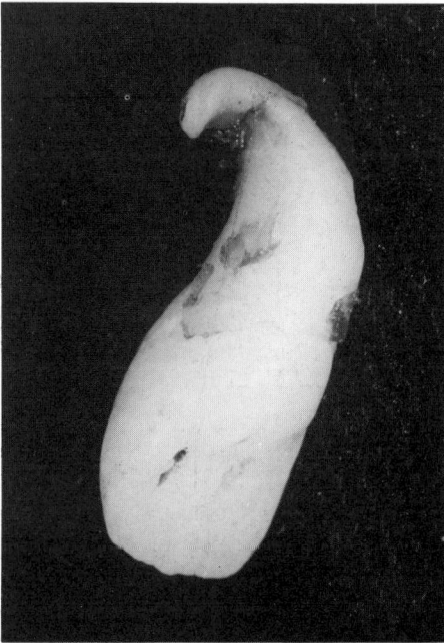

Fig. 9.7. An extracted dilacerated incisor showing distortion of the root.

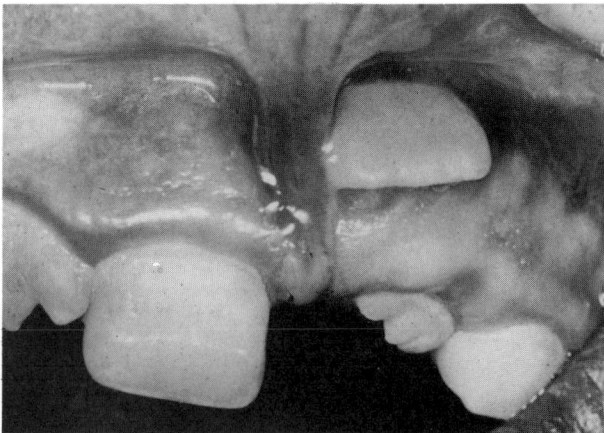

Fig. 9.8. Tilting of lateral incisor where there is a dilacerated central incisor unable to erupt fully.

Supernumerary Teeth

All teeth extra to the normal complement are given the generic name of supernumerary teeth. They occur in about 1 per cent of the population and result from excessive but organized growth of the dental lamina. Most supernumeraries are found in the upper incisor region, but they can occur anywhere in the jaws.[2]

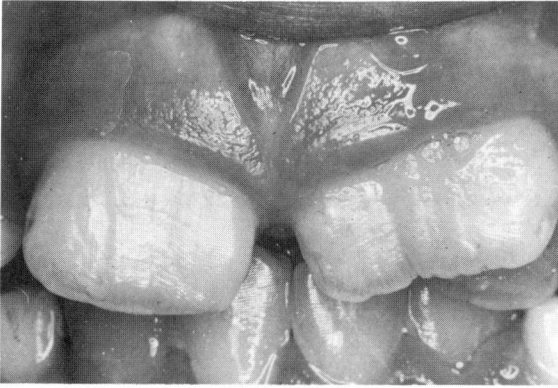

Fig. 9.9. Extra large upper right central incisor, upper left incisor is connate.

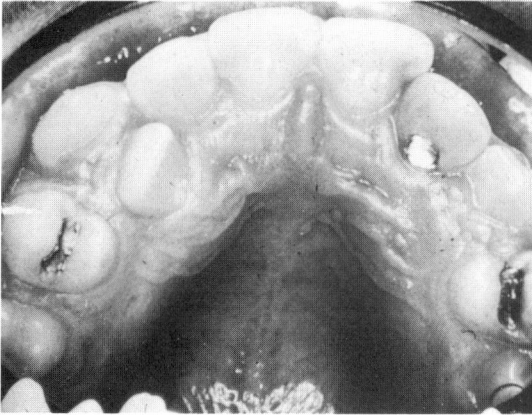

Fig. 9.10. Supplemental upper right lateral incisor.

Supplemental Teeth

As the name implies, this refers to duplication of teeth in the normal series, the most common being the permanent lateral incisor (*Fig.* 9.10). It may be difficult to distinguish the true lateral incisor from its supplemental 'twin'. Usually one of them has to be removed because of crowding and where both are equally well formed, the correct extraction is that of the tooth which is most displaced. A supplemental tooth may have a deep cingulum pit and have a coronal invagination. It is possible that supplemental teeth are an evolutionary throw back (atavism) as the primitive mammalian dentition had three incisors, one canine, four premolars and three molars in each quadrant.

Other Forms of Supernumerary

Other supernumerary teeth differ in shape from the normal series. The term 'mesiodens' is applied to a conical type of supernumerary which is usually found in the midline (*Fig.* 9.11). This either displaces or more commonly prevents

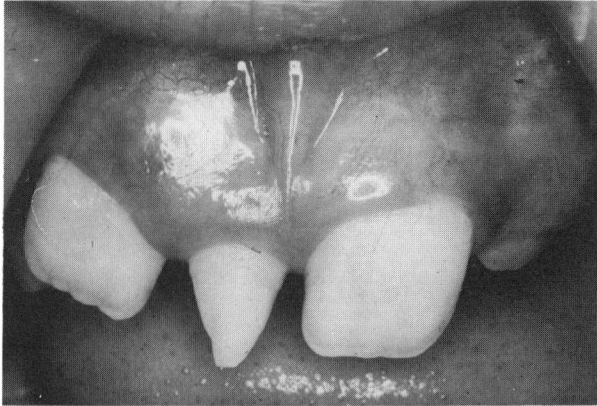

Fig. 9.11. Mesiodens erupted between the upper central incisors.

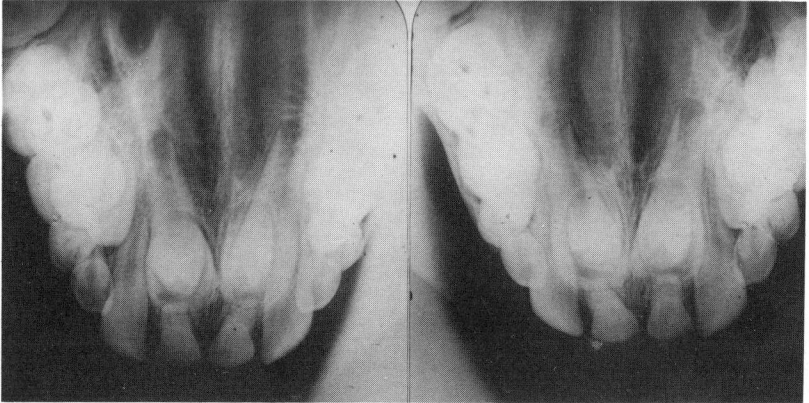

Fig. 9.12. Tuberculated supernumeraries palatal to the upper central incisors preventing their eruption. The two films were taken with a shift of the tube. The teeth furthest from the tube appear to move with it (*see Fig.* 9.13).

eruption of the central incisors. Its calcification may precede that of the permanent central incisor. The presence of a large central diastema or delayed eruption or displacement of a central incisor indicates the need for a radiographic examination. There is usually only a single supernumerary of this type, but sometimes there is a cluster of two or more. On occasion they are placed high and inverted in the palate and have even been known to erupt into the floor of the nose.

The other principal type of supernumerary is tuberculated and is more often paired. They are most commonly located on the palatal side of the central incisors, thus preventing their eruption (*Fig.* 9.12).

Where supernumerary teeth are not deflecting or delaying eruption of the incisors they may be left alone if they are inaccessible; but if there are signs of enlargement of the follicle, with potential cystic formation around the crown, they should be removed. The position of unerupted supernumeraries can be established by the radiographic technique used to locate unerupted canines,

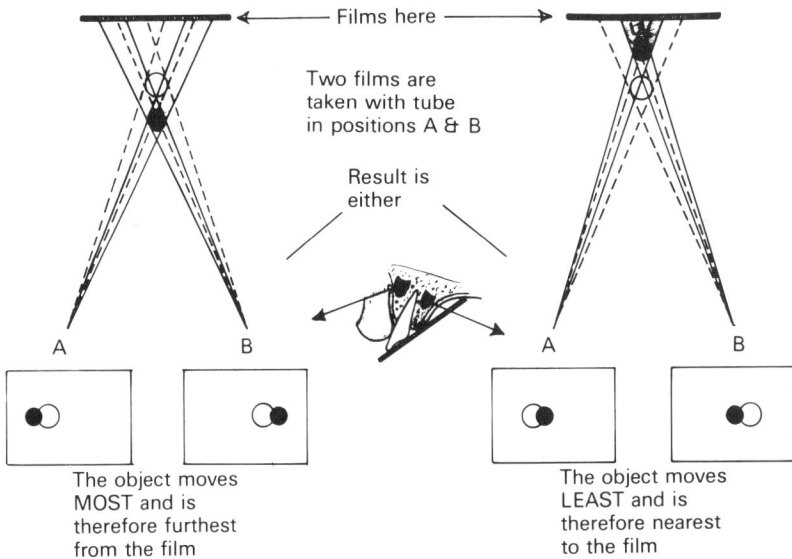

Fig. 9.13. Explanation of the parallax system.

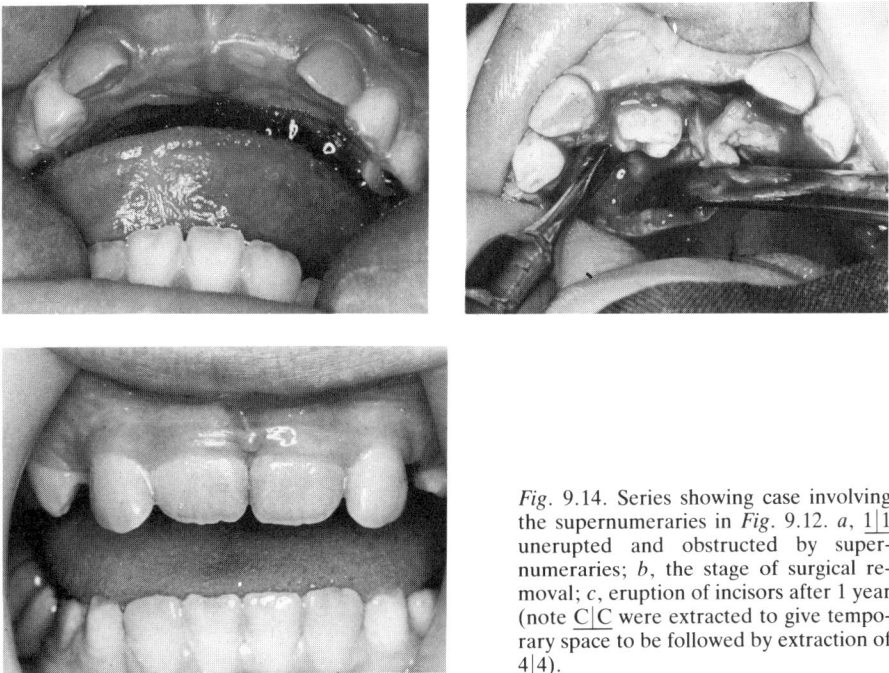

Fig. 9.14. Series showing case involving the supernumeraries in *Fig.* 9.12. *a*, 1|1 unerupted and obstructed by supernumeraries; *b*, the stage of surgical removal; *c*, eruption of incisors after 1 year (note C|C were extracted to give temporary space to be followed by extraction of 4|4).

adopting the principle of parallax (*Figs.* 9.12, 9.13). A true lateral radiograph of the incisor region assists in locating those which are lying deeply in the palate and enables a decision to be made as to whether a buccal, rather than palatal, approach should be made to remove them. Supernumeraries should not be removed surgically before the patient is 6 years of age because there is a danger of displacing the permanent tooth during the operation.

Space requirements must be considered as part of the general orthodontic treatment plan. In a potentially crowded arch, the lateral incisor may encroach on the space for the unerupted central incisor and so the deciduous canines may have to be extracted to provide temporary space. This can be done at the same time as removal of the supernumeraries.

Delayed incisors may take up to 18 months to erupt (*Fig.* 9.14). Where eruption is very delayed due to dense mucoperiosteum, an incision has to be made over the incisal edge.

Supernumeraries may also develop in the premolar or third molar region where they may be similar in form to other teeth in the region or may be conical. Development occurs after most permanent teeth have erupted and thus there is little adverse effect on the occlusion. Multiple supernumeraries occur in cases of cleiodocranial dysostosis, an extremely rare condition.

Surgical Removal

Most mesiodens supernumeraries are removed by a palatal approach, with the flap designed so that the structures in the nasopalatine canal are not severed from their palatal attachment (*Fig.* 9.15). The paraesthesia which may follow sectioning of the nasopalatine nerve to the anterior palate is often unacceptable and occasionally prolonged.

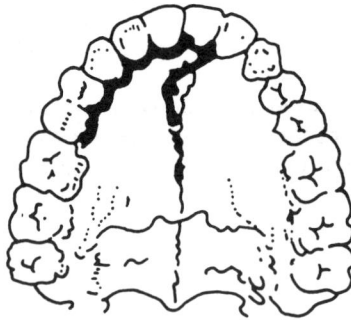

Fig. 9.15. Design of palatal flap for removal of palatally positioned mesiodens.

After flap retraction and before removal of bone, a heavy No. 14 probe should be used to explore beneath the cortical plate in an effort to locate the enamel cap of the mesiodens. The sharp sound of the probe scratching enamel is easily recognized, and precise removal of overlying bone becomes much easier. Sutures that retract the flap by tethering it towards the premolar teeth make access and visibility easier in difficult cases. Occasionally the mesiodens is inverted and the root end is found before the crown. In such cases it is not difficult to confuse the root structure with that of a central or lateral incisor root. Careful exploration with the No. 14 probe or a blunt rotating round bur will usually reveal the crown placed above and posterior to the root, Removal of the buried mesiodens can be achieved by gentle elevation once the bone covering the maximum convexity of the crown has been removed.

When removing supernumerary teeth adjacent to permanent incisors, every effort should be made to retain a collar of bone around the neck of the tooth in the arch. This allows optimal support for the replaced flap and preserves the bony support for the gingival tissue attachment.

In rare instances the route of approach may be found to be inappropriate; i.e., a palatal flap does not provide access to what turns out to be a labially placed supernumerary. When additional flaps must be raised, the area of denuded bone must always be considered: the blood supply to the anterior maxilla can be severely compromised by the elevation of both labial and palatal flaps and occasionally necrosis of a segment of alveolar process can follow. When in doubt, close the inappropriate flap and allow 6 weeks for re-establishment of the blood supply before embarking on the alternative surgical approach.

PREMATURE LOSS OF DECIDUOUS TEETH

One factor that may localize existing crowding is premature loss of deciduous teeth. There is little adverse effect when the jaws are well developed and the dental arches are large. Loss of deciduous incisors through caries does not usually affect the dentition as they will be shed naturally by 5 or 6 years of age. Where the arches are potentially crowded it is the buccal segments that are most severely affected by early loss. The deciduous teeth most commonly extracted prematurely because of caries are the first and second molars. With modern preventive care this loss is becoming less frequent, but it is still a factor to be reckoned with. Space will also close if contact areas are lost due to caries or poor restoration.[3–8]

The earlier the extraction of the deciduous tooth and the greater the tendency to crowding, the more severe the effects will be. Occasionally the occlusion will maintain space, for example due to the intercuspation of the first permanent molars or overeruption of the opposing deciduous tooth.

Early Loss of Second Deciduous Molars

If the second deciduous molar is extracted before eruption of the first permanent molar, the latter tooth will erupt in a more anterior position and total space loss may occur. With later extraction, the upper first permanent molar rotates round its palatal root; while in the lower arch the permanent molar tips mesially with some rotation. The upper second premolar usually erupts into the palate and the lower usually erupts lingually or may impact vertically between first molar and first premolar.

Early Loss of First Deciduous Molars

Where a first deciduous molar is lost prematurely, the first permanent molar and the second deciduous molar drift forwards without rotation or tilting and the anterior teeth spread around the arch. Unilateral loss may cause a shift of the centre line. The consequences depend largely on the sequence of eruption of permanent teeth. In the upper arch, the first premolar usually erupts into the

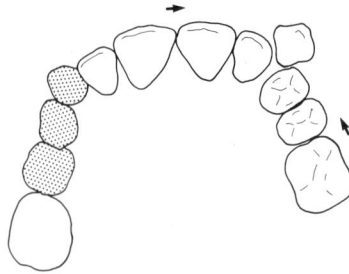

Fig. 9.16. Effect of early loss of |D with forward movement of |5 6 and |3 outlocked.

arch but the canine is outlocked (*Fig.* 9.16); while in the lower arch the canine erupts first and the premolars are short of space.

Early Loss of Deciduous Canines

The deciduous canine is not usually lost early due to caries but because its root is resorbed by a crowded lateral incisor. The lateral incisor encroaches on space previously occupied by the deciduous canine, and the permanent canine is excluded from the arch. With unilateral loss there is a marked shift of the centre line to the affected side.

In general terms, extraction of deciduous canines allows some improvement in incisor crowding.

Space Maintenance

It is impossible to separate the local problem created by early loss of deciduous teeth from the more general problems of crowding, but as a local preventive measure some thought has to be given to maintaining space.

It is questionable whether space maintainers should be fitted, following premature loss of deciduous cheek teeth. There are domestic difficulties in inflicting an appliance on a child at a very early age and in persuading the child to wear it continuously for a number of years, when there is no guarantee that it will prevent the need for later orthodontic treatment. Prolonged use may also hinder good plaque control, with a possible increase in caries. Removable space maintainers fail if not worn adequately, while those that are fixed in the mouth require regular inspection as their distortion or displacement can damage neighbouring teeth.

One situation in which space may be maintained with some advantage is where there is an acceptable alignment of the teeth but with the tendency to mild crowding. In such a case early loss may produce a localized malocclusion for which it is difficult to plan simple orthodontic treatment.

In view of the fact that many children have a potentially crowded mouth and will require extraction of permanent teeth anyway, the use of space maintainers is rarely justifiable. With improved preventive measures, the number of deciduous teeth that have to be extracted because of caries will diminish. The natural tooth forms the ideal space maintainer and it is preferable to root-fill it and to restore it adequately than to extract it prematurely. When a deciduous tooth has to be lost from a mouth in which plaque control is poor, or where there is a high caries rate, compensating, balancing and symmetrical extractions of other deciduous teeth have to be considered. Opinion is divided on the desirability of further extractions as opposed to space maintenance but there is no doubt that in Class I cases with mild crowding, if a first deciduous molar has to be extracted on one side of the upper arch, the contra-lateral tooth should be extracted to prevent centre-line shift and allow some temporary improvement in incisor crowding. This is a 'balancing extraction'.

If one first deciduous molar has to be extracted in the lower arch it may be desirable to balance, extracting the contra-lateral tooth, and this may signal the need for compensating extractions in the upper arch, particularly if the teeth are of poor quality and need extensive restoration.

Where there is gross crowding in the lower arch and a Class II malocclusion with deep overbite, extensive active treatment will be required. It is better therefore to limit the extraction to the offending deciduous molar and not complicate the problem further by compensating or balancing extractions. The reverse is true if one deciduous molar has to be extracted in a Class III case in a crowded upper arch.

As a general rule the loss of second deciduous molars should not be balanced or compensated because the effect on the centre line is minor and a local malocclusion may be created on one side but not on the other.

There is merit in balancing the loss of one deciduous canine by extraction of its antimere, in order to attempt to minimize the displacement of the centre line, although this is not always successful.

LOSS OF PERMANENT TEETH

As was pointed out earlier, one of the most common causes of spacing is the developmental absence of teeth. Similar problems are created if permanent teeth have to be extracted from arches that are of adequate size to accommodate all the teeth in good alignment. Each problem has to be dealt with on its merits; for example, loss of an upper incisor necessitates a temporary bridge or denture during the developmental period as drifting of neighbouring teeth makes the restoration more difficult later (*Fig.* 9.17).

When permanent teeth are lost from the buccal segments, the space may fail to close if the arches are of normal size or are particularly large. Teeth on either side of the extraction space may drift and rotate and unilateral loss will cause centre line shift. Where there is crowding the space may well close, but this may be accompanied by undesirable tilting (*Fig.* 9.18). Therefore, thought has to be given to either maintaining the space, closing it with fixed appliances, or to moving the teeth in preparation for a pontic. Much depends on whether there are other occlusal problems which require orthodontic treatment or whether this is an isolated situation merely requiring attention to local detail.

At one time first permanent molars were very frequently carious and many had to be condemned at an early age. This is now less common but still occurs in certain disadvantaged groups of children.

The results of the extraction of first permanent molars depend greatly upon timing. When they are removed before eruption of the second molars, space

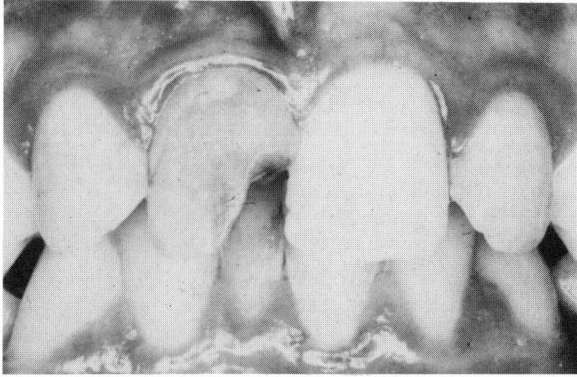

Fig. 9.17. Loss of space in a crowded arch where an upper central incisor has been fractured.

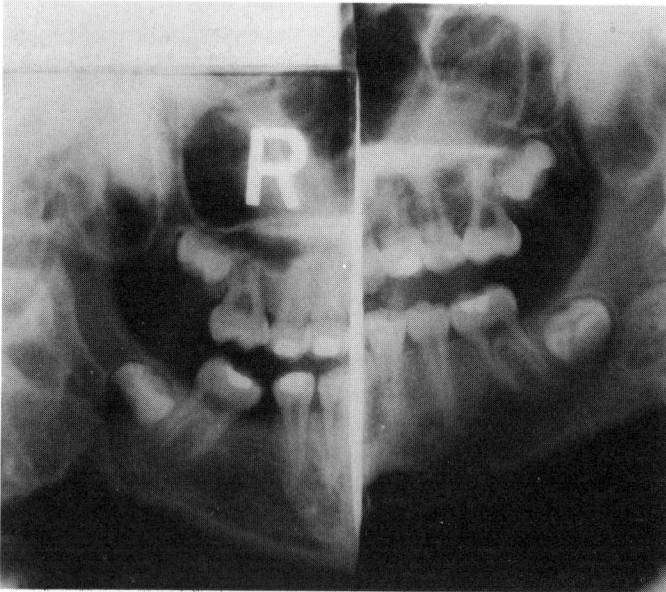

Fig. 9.18. Extraction of all first permanent molars. Note satisfactory positions of 7|7 and |7; but in lower right quadrant the later extraction of 6| leads to an unsatisfactory position of 7|.

closure can be reasonably good, with the second molar erupting more anteriorly (*Fig.* 9.19) and some relief of lower incisor crowding. Particularly in the lower arch, the results are best if the extractions are timed before one-third of the second molar roots have formed and while the crypts are still covered by bone. In the past, some authorities recommended the routine extraction of first permanent molars in Class I cases, to relieve crowding and remove the teeth most susceptible to decay; but this cannot now be accepted because the quality of result is so variable. The second molars may be tipped anteriorly and rotated, and the improvement in incisor crowding may be minimal in some cases.

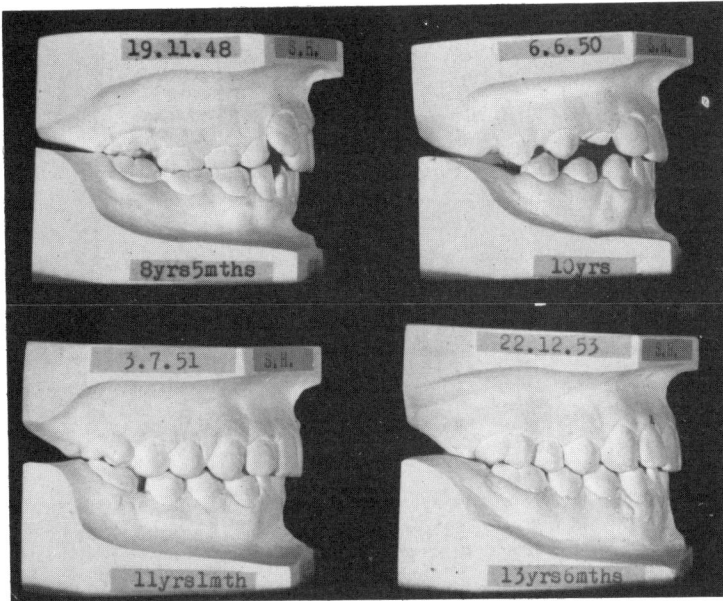

Fig. 9.19. Models showing mildly crowded arches where the extraction of all first permanent molars in a Class I case at the age of 9 years has allowed a satisfactory result and some easement of incisor crowding.

When first permanent molars are extracted after the eruption of second molars, the results are uniformly poor. The second molars tip and rotate mesiopalatally and there may be little change in incisor alignment. Spacing is left at the extraction site and this may give a stagnation area. The occlusion is often disrupted by tipping of teeth adjacent to the extraction site and by overeruption of teeth in the opposing arch. Orthodontic treatment to close the spacing is difficult and tedious, requiring the use of fixed appliances.

For reasons outlined above, first permanent molars are almost never the teeth of choice for extraction for orthodontic reasons. However, if the first permanent molars are in a poor condition at an early age, it will usually be preferable to extract them at a time when the greatest amount of spontaneous improvement can be expected. As it is unusual for a single molar to be of poor long-term prognosis, and as it is desirable to preserve symmetry, consideration should be given to the removal of first permanent molars from the other quadrants according to the following guidelines. These apply only where:

1   The other permanent teeth (apart from third molars) are present, sound and positioned favourably.

2   The second molars have not yet erupted, and preferably root formation is only just commencing.

3   The arches are not spaced.

Class I Cases

$\overline{6}$ is poor:

(*a*) Extract $\overline{6|6}$ at the optimal time. This preserves arch symmetry and will give the most favourable outcome in the lower arch.

(*b*) If the upper arch is mildly crowded, extract 6|6 at the same time. This allows relief of mild upper arch crowding and in these circumstances the results are usually quite acceptable. If the upper arch crowding is more severe and the upper molars are sound, defer a decision on extractions until the upper canines are erupting and then deal with the upper arch crowding on its merits.

One 6 is poor: If crowding in that arch is mild, extract 6|6 early and a reasonable result can be expected. Where upper arch crowding is more severe:

(*a*) Both upper first permanent molars can be extracted early and space to relieve residual labial segment crowding can be provided later by retraction of the upper buccal segments. This is often the best approach to the problem. Or:

(*b*) Extraction of 6|6 can be deferred until 7|7 have erupted and then appliance treatment can be started. This has the disadvantage that treatment is liable to be prolonged, and if removable appliances are to be used, the results can be rather **unsatisfactory with tipping and poor contacts at the extraction sites.**

Planning of treatment in the lower arch can be difficult. 6|6 should not be removed if they are sound. A regular or minimally crowded lower arch should, of course, be accepted. If extractions are required to relieve lower labial **segment crowding, first premolars will be the teeth of choice,** although this does not integrate well with the loss of upper molars.

Class II Cases

The guidlines follow those given above for Class I cases except that if there is a **severe space discrepancy in the upper arch even following the early loss of 6|6** it may be justifiable to extract 4|4 as well, provided that 8|8 are present, of adequate size and are well positioned.

Class III Cases

One 6̄ is poor: Space closure is often very unsatisfactory in the lower arch of Class III cases and so every effort should be made to preserve the lower permanent molars. It will not usually be wise to balance the extraction of one lower molar with the loss of the same tooth on the other side of the arch. The upper arch should be treated on its merits.

One 6 is poor: **The upper arch will often be crowded and the space closure** should be good following early loss of the molar. Consideration should be given to removing the other molar at the same time.

The recommendations outlined above are a compromise aimed to produce an acceptable result with a minimum of therapeutic intervention. They are particularly appropriate where the attitudes of the patient preclude extensive dental or orthodontic treatment; or where orthodontic treatment with fixed appliances is not available. However, they are also useful where these limitations do not apply. It is often more cost-effective to extract badly broken-down first permanent molars at the optimal stage, and deal with any residual occlusal problems with fixed orthodontic appliances, than to go to great lengths to restore the tooth and later to remove other sound teeth as a prelude to a course of fixed appliance treatment.

In a Class I occlusion with mild to moderate crowding where one or more first permanent molars have to be extracted it may be advisable to extract all four. This is really an approach of expediency because the forward movement of the second molars and relief of anterior crowding cannot be relied upon. However, the lower second molars may drift into a good position without tilting, although the result is rarely very good. The best results are obtained if the first permanent molars are extracted at between 8 and 10 years of age so that the second molars can move forwards as they erupt.

The situation becomes more complicated when there is a severe malocclusion and all first permanent molars have to be extracted. Where there is gross crowding in all four quadrants in Class I malocclusion it may be better to retain the upper first permanent molar for as long as possible until the second molar has erupted. This will prevent rapid forward movement of the upper second molar and the space created by the extraction may be utilized to correct the crowding. Where there is urgent need to remove both upper first permanent molars early the space may well close before the second molar drift can be controlled and distal movement of buccal segments or the additional extraction of first premolars may have to be considered in due course. The situation in the lower arch is different, as the lower second molars drift forwards more slowly. Less tilting of the lower second permanent molars will occur if the first permanent molars are extracted by 8–10 years. Where the extraction of the first permanent molars in the lower arch can be delayed until the second molars have fully erupted the use of a fixed appliance may enable the space to be used for anterior alignment.

In Class II cases if the lower first permanent molars have to be extracted early there will be little adverse effect on the inclination of the lower labial segment. If the lower second molars do not come forwards into good position they may have to be uprighted with a fixed appliance, as part of the overall treatment. In the upper arch the extraction of the first permanent molars may be delayed until the eruption of the upper second molars. They can then be held back and the space utilized to retract the anterior teeth.

PROLONGED RETENTION OF DECIDUOUS TEETH

There is appreciable variation in the time at which deciduous teeth are shed naturally. Retention of these teeth is rarely the primary cause of the displacement or impaction of permanent teeth. A marked delay in the natural resorption of a deciduous tooth may indicate that there is no successor or that it is displaced or obstructed. Routine radiographs will reveal the nature of the problem.

Where a deciduous incisor is retained, the permanent tooth will commonly erupt lingually (*Fig*. 9.20) and extraction of the deciduous tooth often allows the permanent incisor to move forwards, obviating the need for an appliance. Where an upper central incisor is already trapped behind the lower labial segment (*Fig*. 9.20), it can be moved forwards with a simple removable appliance in a matter of a few weeks. Alternatively, a thin wooden spatula or the

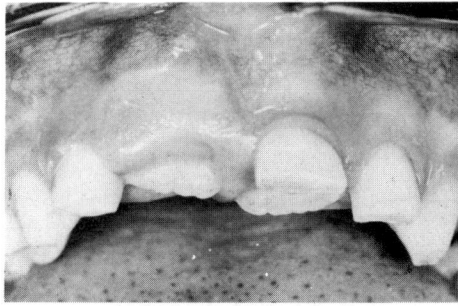

a

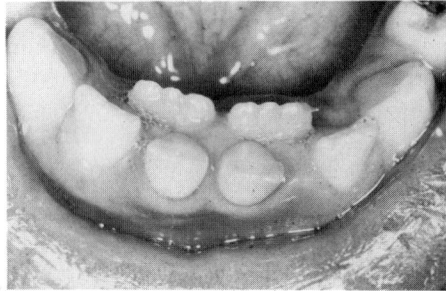

b

Fig. 9.20. Retained deciduous incisors. Lower permanent incisors will move forwards under tongue pressure when the deciduous teeth are lost.

handle of a teaspoon can be used as a lever. The patient should be instructed to use this in front of a mirror for 20 minutes each day (*Fig.* 9.21).

Retention of a deciduous canine may indicate an ectopic position of the permanent successor. When the permanent canine is very displaced or the lateral incisor is missing, the deciduous tooth may be preserved for as long as possible. If the permanent canine is only mildly displaced, the deciduous tooth should be removed as it may exaggerate the displacement of the permanent tooth (*Fig.* 9.22). (The special problem of ectopic canines is dealt with in detail on p. 143).

First and second deciduous molars are not usually retained for any length of time unless their successors are absent. Occasionally they are very persistent and interfere with eruption of the premolar, when they should be extracted. It is difficult to give guidance as to when the second deciduous molar should be removed if it has no successor. It should certainly be extracted if there is potential crowding elsewhere in that quadrant. It should also be removed if it is badly broken down and cannot be restored readily. Where the tooth is contributing to the occlusion and has a good prognosis there is a case for leaving it in place if the arches are large and space closure is unlikely. In some cases these teeth last until the patient is more than 30 years of age.

Where extensive orthodontic treatment is required for other reasons and there is crowding, the extraction of the retained deciduous molar has to be incorporated in the treatment plan.

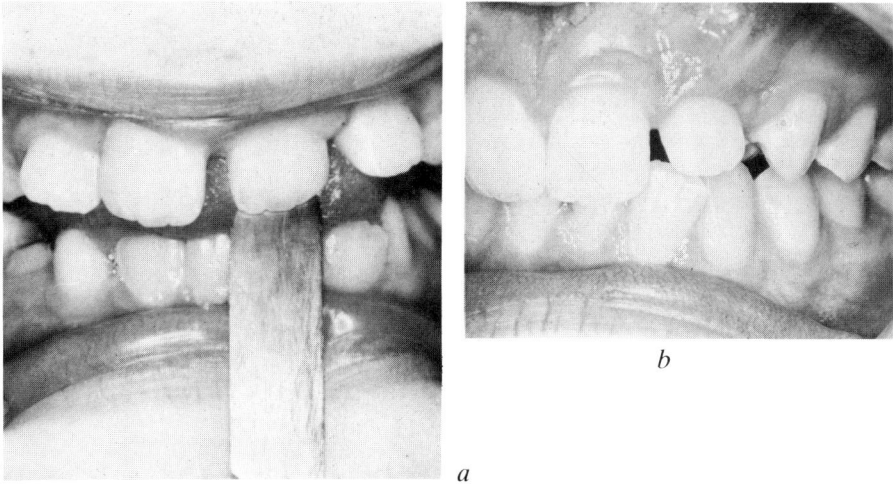

Fig. 9.21. *a*, Use of spatula to lever central incisor over the bite. *b*, The result of treatment.

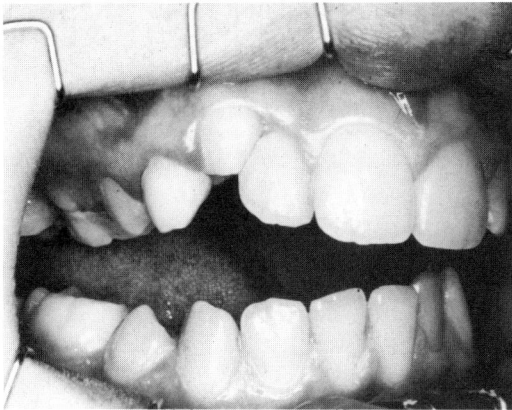

Fig. 9.22. Retained deciduous canine causing displacement of permanent canine. The deciduous tooth should be removed.

Sometimes deciduous molars, particularly second deciduous molars, show signs of relative submergence associated with ankylosis (*Fig.* 9.23). The tooth may erupt normally but later appears to submerge while the rest of the occlusal table rises with growth. The tooth is much firmer than usual and in most cases is probably ankylosed. Submergence is not necessarily connected with the absence of the underlying tooth. In most cases the condition resolves spontaneously, with the deciduous tooth regaining the occlusal level. However, the neighbouring erupted permanent teeth may tilt across the submerging tooth, which should be removed before submergence becomes excessive.

If a tooth is ankylosed it will give a dull note on percussion and the periodontal space may not be visible on a radiograph. Sometimes these teeth are not even visible in the mouth. They have to be removed with care, using a proper surgical approach, with the reflection of a flap and removal of bone.

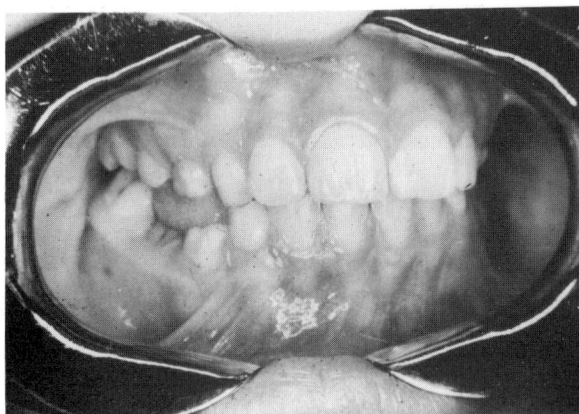

a

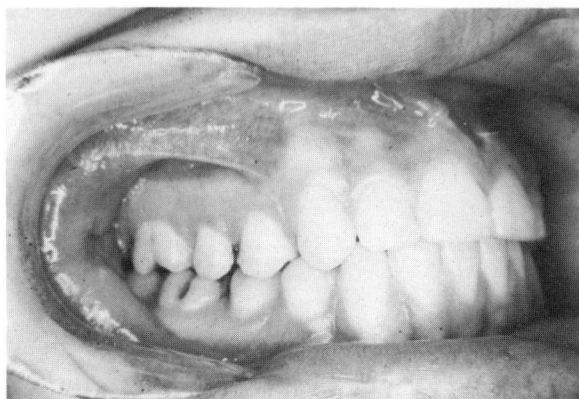

b

Fig. 9.23. *a*, Submerged deciduous teeth in the buccal segment. *b*, The premolars have erupted naturally following extraction of the deciduous molars.

SUCKING HABITS

In the infant various digit- and dummy-sucking habits are extremely common (*see* Chapter 3). They usually produce an anterior open bite or an incomplete overbite and increased overjet (*Fig.* 9.24). The upper arch may be narrowed by pressure from the cheeks on the buccal teeth, which are not supported by the tongue or by occlusion with the lower arch. As both arches are then of equal width, there is often a lateral mandibular displacement into the position of maximum occlusion, causing a unilateral crossbite. These defects may disappear quite rapidly if the habit ceases by 7–8 years and it is the sole causative factor. It is wrong to underestimate the effects of prolonged and persistent sucking habits. The degree of disturbance in the incisor region is in proportion to the amount of time, force and manner in which the digit is sucked.

Few children persist in the habit to the point where the behaviour justifies psychological investigation, and drastic measures to break it are inappropriate. Parents should be discouraged from nagging, as this is often counterproductive.

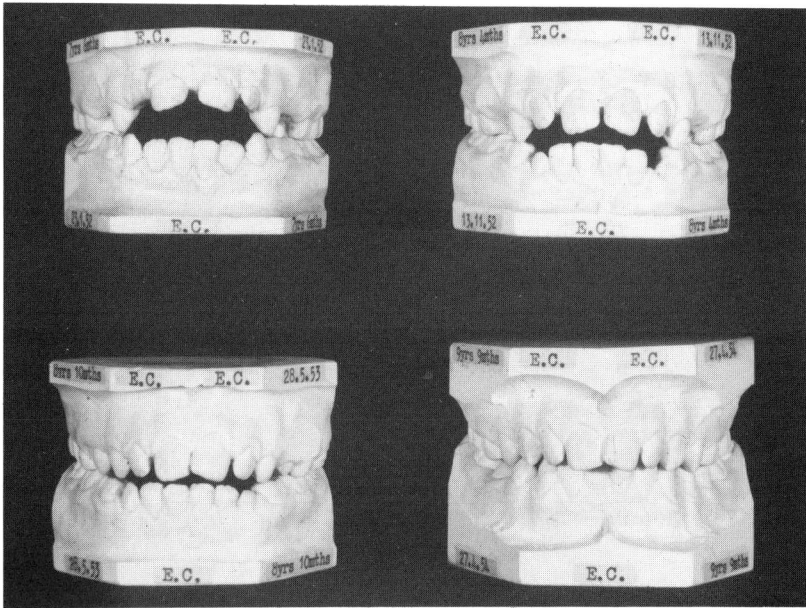

Fig. 9.24. Effects of finger sucking and natural reduction of open bite following withdrawal of the habit.

Simple local treatment to control the habit may not succeed in allowing the open bite to close completely. This is because there may be an adaptive forward tongue posture to effect an anterior oral seal (*see* Chapter 3).

When the habit persists despite a period of observation, some interceptive procedures may be required and many deterrents have been recommended. These include spiked appliances to prick the thumb, fixed bars in the upper arch and other forms of barrier. However, the fitting of a simple appliance which merely covers the palate can be quite effective as it draws attention to the habit and seems to minimize the pleasure. An expansion appliance may be used where there is a narrow upper arch and a displacement in the path of closure.

TRAUMATIC INJURIES

Children are often involved in minor accidents which damage their teeth, particularly when they start to engage in contact sports. Damage to deciduous incisors can be responsible for deformation of permanent incisors and this has already been described (*see* p. 125). Where there is an overjet the upper incisors are more vulnerable and the increased incidence of damage in Class II, division 1 cases is well recognized.

With modern endodontic treatment, most fractured incisors can be retained. Where a substantial proportion of the crown has been destroyed the mesiodistal width of the tooth must be restored otherwise the adjacent teeth will encroach on the space if there is potential crowding in the arch. Teeth that are partially avulsed can be preserved by careful splinting and root treatment where necessary. Where teeth have been extracted or totally avulsed the decision has to be made as to whether they should be replaced by a denture or bridge, taking account of the general state of the mouth and whether there is an existing malocclusion.

Reimplantation is quite successful if done quickly with minimal interference to the supporting tissues once the tooth has been cleansed. A reimplanted tooth may last for several years even if there is a degree of root resorption, and so can be used as a space maintainer with eventual replacement by a bridge or denture. Where the labial segment is very crowded the lateral incisor can be moved mesially and crowned to simulate the central incisor, accepting the fact that there will be some disturbance of centre line (*see Fig.* 8.10). The lateral incisor may require a local fixed appliance to move it bodily. If it is tilted by a simple removable appliance it may not be possible to make a satisfactory jacket crown.

In Class III cases it is usually necessary to maintain space in the upper arch but in Class II cases with a marked overjet there are occasions when this space may be closed by retracting the remaining incisors rather than creating additional space by premolar extractions. This does produce rather a crude arrangement of the three remaining incisors but it may be preferable to extracting sound teeth elsewhere in the arch and eventually replacing the incisor with a bridge or denture.

Traumatic loss of one or more lower incisors is not common, but may result from a fall or following the use of gags in the mouth during general anaesthesia when the teeth are newly erupted. Where there is potential crowding, a lower incisor space may close rapidly but may need controlled tooth movement with a fixed appliance. If the tooth which has been lost was already crowded and the remaining teeth are in good alignment, the space may be allowed to close by natural drift.

It is not a practical policy to try to hold the lower incisor space by fitting a temporary denture as these are very unsatisfactory. If the loss of a lower incisor occurs in a case with a deep overbite, the problem is more complicated and advice should be sought concerning the overall treatment plan in view of the possible deepening of the overbite and adverse effects on the upper arch. The general principle should be that where a lower incisor space is likely to close naturally, it should be allowed to do so.

A LARGE LABIAL FRAENUM

In the newborn the upper labial fraenum is attached at the crest of the gum pad and should be left behind as the alveolar process and teeth develop. It may present a local problem if its attachment remains low on the crest of the alveolar process and with a thick fibrous attachment to the palatal mucosa (*Fig.* 9.25). This is rarely the primary cause of a midline diastema but it may prevent the incisors from coming together naturally following eruption of the upper lateral incisors and canines. There may be a flat table of bone between the incisors and a wide suture.

It may be desirable to carry out a fraenectomy if the fraenum is binding the upper lip down tightly and fostering stagnation in the incisor region, or if it is so bulky as to prevent closure of a diastema. It may also be removed when it shows an ugly fold of tissue. Although a fraenectomy may relieve the stagnation area

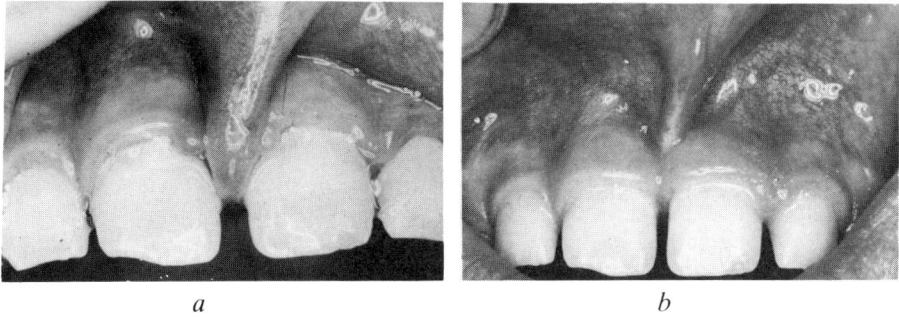

a   *b*

Fig. 9.25. *a*, Persistent low attachment of the upper labial fraenum preventing space closure and causing local stagnation. *b*, Same patient after fraenectomy showing good oral hygiene and space beginning to close.

and improve the appearance, the space cannot always be closed permanently if there is excess spacing in the arch.

Under local anaesthesia a straight mosquito forceps is placed horizontally on the fraenum with the point touching the alveolar mucosa at the junction of the fixed and free investing tissue. Parallel vertical cuts are made with a scalpel from the point of the mosquito forceps down to the palatal gingival attachment on

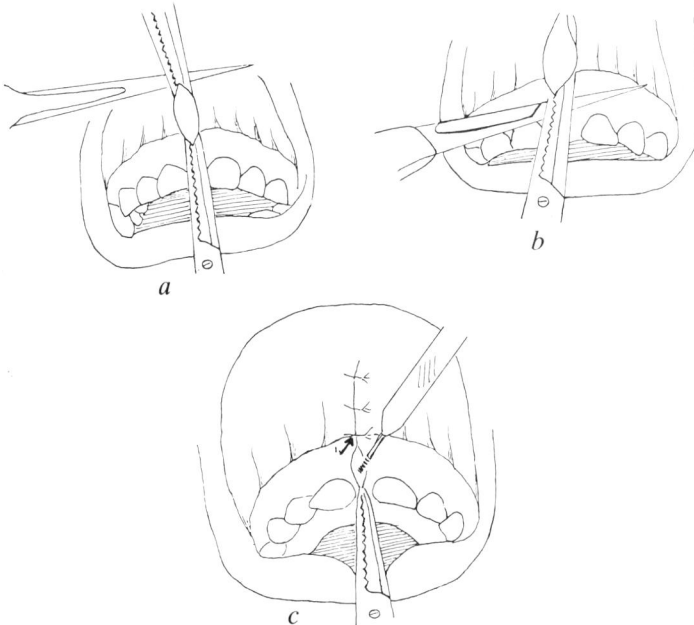

a   *b*

c

Fig. 9.26. *a*, Broad labial fraenum is clipped with horizontal mosquito forceps at junction with lip and vertical clip at attachment to alveolar mucosa between 1|1. Scalpel is used to sever connection between lip and superior surface of fraenum above clip. *b*, Similarly, scalpel cut detaches fibrous fraenum from labial mucosa. *c*, First suture (arrow) fixes level of labial sulcus by uniting both edges of mucobuccal fold to underlying fibrous periosteum. One or more additional sutures close wound in undersurface of lip. A fine straight fissure bur is used to remove fibrous fraenum tissues between 1|1 from gingival crest to apical region.

either side of the fibrous band. By cutting the aspect of the fraenum clamped by the forceps along their superior edge, a wedge of tissue can be dissected out leaving a triangular defect that extends from the lip above to the gingival margin below. The edges of the defect are undermined gently with expanding blunt scissor blades and the first silk suture is placed through the margins of the base of the fraenum and, centrally, through the attached periosteum (*Fig.* 9.26).

This method ensures approximation of the attachment of the lip mucosa to the fixed periosteal tissue at the optimal level; and later contraction and apical drift of the attachment is thus reduced or prevented. The margins of the wound in the lip are closed by one or two silk sutures as required. Finally, where there is a fibrous band in the median suture, the collagenous tissue is removed by a slowly revolving narrow flat fissure bur in a straight handpiece. This excision of collagenous fraenum should extend from the level of the gingival margin to the new point of attachment of the lip to the apical periosteum. This procedure is not necessary when the attachment of the fraenum is superficial, with no extension into the underlying bone. Sutures are easier to remove if left for ten days, and often they are shed within that time.

ABNORMAL POSITION OF CRYPTS

Ectopic Upper Canines

The upper canine is particularly liable to be displaced during its long path of eruption from under the orbital floor. It may lie horizontally; it may be displaced towards the midline of the palate; or may be high in the buccal sulcus. More commonly, it just misses the correct path of eruption and becomes deflected to a lesser extent, either palatally or buccally, and the deciduous canine is retained.

The position of an ectopic canine may be indicated by the position of the adjacent teeth. For example, a labially tilted upper lateral incisor may indicate that the canine is either high and buccal, or low and palatal to its root. If the tooth appears fore-shortened on a pan-oral radiograph, it is tilted either palatally or buccally; and a combination of radiographs will then be required to confirm its exact location. The standard occlusal radiograph does not provide enough information to locate the misplaced canine. A true lateral radiograph of the anterior part of the maxilla is helpful to show the height above the occlusal plane and the relationship of the canine to the incisor roots. This should be viewed in conjuction with a true postero-anterior radiograph which can show the degree of canine crown and root displacement towards the midline.

Some dental surgeons still use a vertex occlusal radiograph (*Fig.* 9.27) taken with the tube in the region of the vertex of the skull and angled along the long axis of the incisors. This method is to be discouraged because of unnecessary irradiation of the pituitary gland, eyes and other structures. It is also unsatisfactory because a long exposure is required with ordinary dental apparatus, and the patient may move and spoil a film which is always rather indistinct owing to the amount and density of the bone through which the X-rays have to pass.

As far as the general practitioner is concerned, two intra-oral views taken with different tube positions give an indication of whether the tooth is palatal or buccal to the line of the arch (*Fig.* 9.28). The tooth furthest from the tube moves in the same direction as the tube according to the principle of parallax. This

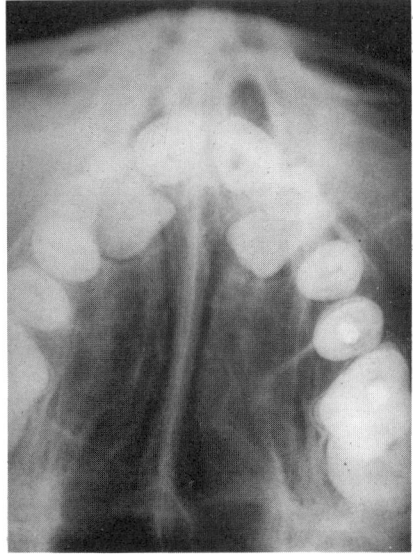

Fig. 9.27. Vertex occlusal radiograph. (*Note:* Not recommended in view of danger to sensitive areas, because of long exposure and often indistinct picture.)

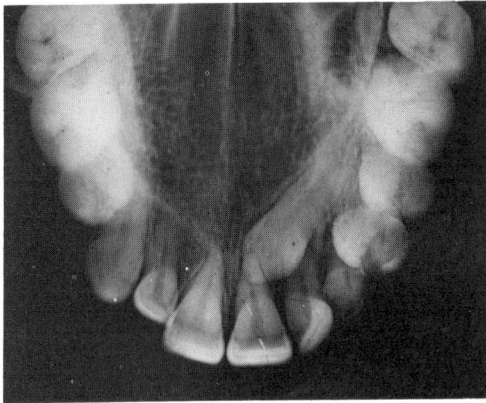

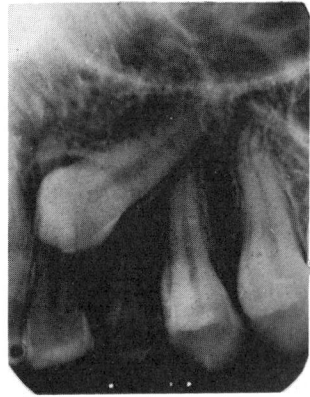

a   *b*

Fig. 9.28. Standard occlusal and intraoral view showing how the unerupted canine has moved with the shift of tube from overlapping the central incisor apex to overlap that of the lateral. The unerupted tooth has moved with the tube; by the principle of parallax it is therefore on a palatal aspect. Two periapical views can also be used.

method is not always satisfactory because it does not deal with a canine which is very high.

It is important to note whether there is any resorption of the root of the lateral incisor or, if this tooth is missing, of the upper central incisor. Root resorption takes place rapidly and may be well advanced by 10 years of age but rarely starts after 14 years. The incisors affected may be completely symptomless and early removal of the canine may prevent loss of the adjacent tooth, which may remain vital and firm even with only one-third to one-half of its root. Where the lateral incisor is a poor risk or surgical removal of the canine might cause further damage, it may be better to extract the lateral incisor and allow the canine to erupt if it is suitably placed.

Simple Treatment where the Canine is not markedly Displaced.

Where sufficient space is not available for the tooth, space must be made either by extracting the first premolar, which is slightly smaller than the canine, or by distal movement of the buccal segment on that side. The canine may not be very displaced and if its apex is in a good position, it may erupt into the palate without help (*Fig.* 9.29). If after a period of observation it does not appear to be erupting, overlying bone and soft tissue can be removed.

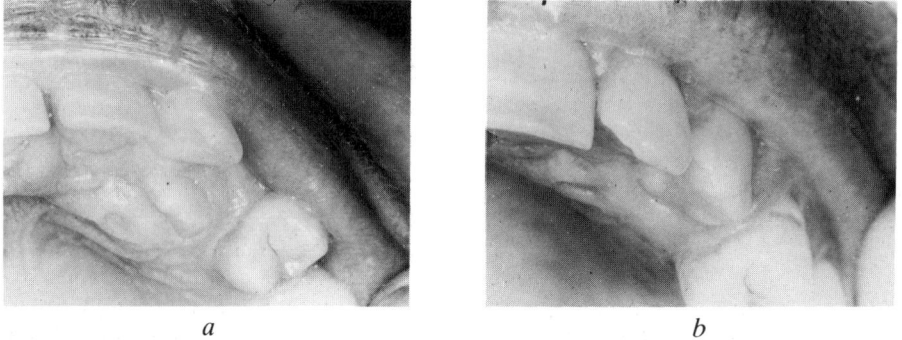

a   *b*

Fig. 9.29. Palatally erupting canine moved into the arch with a simple removable appliance following loss of the deciduous canine and local tooth movement to accommodate it. *a*, Before and, *b*, After treatment.

Where the unerupted canine is in the line of the arch or slightly buccally placed but with a good axial inclination, it may erupt and require no appliance guidance if adequate space has been created as described previously. The more mesially displaced canine, which may or may not cause resorption of the lateral incisor, can sometimes be allowed to erupt into the position of the lateral if that tooth is extracted (*see* p. 117).

Treatment when the Canine is markedly Displaced

In deciding whether a tooth should be brought into the arch from a difficult position, the most important factor is whether the patient is prepared to accept treatment and appreciates the time involved. The procedure should be explained in detail and the patient should not be unduly encouraged since voluntary cooperation over at least 18 months is essential for success. The patient may prefer to accept some form of compromise.

If it is decided to leave the buried canine it should be reviewed by radiographic examination to check there is no enlargement of the crypt with cystic formation. Its extraction can be delayed and sometimes it is possible to combine this with extraction of third molars if they are impacted. In some cases where the tooth is distant from the arch and where there is considerable crowding, the first premolar and the lateral incisor may be in contact and give an acceptable appearance and function. In other cases the deciduous canine may be in place for many years if its crown is intact and it is aesthetically acceptable (*Fig.* 9.30).

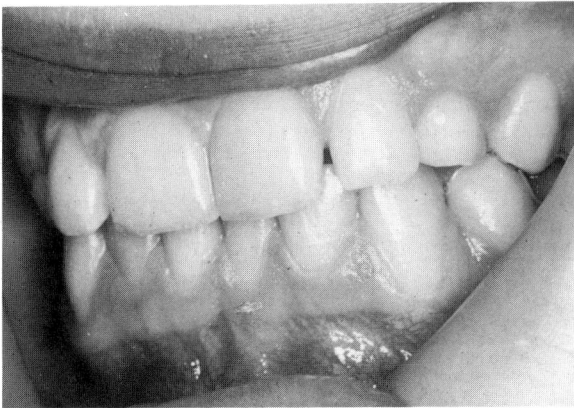

Fig. 9.30. Retention of deciduous canine is aesthetically pleasing when permanent canine is grossly displaced.

Where the deciduous canine is not viable or its crown has been subjected to considerable attrition or caries, some distal movement of the buccal segment may be required to make adequate space for a pontic of reasonable size. A small amount of additional space can often be obtained by local tooth movement.

Where there is a reasonable prognosis for bringing the canine into the arch (*Fig.* 9.31), traction can be applied to its crown once space has been provided and the tooth has been exposed. Where space requirements are minimal some distal movement of the buccal segments may be carried out but often the first premolar is extracted.

One of the best ways of linking the attachment to an appliance is by a length of gold chain. This can be tied to the attachment and when the flap is closed and sutured into place the chain can be left curled up until healing has occurred when it can be unwound and attached to the appliance. The essential feature of the appliance used to apply traction is a long arm, which can be either soldered to the bridge of an Adams crib on a removable appliance or to a palatal arch of a fixed appliance. The patient must be able to attach the spring to the protruding links of chain. In many ways a removable appliance, which can be taken out to clean the mouth, is preferable. As the tooth erupts, links of the chain can be removed. It may take 12–18 months to align a difficult canine and during this time other aspects of treatment may have to be deferred.

Surgical Management

On many occasions it is difficult to obtain access to the crown of the buried canine without the removal of excessive amounts of palatal bone, to the detriment of the adjacent incisor teeth. When sufficient space exists betwen the roots of the adjacent teeth, a punch may be inserted in the labial alveolar process and directed downwards and backwards on to the enamel of the buried canine. Provided that sufficient bone has been removed on the palatal aspect to uncover the maximum convexity of the crown of the buried canine, the tooth can be tapped into the palatal opening by gentle force on the punch with a surgical mallet. During this procedure the assistant must support the adjacent incisor teeth to prevent unwanted displacement.

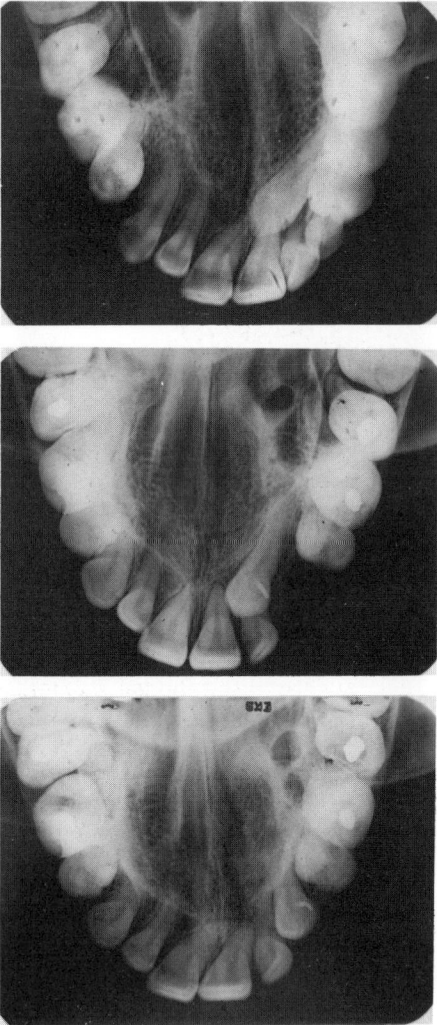

Fig. 9.31. Radiographs showing displaced canine brought into position by traction following the extraction of |C and |4.

When the canine is resistant to efforts to disimpact it, the crown may be separated from the root with a large flat fissure bur; the space created between crown and root often facilitates the elevation of the crown or root section without prejudice to adjacent structures.

While it is important to complete the cut between crown and root with no ragged overhang, it is also important not to perforate the bone and mucosa of the nasal floor.

At the completion of all open flap procedures for the surgical removal of displaced maxillary canines, the soft tissues investing the crown of the buried tooth should be gently curetted from the cavity, other debris should be removed by irrigation, and the wound closed with sutures that pull the flap firmly into position. This is particularly important on the palatal aspect, where poor

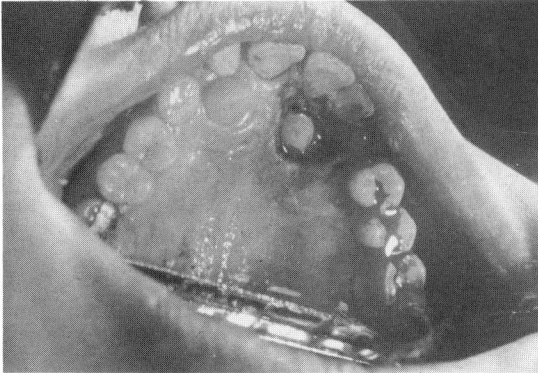

Fig. 9.32. Adequate exposure of crown of canine buried in palate. After clearance of soft and hard tissues a soft dressing is placed to cover the operative site and prevent undue proliferation of marginal tissues.

suturing may lead to distension of the palate by haematoma formation: this can lead to the complications of infection and delayed healing.

In certain circumstances the orthodontist will wish the oral surgeon to uncover the crown of the buried canine so that it will erupt spontaneously, or under traction, into the dental arch. Successful uncovering for eruption depends on two principal points of technique. First, the crown of the tooth being uncovered should be cleared of soft tissue and bone in such a way that the maximum convexity of the crown is exposed from the tip to the cervical region (*Fig.* 9.32). Secondly, the overlying soft tissue should be keratinized gingival or palatal mucosa if a satisfactory gingival attachment is to be obtained on completion of eruption. When access is through mobile tissues in the sulcus a satisfactory result is rarely obtained. Vanarsdall and Corn[9] have shown that severe tissue loss occurs when labially displaced teeth are brought into the arch without the presence of attached gingiva.

Following adequate exposure of the crown of the canine, a soft surgical pack is placed in the wound and held in place by sutures for at least 2–3 weeks. It may be replaced at intervals, over a longer period, if eruption is slow.

Maxillary canines that are surgically accessible and of a crown size which will fit the available space in the dental arch may be transferred from their impacted position into the definitive site by repositioning or transplantation.

In the repositioning procedure, after adequate exposure, the tooth is manipulated in the alveolar space in such a way that the crown is aligned with the adjacent teeth and in a suitable occlusal position to make light contact with the opposite number in the lower arch. The repositioned tooth is supported by sutures in the replaced soft tissues and splinted by a removable retainer for about 2 weeks. After this period gentle masticatory forces are used to enhance the development of a normal tooth–socket relationship.

Transplantation of a displaced canine is an extension of the repositioning technique, and the same general principles of assessment and the preparation of space in the arch should be adopted. In repositioning, there is usually room to move the canine into a suitable position within the existing space in the alveolar process. In the transplantation procedure a new socket must be created by

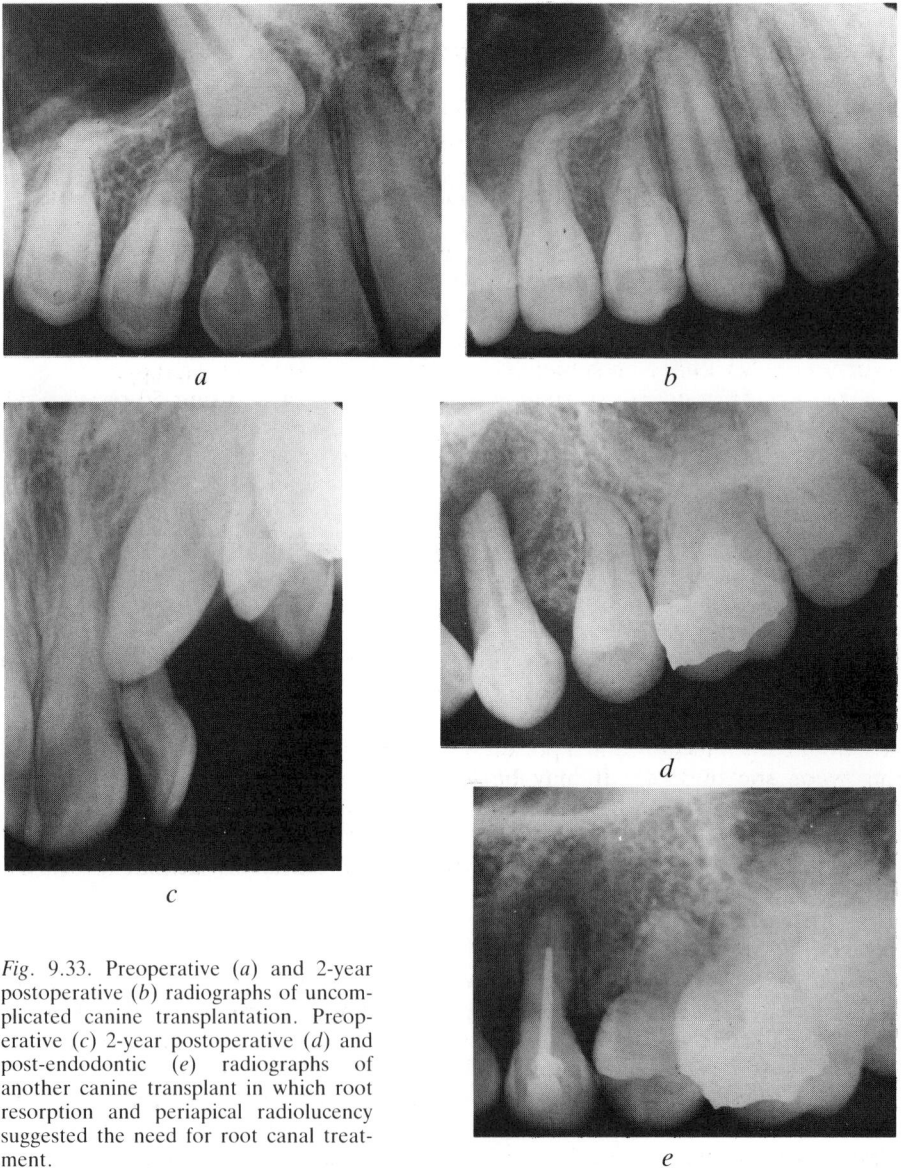

Fig. 9.33. Preoperative (*a*) and 2-year postoperative (*b*) radiographs of uncomplicated canine transplantation. Preoperative (*c*) 2-year postoperative (*d*) and post-endodontic (*e*) radiographs of another canine transplant in which root resorption and periapical radiolucency suggested the need for root canal treatment.

careful removal of bone with large acrylic-cutting burs under adequate irrigation. Ideally, the mesiodistal width of the tooth to be transplanted should fit the space available. The tooth to be transplanted should, whenever possible after atraumatic removal, be retained within the bleeding soft tissues until finally positioned in the new socket. Root canal treatment is not indicated at the time of transplantation but may be required at some later period during follow-up if apical infection or severe root resorption is observed (*Fig.* 9.33). Andreasen[10] has explored many clinical factors that may compromise the success of transplantation, and the success rate with maxillary canines has, in recent years, been encouragingly high.[11]

Immobilization of the transplanted tooth may be achieved by attaching it to an existing fixed upper arch or splinting with a removable appliance. The period of fixation is generally limited to 2–3 weeks following transplantation: early return to functional forces enhances the establishment of a normal periodontal attachment.

Vitality in transplanted teeth is less important, in the assessment of success, than viability; while there may be some darkening of the crown and little or no response to electrical or other pulp tests for a considerable period, the transplant that is firm, showing no radiological signs of apical infection and little or no root resorption, should not be subjected routinely to endodontic therapy.

After 2 years a degree of root resorption is evident in about 50 per cent of cases. The overall success rate of canine transplantation depends on many factors, not least of which is the age at which transplantation is carried out. Teeth with patent apices are obviously likely to achieve a new pulpal blood supply more rapidly than those with closed apices. Nevertheless, most recent series reporting results of canine transplants in adolescents and young adults show success rates in the region of 70 per cent. With results of this order, the procedure must be given more serious consideration when all other treatment avenues appear closed.

Occasionally it is necessary to remove a buried maxillary canine from the palate before adequate space can be created for transplantation of the tooth into the dental arch. In these circumstances the canine tooth may be removed atraumatically and stored in a pocket in the buccal soft tissues above and behind the zygomatic buttress. It may be left there, without inconvenience to the patient, until conditions are suitable for transplantation. While lodged in the transfer site the canine root usually becomes enclosed in a sheath of periodontium and new bone. The whole cylinder of tooth and attachments may be transferred into the new socket in the alveolar process.

Impacted First Permanent Molars

The impaction of the first permanent molar under the distal bulge of the second deciduous molar may escape notice during routine inspection (*Fig.* 9.34). Mild cases of impaction may be self-correcting, but plaque control can be difficult in this area. Caries and/or root resorption of the second deciduous molar may cause the patient to present with pain. Under these circumstances the deciduous tooth has to be extracted and, if necessary, the first molar can be uprighted later. Where there is severe space loss, a premolar extraction will be required in that quadrant.

In cases of moderate impaction it is possible to move the first molar distally by passing a piece of 0.5 mm brass ligature wire around the contact point. The free ends of the wire are twisted firmly together, tightening the noose, and the twisted end is cut, leaving a short tag, which is bent to lie against the gingival margin. The wire has to be replaced at intervals, but unless there is a measurable improvement it should be discontinued after three visits. Discing the distal surface of the second deciduous molar may provide extra space for the first molar eruption.

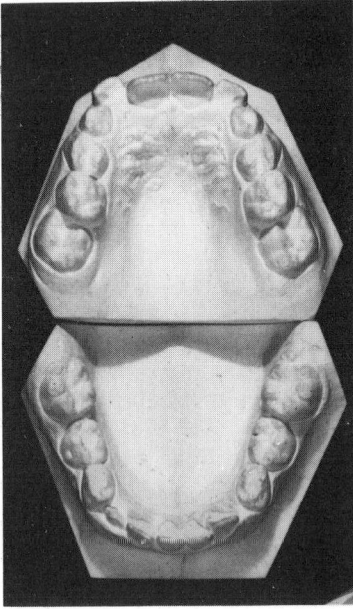

Fig. 9.34. Impacted upper first permanent molars.

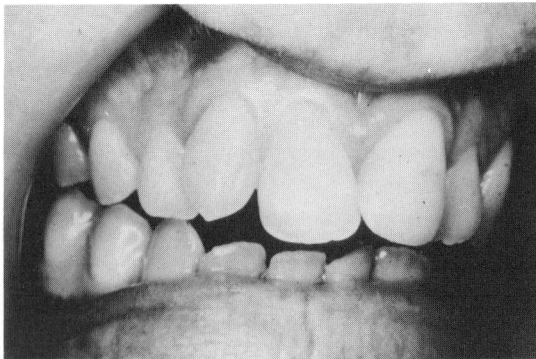

Fig. 9.35. Total transposition of upper canine and lateral incisor.

Total Transposition

On rare occasions there is a total transposition of teeth, such as the lower lateral incisor and canine, or upper canine and first premolar (*Fig.* 9.35). Orthodontic treatment to correct the transposition is not indicated and the position has to be accepted unless crowding makes the extraction of one or other tooth necessary.

REFERENCES

1. Gardiner J. N. (1955) A survey of malocclusion and some aetiological factors in 1000 Sheffield school children. *Dent. Practit.* **6**; 187–8.
2. Taylor G. S. (1972) Characteristics of supernumerary teeth in the primary and permanent dentition. *Dent. Practit.* **22**; 203–8.
3. Breakspeare E. K. (1960) Further observations on early loss of deciduous molars. *Dent. Practit.* **11**; 233–50.
4. Breakspeare E. K. (1951) Sequelae of early loss of deciduous molars. *Dent. Record* **71**; 127–35.
5. Clinch L. M. (1959) A longitudinal study of the results of premature loss of deciduous teeth between 3–4 and 13–15 years of age. *Dent. Practit.* **9**; 109–26.
6. Linder–Aronson S. (1960) The effects of premature loss of deciduous teeth. A biometric study in 14 and 15 year olds. *Acta. Odont. Scand.* **18**; 101–22.
7. Lundström A. (1955) The significance of early loss of deciduous teeth in the aetiology of malocclusion. *Am. J. Orthodont.* **41**; 810–26.
8. Richardson M. E. (1965) The relationship between the relative amount of space present in the deciduous dental arch and the rate and degree of space closure subsequent to the extraction of a deciduous molar. *Dent. Practit.* **16**; 111–8.
9. Vanarsdall R. L. and Corn H. (1977) Soft tissue management of labially positioned unerupted teeth. *Am. J. Orthodont.* **72**; 53.
10. Andreasen J. O. (1981) Ex-articulations. In: Andreasen J. E. (ed) *Traumatic Injuries of the Teeth.* Copenhagen, W. B. Saunders, pp. 203–42.
11. Moss J. P. (1975) The indications for the transplantation of maxillary canines in the light of 100 cases. *Br. J. Oral Surg.* **12**; 268–74.

Chapter 10

Class I Malocclusions

Class I malocclusions include all those anomalies where the anteroposterior relationship of the lower and upper arches is within normal limits. There may, however, be transverse or vertical arch malrelationships. Crowding and local irregularities (*see* Chapter 9) are common causes of Class I malocclusion. Generalized spacing is unusual. All of these irregularities may be found in association with the other classes of malocclusion.

OCCLUSAL FEATURES

The incisor relationship is Class I (*Fig.* 10.1). This does not imply an ideal incisor relationship because there may be an anterior open bite or a bimaxillary proclination with an increase in overjet and a reduction in overbite (*Fig.* 10.2). The buccal segment relationship is often Class I, but there may have been drift of first permanent molars following premature loss of deciduous teeth; and if the canines are crowded, they may not be in a Class I relationship.

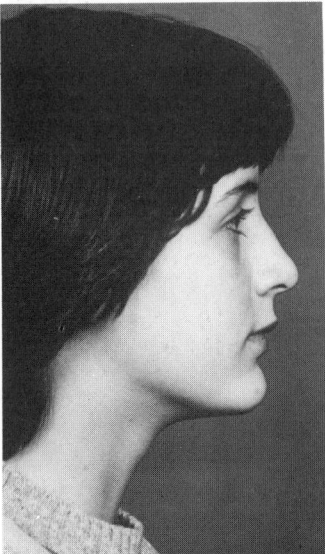

a

b

Fig. 10.1. A typical Class I malocclusion. The patient has a Class I skeletal profile.

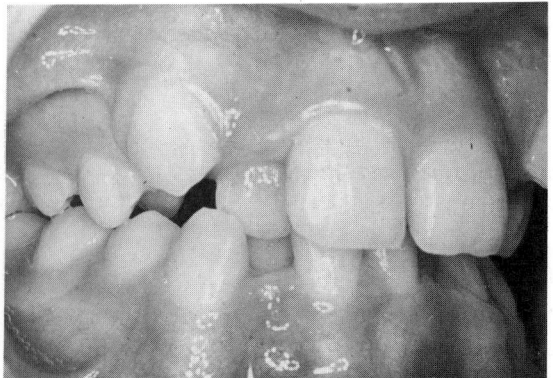

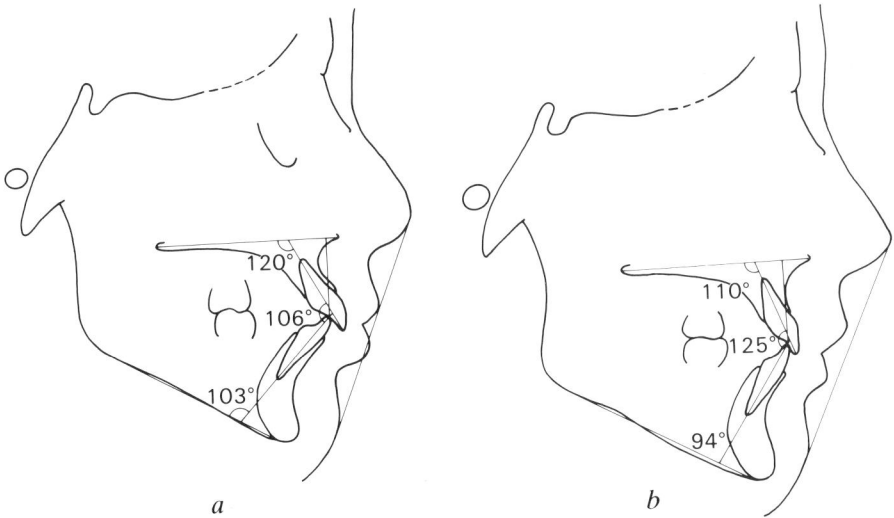

Fig. 10.2. *a*, A Class I malocclusion with bimaxillary proclination. Note that although the overjet is somewhat increased, it cannot satisfactorily be reduced by simple retroclination of the upper incisors because the incisor relationship is already Class I. *b*, The bimaxillary proclination has been reduced and is now stable: the soft tissues have adapted to the new position of the teeth. Although the bimaxillary proclination was reduced completely during treatment, the incisors have come forward a little: note that the lower incisor edge is still in advance of the upper root centroid.

It may be difficult to decide how to classify a borderline case. For example, if several of the upper incisors are instanding, should the patient be described as having a Class III malocclusion? It is probably reasonable to be guided by the general features: if at least two upper incisors are in a normal relationship and if the other occlusal features are in harmony, the occlusion is Class I. It should be remembered that classification is merely an aid to description and the treatment of a borderline case should not be affected by its categorization.

SKELETAL RELATIONSHIPS

The skeletal pattern is usually Class I, but mild skeletal malrelationships accompanied by dento-alveolar compensation are often associated with Class I malocclusions. With a Class II skeletal pattern, compensation is usually by lower incisor proclination.

Vertical and transverse skeletal malrelationships may be associated with anterior open bites and crossbites respectively, although these are found more commonly where there is a Class III malocclusion.

FACIAL GROWTH

In Class I cases, the anteroposterior jaw relationship is generally favourable and this does not usually change appreciably with facial growth: any minor changes are absorbed by dento-alveolar adaptation. Skeletal open bites tend to become more severe because dento-alveolar compensation for the increased anterior intermaxillary height is already at its limits and vertical dento-alveolar growth may not keep pace with any further facial growth.

SOFT TISSUE AND SWALLOWING BEHAVIOUR

The soft tissue pattern is favourable in the great majority of Class I cases and does not impose limitations on treatment objectives. Incomplete overbites associated with digit-sucking habits tend to improve, unless they are maintained by an adaptive swallowing pattern. In cases of bimaxillary proclination, the lips are full and everted and this is a major factor in determining the tooth positions (*Fig.* 10.2).

MANDIBULAR POSITION AND PATH OF CLOSURE

There are no characteristic mandibular postures. However, occlusal irregularities such as instanding incisors and unilateral crossbites are frequently associated with mandibular displacements and so it is important that the path of closure is checked during the initial assessment.

TREATMENT OBJECTIVES

Clearly the primary objective is to deal with the patient's main concern, which will usually be irregularity of the incisors. However, it is important to deal with any other aspect of the malocclusion that might subsequently give problems, and to leave the patient with a healthy, functional occlusion. Particularly where removable appliances are to be used, treatment objectives are limited by the tooth movements that can be achieved. An overambitious treatment plan may leave the patient worse off than before, with unclosed extraction spaces, tilted teeth and a disrupted occlusion. This can be a major problem in the milder cases where only a small amount of space is required and where extraction spaces are difficult to close. The potential benefit of orthodontic treatment to the patient may be minimal and it is a serious matter if they are left with a poorer occlusion than before.

Good results can be obtained with removable appliances in carefully selected cases. Severe problems requiring complex tooth movements, and minor irregularities where active space closure following extractions will be required, should be treated with fixed appliances.

TREATMENT

The management of local irregularities is discussed in Chapter 9, and the indications for extraction of teeth in crowded cases are described in Chapter 8.

Crowding

This is due to disproportion between tooth size and arch size. Expansion of arch size to relieve crowding was recommended by Angle but all the long-term studies published have found that relapse is very common. Expansion of lower intercanine width and labial movement of lower incisors are particularly unstable.[1] Thus, in general, crowding has to be dealt with either by distal movement of buccal segments, which gives very limited space, or by extractions (*see* Chapter 8).

Crowding is often first apparent on eruption of the incisors, but may sometimes improve with arch growth and by utilization of the leeway space. Moorrees[2] found that many cases with a good occlusion in the permanent dentition had previously shown some signs of crowding. On the other hand, there is little hope that moderate to severe crowding in the mixed dentition will improve to any appreciable extent; and in the permanent dentition the tendency is for crowding to become more severe rather than to improve (*see* Chapter 2).

Spacing

Spacing may occur because the teeth are small in relation to the size of the arch or because teeth are missing (*see* Chapter 9). Sometimes this is acceptable to the patient. Complete closure of appreciable spacing may not be possible and it is often best to concentrate the space in the premolar region, using fixed appliances, and to fit bridges.

Bimaxillary Proclination

Bimaxillary proclination may be a feature of Class II, division 1 malocclusion, but quite often the incisor relationship is Class I, which may mistakenly be diagnosed as Class II, division 1 because of the increase in overjet (*see Fig. 10.2*). The distinction is very important because the overjet cannot satisfactorily be reduced in Class I cases with bimaxillary proclination unless the lower incisors are also retracted.

The proclination of the upper and lower incisors is due to the soft tissue pattern. Usually the lips are full and everted and the tongue acts to mould the dental arches as the teeth erupt. Occasionally the tongue itself is very large and is the primary cause of the bimaxillary proclination, but this is unusual.

A mild degree of bimaxillary proclination can be pleasing, and it should be remembered that the lower face fullness will often become less marked in the adult because growth of the nose and increased prominence of the chin change the character of the face. In some racial groups the incisors are typically more proclined than in the Caucasian norms (*see Table* 6.2). The individual values must be compared with the appropriate norms; and even having done so, treatment should not be suggested solely because of a deviation from these average values. Treatment is justified only if the individual would be considered to be facially disadvantaged within his own racial group because of the malocclusion. Even if this is the case, it may still not be possible to achieve a stable improvement in the occlusion because of the soft tissue pattern.

It is sometimes suggested that bimaxillary proclination should not be treated because of its potential instability. This is too sweeping a conclusion, because in some cases the soft tissues adapt to the corrected incisor positions. It should be remembered that to a large extent the position of the incisors reflects the soft tissue pattern at the time they erupted, and this may subsequently have matured.

If the tongue is very large and appears to fill the oral cavity as far as can be judged clinically or from a lateral skull radiograph, incisor retraction will probably not be stable, or at least not without a surgical reduction in tongue size which is justifiable only in the most severe cases. The fundamental question is whether the lips will drop back with the retraction of the incisor teeth, establishing a new position of soft tissue balance. This is most likely to happen where the patient has to make an appreciable effort to obtain a lip seal over the proclined incisors but could be expected to achieve a habitual lip seal after they had been retracted. If the lips are very full and are long enough to obtain a seal easily in spite of the bimaxillary proclination, they may drop back less when the incisors are retracted and so stability is problematical.

The lower incisors have to be tipped back far enough to allow an acceptable inclination of the upper incisors. If there is a Class II skeletal pattern, the lower incisors will still have to compensate for this. The correct position of the lower incisor edge is readily assessed from the edge–centroid relationship: the lower edge in these cases should be positioned to lie directly below the upper incisor centroid (*see Fig.* 10.2). The need for extraction of teeth in the lower and upper arches can then be evaluated. It is important to allow enough space for full retraction of the upper and lower incisors because if the bimaxillary proclination is reduced only partially, relapse is more likely. The height of the upper incisor edge is important: the lower lip should cover at least the incisal third of the labial surface of the retracted upper incisors when a lip seal is obtained. If this is not the case, relapse is to be expected.

Although the incisors will be tipped lingually, this is best achieved with fixed appliances which can give more precise anteroposterior and vertical control of tooth positions, and are well tolerated in the lower arch.

Vertical Anomalies

By definition, deep overbites are not found in Class I incisor relationships: they are discussed in the chapters on Class II malocclusions. An anterior open bite is present when there is no anterior incisor contact and no vertical overlap of the lower incisors by the uppers. An incomplete overbite is a minor variant of an anterior open bite. Isolated posterior open bites are rare and there is seldom any obvious cause. They are usually attributed to localized failure of alveolar process development.

Anterior Open Bite

An anterior open bite may be caused by digit-sucking habits (*see* p. 140); by atypical swallowing patterns (*see* p. 25); or by skeletal factors (*Fig.* 10.3). Atypical swallowing patterns are commonly associated with anterior open bites, but they are often secondary: the tongue tends to come forwards to seal off the gap between the incisors. Such an adaptation commonly perpetuates an anterior open bite due to digit-sucking even after the habit has been discontinued. Adaptations in swallowing behaviour to obtain an anterior oral seal in Class II, division 1 cases are associated with an incomplete overbite rather than an anterior open bite; but a primary tongue thrust can be a rare cause of anterior open bite.

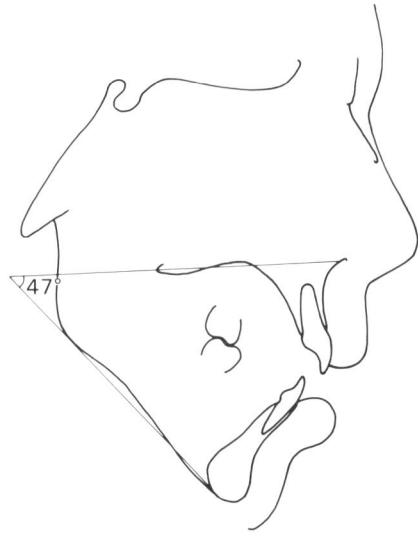

Fig. 10.3. A skeletal open bite. The height of the intermaxillary space is increased anteriorly and there is an associated anterior open bite.

Skeletal Anterior Open Bites (Fig. 10.3)

These are usually due to an increase in anterior intermaxillary height but can occasionally be attributed to localized failure of maxillary dento-alveolar development. The latter can occur in patients with clefts of the lip and palate, and rarely in other cases for no apparent reason.

When the anterior intermaxillary height is excessive, the teeth and alveolar processes may grow to their full extent but fail to achieve an overbite (*Fig.* 10.3). This is more common in Class III cases but can be found with Class I malocclusions. In the more severe cases, the open bite extends into the buccal segments and only the most distal teeth may meet in occlusion. There is generally a posterior mandibular growth rotation and the open bite tends to become worse with growth.

A skeletal open bite is often of little concern to the patient and it may be the dental practioner who is the first to draw attention to it. Occasionally the patient will complain of difficulty in incising food but this is rarely a serious problem. There are no periodontal problems typically associated with an anterior open bite but there have been reports of a slightly increased prevalence of tenderness in the muscles of mastication.[3]

It is important to recognize that in cases of skeletal open bite, the posterior teeth are not 'propping open' the bite: these teeth have succeeded in establishing an occlusion at a position where the intermaxillary height is less, without encroaching on the rest position of the mandible. Thus grinding or extraction of posterior teeth is not helpful—it merely means that the patient has to overclose to obtain an occlusion and is even more liable to suffer from muscle pain. Extrusion of anterior teeth is also ill advised: the alveolar bone will not usually grow with the teeth and so tooth support is reduced; and the incisors are already at a reasonable height relative to the lips and may look very unsightly if they are extruded.

The only satisfactory treatment of a skeletal open bite is by surgery, usually to the mandible (*see* Chapter 19). However, because a skeletal open bite is in itself rarely of serious concern to the patient, surgery may not be indicated unless there is some co-existing anomaly, such as a Class III skeletal pattern, to be dealt with at the same time. It should be noted that surgical correction of skeletal open bite is particularly liable to relapse due to the action of the musculature and careful presurgical planning and postsurgical fixation are essential.

Transverse Anomalies

Scissors bites (*Fig.* 10.4) and crossbites are found most commonly in Class II and Class III cases respectively, but they do arise in Class I cases and will be discussed here.

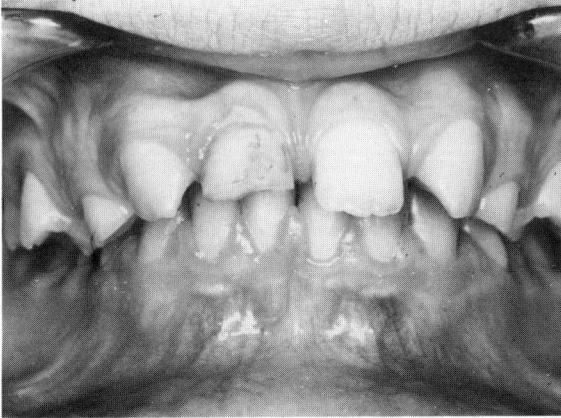

Fig. 10.4. A bilateral scissors bite.

Scissors Bite

This occurs when the upper arch is too broad relative to the lower, and usually reflects an underlying skeletal mismatch. The milder cases involve only a few teeth. Complete unilateral scissors bite is seldom found and bilateral cases are very rare.

A scissors bite, even of quite a minor extent, can cause severe occlusal dysfunction and should be corrected. There will often be a mandibular displacement on closure into occlusion. If only a few teeth are involved, correction may be straightforward.

A complete unilateral scissors bite with a displacement can be treated by expansion of the lower arch and possibly some contraction of the upper arch using removable appliances or fixed arches. Stability depends on a good intercuspation of the teeth. A complete unilateral scissors bite without displacement and the bilateral condition are very rare and may require surgical intervention.

Crossbites

These may be unilateral or bilateral and often reflect some discrepancy in the widths of the dental bases.

a

b

c

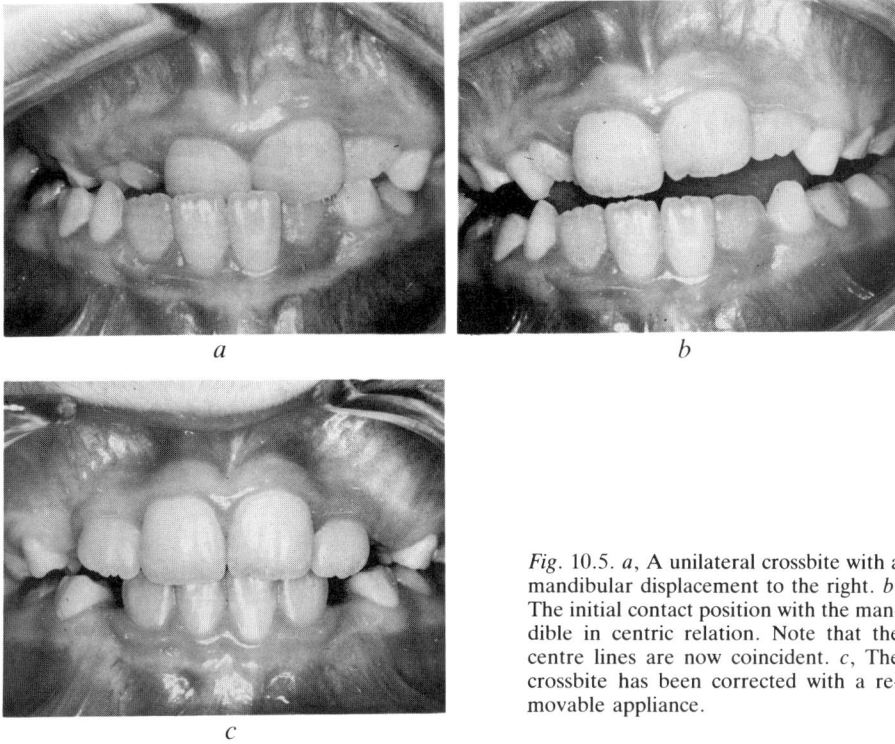

Fig. 10.5. *a*, A unilateral crossbite with a mandibular displacement to the right. *b*, The initial contact position with the mandible in centric relation. Note that the centre lines are now coincident. *c*, The crossbite has been corrected with a removable appliance.

Unilateral crossbite with lateral displacement (*Fig.* 10.5)   Where the arches are symmetrical and of equal width, the mandible will usually be displaced to one side in order to obtain maximal intercuspation, producing a crossbite. This type of crossbite may be due to a mild discrepancy in dental base widths, but commonly is associated with a digit-sucking habit: when the finger or thumb is being sucked, the teeth are parted, the tongue is low and the contraction of the buccinator muscles narrows the upper arch slightly.

Unilateral crossbites with displacement should be treated by maxillary arch expansion in order to eliminate the displacement. A removable appliance with posterior bite planes has the merit that secondary expansion of the lower arch through intercuspation of the teeth is avoided, but expansion can also successfully be achieved with a fixed palatal arch (*Fig.* 10.6).

In some cases where the buccal inclination of the upper teeth is already partly compensating for the underlying dental base discrepancy, further buccal tipping would not give a satisfactory or stable occlusion and rapid maxillary expansion may be indicated. The objective is to widen the maxillary base by expanding the mid-palatal suture. The maxilla hinges around its other sutural attachments with the upper facial skeleton and so this procedure is not feasible after the late teens when some of these sutures may have started to fuse. Bone is laid down at the expanded sutural margins in the usual manner and the dental base expansion is stable. However, the teeth tend to relapse partially, under the influence of the facial musculature, and so some degree of overexpansion is desirable.

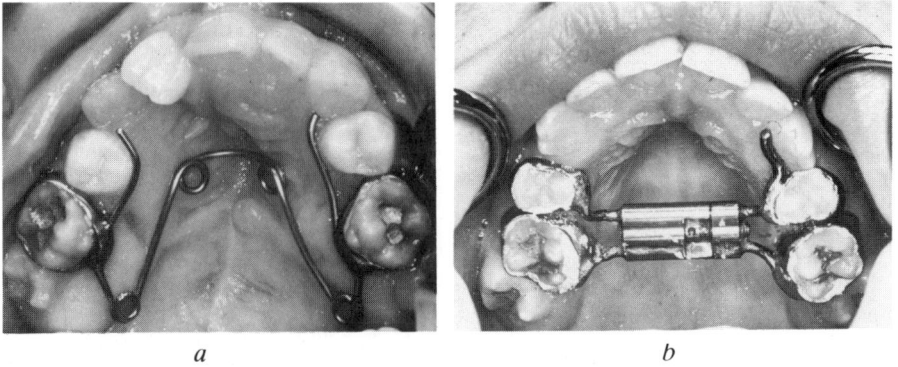

a   *b*

Fig. 10.6. *a*, A quad-helix appliance for expansion of the maxillary arch. *b*, A Hyrax screw for rapid maxillary expansion.

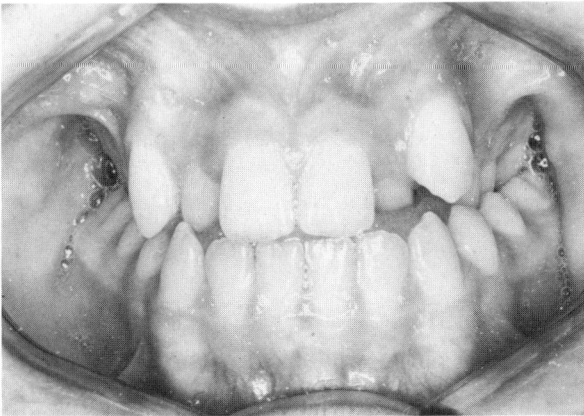

Fig. 10.7. A bilateral crossbite.

The appliance used is a heavy screw attached to bands or splints (*Fig.* 10.6). The parent is instructed to turn the screw twice a day over a period of about two weeks, producing an expansion of up to 7 mm. The key should be attached to a length of thread so that there is no risk of its being dropped down the patient's throat. Rapid maxillary expansion is indicated in only a few cases and must not be used indiscriminately. Where the maxilla is very narrow, the patient's nasal airway may be improved, but treatment is not indicated for this reason alone.

Unilateral crossbite without lateral displacement   These patients usually display an underlying skeletal asymmetry. This may be pathological in origin (e.g. unilateral cleft palate, unilateral condylar hyperplasia). Correction of the crossbite is seldom indicated: in the first place there may be no functional or aesthetic disadvantage to the patient; and stability of correction is doubtful.

Bilateral crossbite (*Fig.* 10.7)   This is always associated with a maxillary dental base that is narrow relative to the mandibular base. Usually there is no displacement and so the patient suffers no functional or aesthetic problems. A danger of treatment is that correction followed by partial relapse could give rise to a unilateral crossbite with an associated mandibular displacement, which in turn might lead to muscle and joint dysfunction. Where there are special circumstances that make upper arch expansion desirable, rapid maxillary expansion is generally to be preferred; but even with overexpansion and prolonged retention, stability cannot be guaranteed.

REFERENCES

1. Little R. M., Wallen T. R. and Reidel R. A. (1981) Stability and relapse of mandibular anterior alignment–first premolar extraction cases treated by traditional edgewise. *Am. J. Orthodont.* **80**; 349–65.
2. Moorrees C. F. A. (1959) *The Dentition of the Growing Child.* Cambridge, Mass., Harvard University Press.
3. Mohlin B., Ingervall B. and Thilander B. (1980) Relation between malocclusion and mandibular dysfunction in Swedish men. *Eur. J. Orthodont.* **2**; 229–38.

Chapter 11

Class II, Division 1 Malocclusions

Class II, division 1 malocclusions are the most common of arch malrelationships (*see* p. 5). The prominence of the upper incisors is frequently a cause of concern to the patient and parents and the risk of incisor fracture is appreciably greater than in other cases.

OCCLUSAL FEATURES '

There is a Class II incisor relationship with proclination or an average inclination of the upper incisors and an increased overjet (*Fig.* 11.1). The overbite is frequently deep and is often incomplete because of an adaptive pattern of swallowing behaviour or where there is a digit-sucking habit.

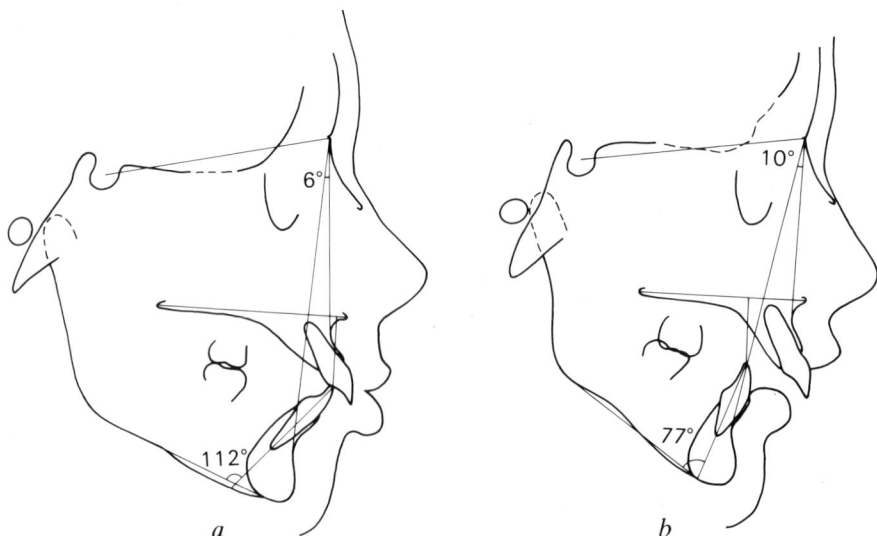

Fig. 11.1. Typical Class II, division 1 cases showing dento-alveolar compensation and exacerbation. *a*, In this case, the Class II skeletal pattern is more than compensated by the proclination of the lower incisors so that the lower incisor edge lies in advance of the upper root centroid. Indeed, establishment of a Class I incisor relationship by palatal tipping of the upper incisors will leave a mild bimaxillary proclination and a slightly increased overjet. *b*, The rather severe Class II skeletal pattern together with the retroclination of the lower incisors makes this a very difficult case to treat (*see Fig.* 11.11.)

The buccal segment relationship is usually Class II, but it can be Class I where the incisor malrelationship has been produced by a digit-sucking habit or by an unusual soft tissue pattern. Crossbite and scissors bite may occasionally be found in association with Class II, division 1 malocclusions.

SKELETAL RELATIONSHIPS

The skeletal pattern is generally Class II (*Fig.* 11.1), the severity of the arch malrelationship being associated with the degree of the skeletal discrepancy. Dento-alveolar compensation by proclination of the lower incisors may make the malocclusion less severe than the skeletal pattern would have led one to expect. In some Class II, division 1 cases, there is a receding chin which gives a poor facial profile. The Class II, division 1 cases associated with a Class I skeletal pattern are usually rather mild and are due either to a local factor, such as a digit-sucking habit, or to the relationship of the teeth and alveolar processes to their dental bases.

The lower facial height is generally average or reduced. In some cases there is a rather high maxillary–mandibular planes angle (*Fig.* 11.2).

FACIAL GROWTH

The wide range of facial morphology that can be associated with Class II, division 1 malocclusions (*Fig.* 11.2) is a reflection of the varying patterns of facial growth. An anterior direction of mandibular growth with signs of an anterior

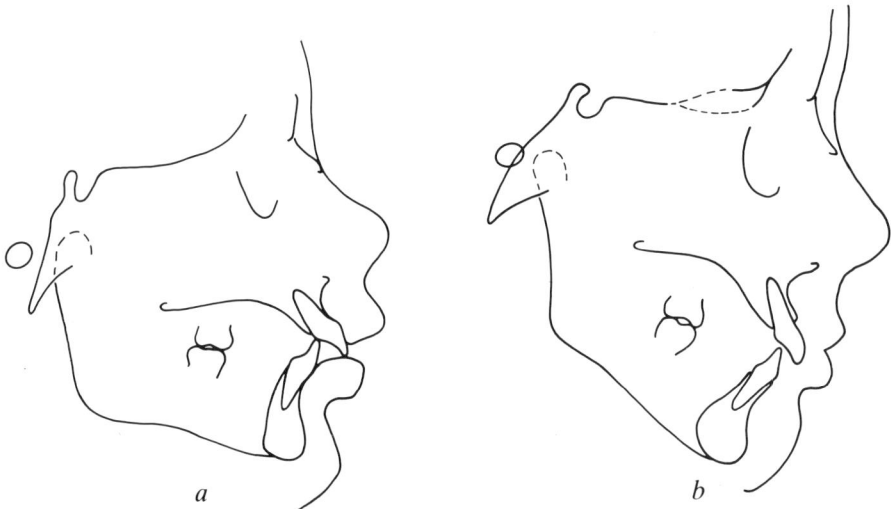

Fig. 11.2. *a*, In this case the maxillary–mandibular planes angle is low, the anterior intermaxillary height is reduced and there are signs of an anterior pattern of growth rotation. *b*, A rather high maxillary–mandibular planes angle and signs of a posterior pattern of growth rotation indicate that this patient will probably have a trend towards a vertical growth pattern.

mandibular growth rotation (*Fig.* 11.2*a*) is generally favourable because the skeletal relationship will tend to improve, as will the soft tissue pattern.

Cases with signs of vertical growth and a posterior mandibular rotation present many difficulties (*Fig.* 11.2*b*). The skeletal pattern may deteriorate if treatment encourages further posterior mandibular rotation by extrusion of molar teeth. In these cases the lips are often already incompetent and this may not improve appreciably with maturation. The facial appearance is also poor, with a receding chin, and this may not be helped by treatment directed towards retracting the upper labial segment.

SOFT TISSUES

Many mild Class II, division 1 cases can obtain a lip seal without undue effort, or could do so but for the interposition of the upper incisors (*Fig.* 11.3). At the other extreme the lips are grossly incompetent and there is little prospect of obtaining a lip seal, even after reduction of the overjet. Lip pattern is important because stability of overjet reduction depends upon the patient maintaining a lip seal, with the lower lip controlling the upper incisor positions.

Swallowing behaviour is related to lip morphology. Where it is possible to obtain a lip seal without undue effort this is usually done and swallowing is normal. In some cases the mandible is postured forwards habitually, which facilitates a lip seal, and swallowing takes place with the teeth parted. Where undue muscular effort is required to obtain a lip seal, either because of the degree of lip incompetence or because of the size of overjet, an anterior oral seal is obtained between the lower lip, the tongue and the alveolar mucosa (*Fig.* 11.3). When the tongue habitually lies above the lower incisor edges, the overbite is incomplete, although often only to a minor extent.

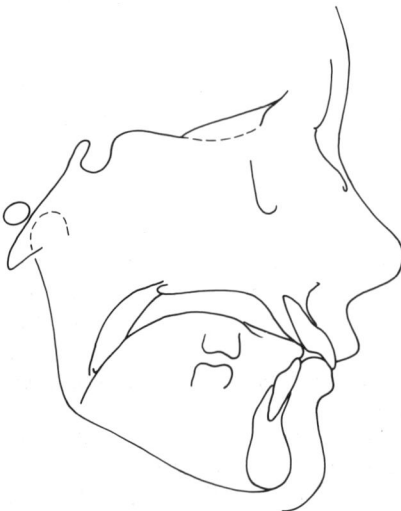

Fig. 11.3. The lower lip falls behind the upper incisors and an anterior oral seal is formed by contact between tongue, palate and lower lip. Note that there is also a posterior oral seal between tongue and soft palate.

SWALLOWING BEHAVIOUR

Atypical swallowing is particularly common in Class II, division 1 cases. Usually these adaptations are necessitated by variations in the incisor relationship. For example, when there is a tongue to lower lip seal, swallowing will normally take place with the teeth parted, as is the case when there is a forward posture of the mandible to allow a lip seal. In cases where the overbite is markedly incomplete, due, for example, to a digit-sucking habit, the tongue will again come forwards into contact with the lower lip. These adaptive patterns are generally of little clinical importance because they are modified spontaneously when the overjet is reduced and the patient is able to achieve a lip seal. The major exception is where the lips are too short to obtain a lip seal even after the overjet has been reduced: a tongue to lower lip seal will persist, and the overjet will relapse.

It is important to distinguish an adaptive pattern, which is common in Class II, division 1 malocclusions, from a primary tongue thrust, which is rare. Primary tongue thrust was discussed in Chapter 3: the overbite is always substantially incomplete and the circumoral contraction during swallowing is greater than would be expected from the degree of lip incompetence. This pattern does not modify on retraction of the incisors, and so it is prudent not to attempt to change the incisor relationship. Any treatment should be directed towards relief of crowding and alignment of the teeth.

THE SOFT TISSUES AND INCISOR POSITIONS

Where the overbite is incomplete and in the absence of a digit-sucking habit, the lower incisors reflect the position of soft tissue balance.

If the overbite is deep and complete, it is possible that the occlusion of the lower incisors may have held them back during favourable mandibular growth so that their true position of muscle balance is further forward. This is much less common in Class II, division 1 than in Class II, division 2.

In cases where, before treatment, the lower lip lies between the upper and lower incisors, a small amount of lower incisor advancement may be stable because the muscle balance changes once the overjet has been reduced. If the lower lip does not cover at least the incisal third of the upper incisor crown, the overjet is liable to increase: and if the lips are parted habitually, complete relapse may follow because the patient reverts to a tongue to lower lip seal.

MANDIBULAR FUNCTION

A number of individuals with Class II, division 1 malocclusions posture the mandible forwards habitually. In mild to moderately severe cases, this enables a lip seal to be obtained without undue circumoral contraction. In other cases the posture may have been adopted initially for aesthetic reasons and has become habitual. Cases like this generally swallow with the mandible in the postured position, and some have an anterior position of occlusion.

It is important to determine true centric relation and to recognize that these patients do have an upward and backward path of closure to true centric occlusion. It is also important not to mistake this for a distal displacement of the mandible with overclosure: this is very unusual in an unmutilated dentition. Treatment must be planned to centric relation, not to the postured position, because this will be lost when the upper incisors are retracted.

Correction of the incisor position and the establishment of centric relation reveals the true severity of the skeletal pattern, and this may result in a deterioration in facial appearance. The patient, and parents of a child patient, must be warned of this. Acceptance of postures is not recommended because they may be lost later in life as the patient ages.

TREATMENT OBJECTIVES

In Class II, division 1 malocclusions major objectives of treatment are to relieve crowding and irregularity of the teeth and to establish a stable Class I incisor relationship in harmony with the other facial features. If the lips are grossly incompetent, a stable reduction in overjet may not be attainable. Where there is an appreciable incisor edge–centroid discrepancy (*see Fig.* 11.11) it may not be possible to obtain a stable overbite reduction because there is insufficient bone to allow the required amount of palatal movement of the upper incisor roots; and the lower incisors cannot be advanced far enough to compensate for the skeletal pattern. In these circumstances a combined surgical and orthodontic approach may be the best way to provide an acceptable result (*see* Chapter 19). Even where it is possible to correct the overjet by orthodontic treatment in the severe Class II case, the facial appearance may still be poor and surgical correction of the jaw relationship may be preferable.

TREATMENT

Early Mixed Dentition Stage

Treatment of a Class II, division 1 malocclusion may be sought in the early mixed dentition, because of the unsightly facial appearance or the vulnerability of the upper incisors to trauma (*Fig.* 11.4). Unless the overjet is corrected fully, there is little prospect of stability. Although the incisors may be spaced, there is rarely sufficent room to retract them fully. Sometimes it is possible to create space by extraction of the upper decidous canines, provided that the upper

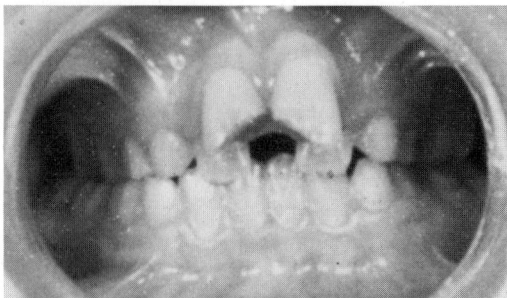

Fig. 11.4. Where the lips are habitually parted and the upper incisors are prominent, they are particularly vulnerable to trauma.

permanent canines are high and buccal and are well clear of the lateral incisor roots, remembering that the incisor roots will move labially as the teeth are tipped back. In other cases, correction of the arch malrelationships with a functional appliance may be possible and this may be particularly valuable in cases where the severity of the malocclusion necessitates early intervention in order to obtain the maximal help from facial growth (*see* Chapter 17).

While it may be feasible to correct the incisor malrelationship in the early mixed dentition, a number of problems may arise, and so this should be attempted only where there are strong indications for doing so. In many younger children the lips are parted habitually and so overjet reduction may not be stable. Prolonged retention while waiting for the soft tissues to mature is very undesirable, both for dental health and for patient cooperation. In most cases which are treated early, a further appliance is required in the late mixed or early permanent dentition, and thus treatment is liable to extend over many years.

Late Mixed and Permanent Dentition Stages

The difficulty of correction of the incisor malrelationship is directly related to the severity of the incisor edge–centroid discrepancy. However severe the skeletal malrelationship may be, if there is full dento-alveolar compensation by lower incisor proclination so that the lower incisor edges lie 2–4 mm in advance of the upper incisor root centroid (*Fig.* 11.1*a*), the upper incisors can be tipped back to achieve a Class I incisor relationship with a stable overbite. There may still be other difficulties, for example inclinations of other teeth may be unfavourable, or the overbite may be difficult to reduce, but in general, treatment is comparatively straightforward.

Where the lower incisor edges lie behind the upper centroid (*see Fig.* 11.11), this relationship must be corrected to avoid the risk of creating a Class II, division 2 incisor relationship with a deep overbite.

Favourable Incisor Edge–Centroid Relationship

Treatment with removable appliances   Many of these mild cases can be treated with removable appliances.

The lower arch: The best results are obtained where the lower arch can be accepted without extractions, except perhaps of third molars (*Fig.* 11.5) or where there is moderately severe crowding with favourable inclinations of the teeth so that spontaneous alignment and space closure can occur following extraction of lower first premolars (*Fig.* 11.6). If possible, the teeth should be extracted before the second permanent molars have erupted, and certainly while the face is still growing, when spontaneous alignment and space closure are more satisfactory. Overbite reduction depends on accelerated eruption of the buccal segments while the lower incisors are restrained by a bite plane. If this is to be stable, sufficient growth in facial height must occur to restore the relationship of the mandible to the upper face (*Fig.* 11.7*c*).

It has been pointed out that the posterior rotation of the mandible produced by a bite plane (and many by fixed appliances particularly when Class II elastics

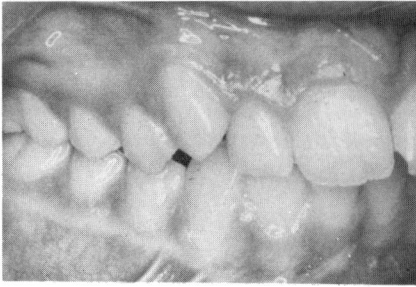
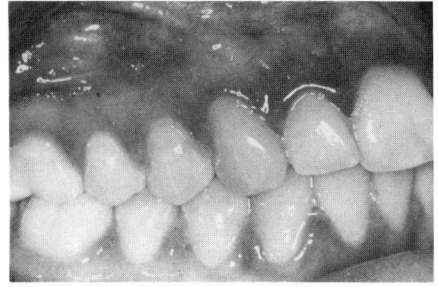

a   *b*

Fig. 11.5. A Class II, division 1 malocclusion treated by distal movement of the upper buccal segments using an 'en masse' appliance, with no extractions in the lower arch.

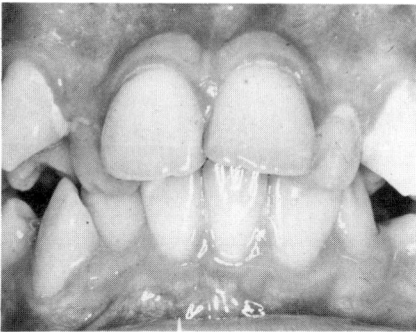
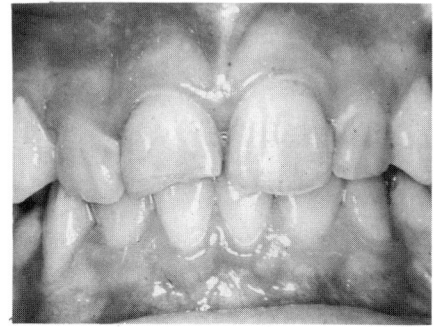

a

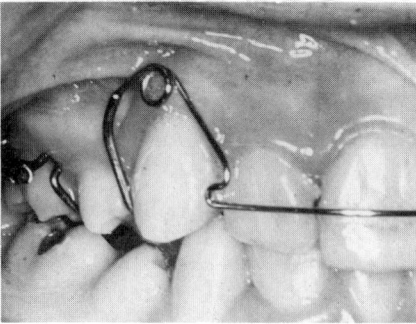

Fig. 11.6. A mild Class II, division 1 case with crowding treated by the extraction of four first premolars and an upper removable appliance. The lower arch has aligned spontaneously to a satisfactory extent.

b

are used) exaggerates the Class II skeletal tendency and increases lip incompetence, both of these changes being particularly unfavourable in Class II, division 1 cases. Provided the face is still growing, however, these ill effects are transient.

In adults, overbite reduction with a bite plane is very difficult. In some patients who have had a tendency to posterior mandibular rotation and a high maxillary–mandibular planes angle, a permanent opening of the intermaxillary space may be achieved, with long-term undesirable effects on the skeletal pattern and lip incompetence. In others, and particularly where there has been an anterior growth rotation, the maxillary–mandibular planes angle will gradually close after treatment, with intrusion of the buccal teeth. In these cases,

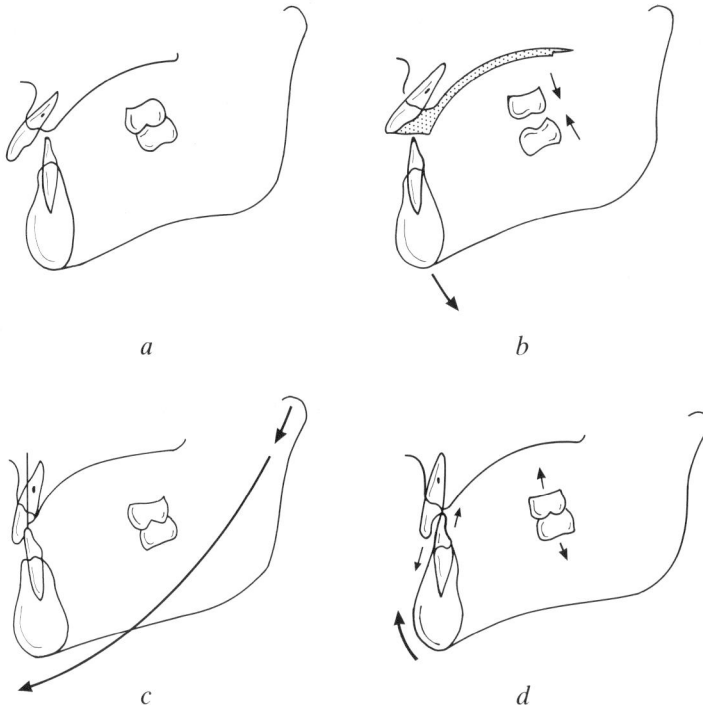

Fig. 11.7. Effects of an anterior bite plane (*a, b*). The immediate effect is to rotate the mandible posteriorly so that the molars are free to erupt. *c*, In the growing child, growth in posterior face height catches up and so the mandible rotates anteriorly again. Thus there is no net increase in the anterior intermaxillary height and provided a satisfactory inter-incisor relationship has been achieved, the overbite should be stable. *d*, In the adult, the intermaxillary height is liable to regress towards its original value, with gradual intrusion of buccal teeth. The occlusal stop on the incisors will rarely be secure enough to prevent them from sliding past one another as the face height reduces, and the overbite tends to deepen.

however, the incisors may not intrude but rather slide past one another with some increase in overjet and overbite (*Fig.* 11.7*d*). For these reasons, active intrusion of the labial segments with fixed appliances is indicated in adults.

The upper arch: As a general rule in Class II cases, teeth should be removed from the upper arch at least as far forwards as from the lower. When the lower arch is treated without extractions, or where lower second or third molars are to be removed, upper arch treatment depends to a great extent on the amount of space that is required to relieve crowding and reduce the overjet. Retraction of upper buccal segments with headgear (*see Fig.* 11.5) may be appropriate where less than one-half premolar width of space is needed. This is achieved more readily before the second permanent molars have erupted, or following their extraction: on the other hand, if more space is required in the upper arch, or if lower premolars are to be removed, extraction of upper first premolars is the simplest way of providing the space necessary to establish a Class I canine relationship.

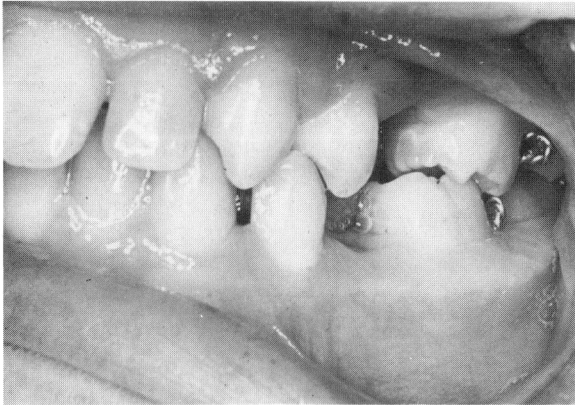

a

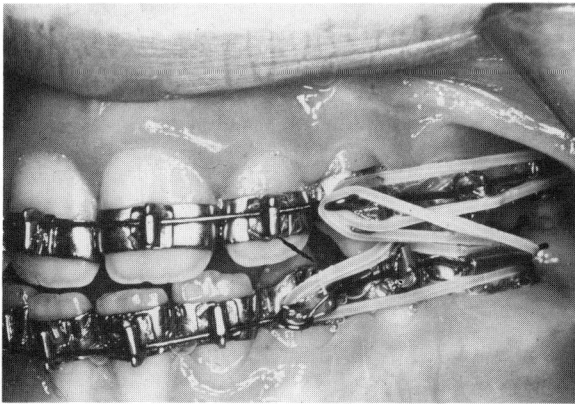

b

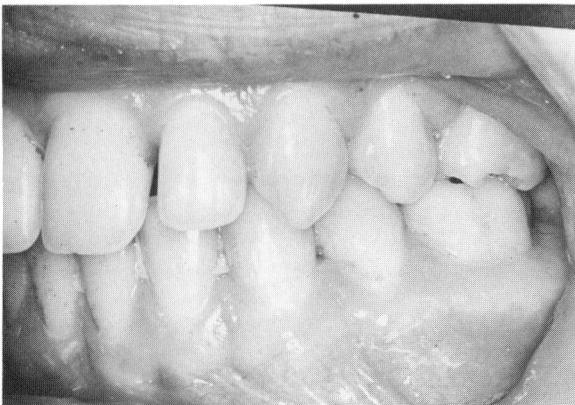

c

Fig. 11.8. A mild Class II, division 1 case with no crowding treated by the extraction of second premolars and fixed appliances.

Treatment with fixed appliances   Mild cases present few difficulties when fixed appliances are used. Where there is no crowding, the lower arch is accepted and the upper arch is retracted. This can often be done with removable appliances, but incisor rotation or other dental irregularities may necessitate the use of a fixed appliance. Mild to moderate crowding is best dealt with by extraction of second premolars (*Fig.* 11.8). It is particularly important not to retract lower incisors in Class II cases, and the risk of doing so is less when second rather than first premolars are removed, because the anchorage balance favours closure of residual space by forward movement of the molars rather than by undue retraction of the labial segments. Cases with severe crowding are treated more readily with loss of first premolars, and it should be remembered that reduction of a deep overbite also requires some space. Extractions in the upper arch generally correspond to those in the lower.

Overbite reduction, even with fixed appliances, is obtained at least in part by elevation of the buccal segments. This is of little consequence in the child where the face will grow, but every attempt should be made to achieve as much incisor intrusion as possible in the adult. This is difficult. It is essential that the apices of the lower incisors are clear of the lingual cortical plate of the mandibular symphysis (*Fig.* 11.9), otherwise intrusion will be almost impossible. Intermaxillary elastics favour molar extrusion.

In some Class II, division 1 cases there is excessive vertical development of the upper labial segment and the patient displays an undue amount of gingivae, especially when smiling. In these cases, if the upper labial segment is merely retracted, the patient will be left with a 'gummy smile' at the end of treatment

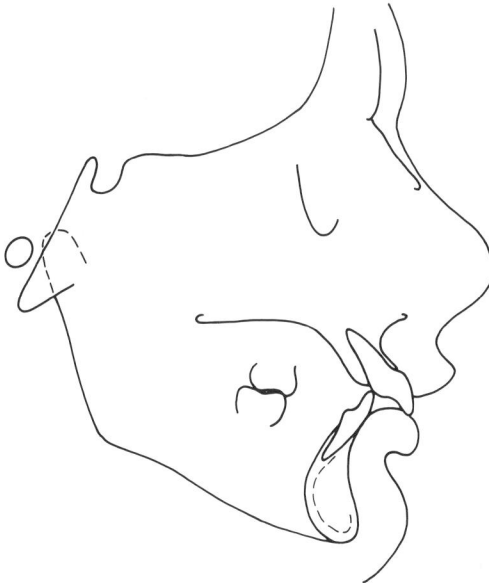

Fig. 11.9. Intrusion of lower incisors is possible only if the apices are clear of the mandibular cortex. In this case the apices would have to be torqued labially before the teeth could be intruded.

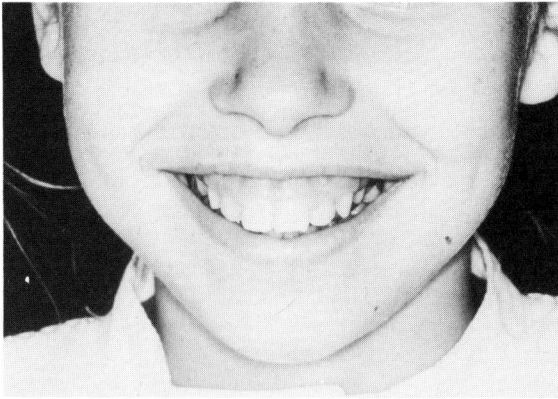

Fig. 11.10. A 'gummy' smile. For a good aesthetic result the upper incisors would have to
be intruded as well as being retracted.

(*Fig.* 11.10). Provided that they will still be controlled by the lower lip, some
intrusion of the upper incisors during their retraction is desirable: this is best
achieved using high-pull headgear to the labial segment during its retraction.
Once again Class II elastics should be avoided because they tend to extrude the
upper labial segment.

Unfavourable Incisor Edge–Centroid Relationship
The incisor edge–centroid relationship must be corrected if a stable reduction in
overbite is to be obtained, and these cases are not suitable for treatment with
removable appliances (*Fig.* 11.11).
   By far the simplest method of correcting the edge–centroid discrepancy would
be to advance the lower incisor edges, but even where there are signs that the
lower incisors have been restrained, or where it is expected that favourable
growth of the mandible will reduce the skeletal discrepancy, the amount of
advancement of the lower incisors that will be stable is questionable. Thus the
incisor edge–centroid relationship should be corrected where possible by palatal
movement of the upper incisor roots using a fixed appliance.
   In more severe cases, it is not feasible to correct the incisor edge–centroid
relationship completely by palatal movement of the upper incisor roots. This
may be because there is insufficient bone palatal to the upper incisors, and little
alveolar bone remodelling can be expected at apical level. A further factor may
be that extensive palatal movement of the upper incisors might result in an
unacceptable facial appearance, with the dentition set too far back relative to the
upper face. In these cases it is necessary to explore the possibility of lower
incisor advancement. If this is not feasible, surgical correction of the skeletal
malrelationship will be necessary.
   Some stable lower incisor edge advancement can be obtained in the following
circumstances:
   1 If there has been persistent finger- or thumb-sucking, the lower labial

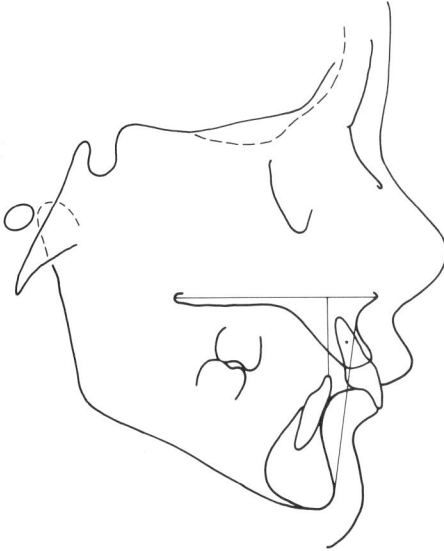

Fig. 11.11. A severe Class II division 1 incisor malrelationship. The lower incisor edge is 6 mm behind the upper centroid and for a stable reduction in overbite, it should be 2 mm in advance of it. It would be neither possible nor aesthetically acceptable to retract the upper centroid by this amount. Some advancement of the lower incisor edge should occur with favourable growth in this 9-year-old boy, and with a change in lower lip position, some proclination could be stable. However, if growth were not favourable, orthodontic correction of this malocclusion would not be possible.

segment may have been retroclined. Some spontaneous correction may follow cessation of the habit but, particularly if the lower lip falls between the upper and lower incisors, full recovery may not have occurred.

2   Some lower incisor proclination may be stable in cases with a tongue to lower lip anterior oral seal, when a lip seal can be established following upper incisor retraction and the soft tissue balance changes.

3   In cases with a deep, complete overbite and the morphological signs of an anterior mandibular growth rotation, full dento-alveolar adaptation may have been prevented by contact of the lower incisors with the palate and some advancement may be stable. Particularly in cases showing signs of a forward mandibular growth rotation, the skeletal relationship may be expected to improve with further growth and this in turn may enable the lower incisor edges to be advanced relative to the upper face.

Lower incisor advancement should be undertaken only where there are no reasonable orthodontic alternatives and where there are signs indicating that they have been held back. The problem for the clinician is that all these signs are fallible and there are no secure guidelines as to how much advancement will be stable. This is discussed in more detail with Class II, division 2 malocclusions. Relapse with crowding is common in cases where lower incisors have been proclined, even following long-term retention.

Following evaluation of the possibilities of dealing with the incisor mal-relationship, attention can be focused on relief of crowding and correction of other aspects of the malocclusion. The principles here are identical with those discussed previously for the milder cases, except that fixed appliance treatment will always be required.

Chapter 12

Class II, Division 2 Malocclusions

Class II, division 2 malocclusions (*Fig.* 12.1) occur in about 10 per cent of children. In milder forms they may be perfectly acceptable functionally, and the facial appearance can be pleasing. In severe cases the overbite is very deep, possibly associated with periodontal trauma palatal to the upper, and labial to the lower incisors. A Class II, division 2 incisor relationship is generally the result of dento-alveolar compensation for a Class II skeletal pattern by retroclination of the upper central incisors (*Fig.* 12.1). The more severe the skeletal malrelationship and the more that compensation occurs by retroclination of the upper, rather than by proclination of the lower incisors, the deeper the overbite will be.

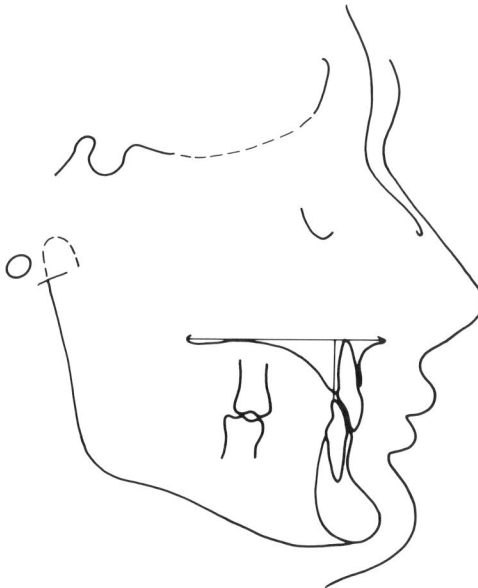

Fig. 12.1. A moderately severe Class II, division 2 case. The deep overbite is in part due to retroclination of the upper incisors which is compensating for the mild Class II skeletal pattern. The lower incisor edge lies behind the upper root centroid. The lips are competent with a high lip line and prominent lower labiomental fold.

OCCLUSAL FEATURES

Class II, division 2 malocclusions are characterized by a Class II incisor relationship with retroclination of the upper central incisors. The upper lateral incisors may also be retroclined, but typically they are proclined, mesially inclined and mesiolabially rotated (*Fig.* 12.2). The overbite is deep and complete and the overjet is average or only slightly increased. Overbite depth is strongly associated with the anteroposterior relationship between the lower incisor edges

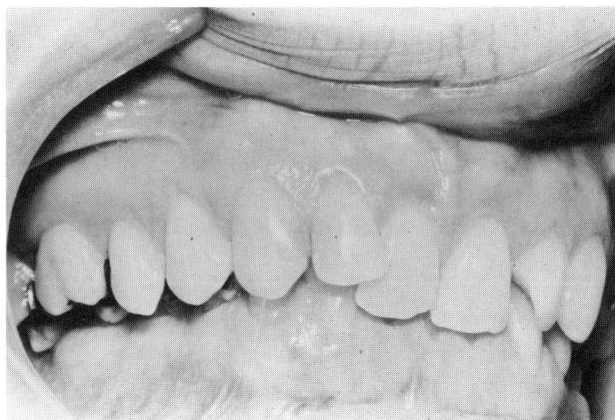

Fig. 12.2. A Class II, division 2 malocclusion with a scissor bite. The overbite is deep and potentially traumatic.

and the upper incisor root centroid (*Fig.* 12.1): the greater the discrepancy, the more difficult is stable correction of the overbite. In some cases there is an increased crown–root angle of the upper incisors, so that although the inclination of the tooth is within average limits, the crown is retroclined and the overbite is correspondingly deep. Sometimes the lower incisors are proclined, helping to compensate for the skeletal pattern, but in other cases they are retroclined.

The anteroposterior buccal segment relationship is usually mild Class II, although it can be Class I in cases of bimaxillary retroclination. A full unit Class II buccal segment relationship is not common. Transversely, there may be a scissors bite (buccal crossbite) (*Fig.* 12.2), which is often confined to the premolars. A bilateral complete scissors bite is rare, which is fortunate because correction is difficult.

SKELETAL RELATIONSHIPS

The skeletal pattern may be Class I, but is generally mild Class II, and the chin is well developed so that the facial profile is good (*Fig.* 12.1). A severe Class II skeletal pattern is rarely found because this would usually lead to a Class II, division 1 incisor relationship.

The lower anterior face height is often smaller than average and characteristically the maxillary–mandibular planes angle is low, with a well-developed mandibular angle.

Transversely, the maxillary base may be broad relative to the lower but this is usually compensated for by the angulation of the teeth, although a scissors bite involving the premolars is not rare.

FACIAL GROWTH

In many Class II, division 2 patients, facial growth is favourable, and there is an anterior mandibular rotation, as might be expected from the diminished anterior face height and the form of the chin. Even where the skeletal pattern improves with growth, the malocclusion will generally not change because dento-alveolar adaptation maintains the pre-existing incisor relationship. However, favourable growth is very important in helping the orthodontic correction of a severe Class II, division 2 incisor malrelationship.

SOFT TISSUES

The lips are almost always of adequate length to meet without strain. Frequently the lip line is high relative to the upper incisor crown, and the higher the lip line the more retroclined the upper incisors are liable to be. There is often a well-developed labiomental fold (*Fig.* 12.1). Rix described a teeth-apart swallowing behaviour in Class II, division 2 cases, but this is rarely of clinical importance.

MANDIBULAR FUNCTION

Mandibular posture and path of closure are generally normal. The deep overbite may prevent free lateral excursion of the mandible, but symptoms of muscle or facial pain seldom result from this. If many posterior teeth have been lost, there may be a posterior displacement of the mandible and overclosure, which are associated with muscle and joint pain.

TREATMENT OBJECTIVES

In mild cases the occlusion may be aesthetically and functionally satisfactory, and so treatment is not indicated. The position of the upper lateral incisors may be very unsightly if they are proclined, and this is the commonest of these patients' complaints. Where the overbite is not very deep, it may be accepted and treatment directed towards alignment of the lateral incisors. A deep and potentially traumatic overbite must be corrected, although this can be difficult, particularly in the adult.

TREATMENT

The Overbite is to be Accepted

In these cases, treatment is directed towards relief of crowding and alignment of the teeth, particularly of the upper lateral incisors. If the lower arch is well aligned or only mildly crowded, it should be accepted in spite of the fact that crowding may well increase during the later stages of facial growth (*see* p. 46). The extraction of lower premolars in these cases may be followed by a small amount of lingual tipping of the lower incisors as they align, and this can be sufficient to precipitate a serious deepening of the overbite.

Severe lower arch crowding is not common, but when it is found, extraction of first premolars is required, provided that all the lower permanent teeth are present, sound and in favourable positions. Spontaneous alignment of the lower labial segment and closure of the extraction spaces may be expected. However, if the overbite is already deep, there is the risk of its becoming worse and these cases are better treated with fixed appliances as described below.

Distal movement of the upper buccal segments following removal of second

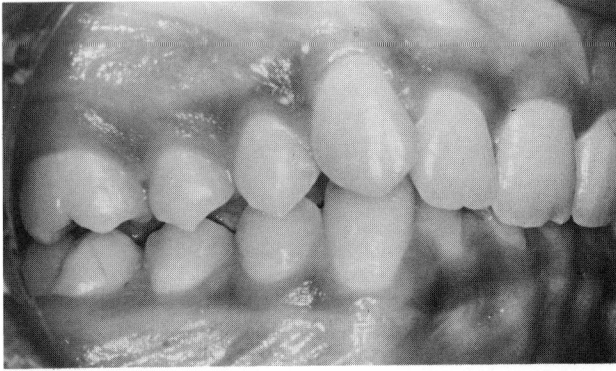

a

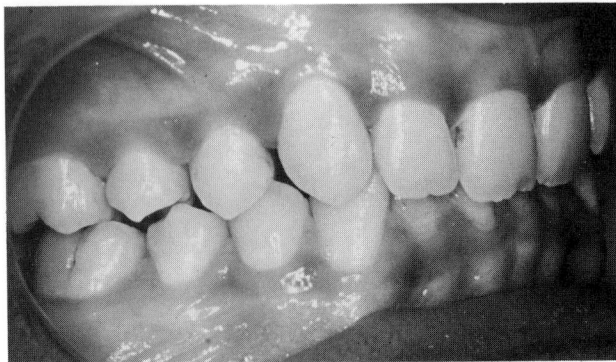

b

Fig. 12.3. A mild Class II, division 2 malocclusion treated by retraction of the upper buccal segments with headgear. *a*, Start of treatment. *b*, Completion of treatment. The buccal segment relationship has been corrected and the prominence of the lateral incisors and canines has been reduced.

permanent molars is generally the best approach to treatment (*Fig.* 12.3) where the buccal segments are less than one-half premolar width in distocclusion and provided that lower premolars are not to be extracted. With a more severe Class II buccal segment relationship, or when lower first premolars are to be lost, upper first premolars should be removed. In many cases adequate alignment of the upper arch can be obtained with removable appliances. The lateral incisor position is particularly liable to relapse to a small extent, but this can be quite acceptable. Where these teeth are rotated severely, fixed appliances are necessary and all possible measures should be taken to prevent relapse to an unacceptable degree. Over-rotation, pericision and prolonged retention are all helpful (*see* Chapter 17).

Because the upper incisors are retroclined, they need less space than would be the case if they had average inclinations. The reason is that the contact areas are positioned more labially, and if the teeth were at average inclinations with these contact positions, the overjet would be increased (*Fig.* 12.4). Thus, even if the lower incisors are slightly crowded, it may still be possible to align the upper incisors around them with the canines in a Class I relationship.

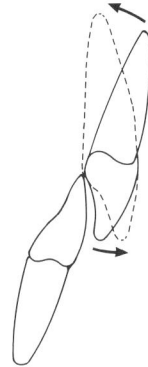

Fig. 12.4. In a Class II, division 2 incisor relationship the contact areas of the upper central incisors lie too far forward relative to the lower incisor edges but this is masked by their retroclination. If the inclination of the upper incisors were corrected by rotating them around their contact areas, this would be revealed by the increase in overjet.

The Overbite is to be Corrected

The first step is to consider how the incisor relationship is to be dealt with, and then decisions can be made about other aspects of treatment.

Overbite Control

In a growing child, the overbite may be corrected by restraining the lower labial segment while allowing growth of the buccal segments, so levelling the curve of Spee. The mandible is rotated posteriorly but, with growth, posterior facial height catches up (*see Fig.* 11.7). In many Class II, division 2 cases the upper labial segment also has to be prevented from erupting in order to correct the relationship between the incisor edges and the lower lip (*Fig.* 12.1). In adults, active intrusion of the labial segment is required, and this is difficult. Class II, division 2 cases do not often tolerate a permanent increase in intermaxillary height and if this happens, due to elevation of the buccal segments in an adult, the buccal teeth will be intruded gradually by the forces of the occlusion. The

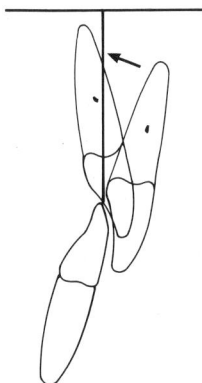

Fig. 12.5. A stable reduction of the over-bite requires correction of the edge–centroid relationship.

incisors are liable to slide past one another, rather than to intrude, with consequent deepening of the overbite.

The crucial factor in overbite stability in all treated cases is correction of the incisor edge–centroid relationship (*Fig.* 12.5). Stability can be ensured by sufficient retraction of the upper centroid using fixed appliances with palatal root torque, but in severe cases the alveolar process may not be thick enough to allow full correction in this way, because little periosteal bone remodelling occurs on the palate at the level of the incisor apices. Thus, in severe cases, it may be necessary to advance the lower incisor edges. This is achieved much more simply than is upper palatal root torque, but stability is uncertain. If the lower incisors drop back again due to soft tissue imbalance, the overbite will deepen and the lower labial segment will become crowded. A further danger is that the alveolar bone labial to the lower incisors is thin and with injudicious or rapid proclination of these teeth, crestal bone loss and gingival recession may occur.

Before the decision is taken to advance the lower labial segment, there must be a definite indication that this will be stable. In many Class II, division 2 cases, mandibular growth following eruption of the incisors has been favourable with improvement in the skeletal pattern, but this has not been reflected in a change in the incisor relationship because of dento-alveolar adaptation resulting from the incisor contact. Further favourable growth may occur during and following orthodontic treatment.

Indications of earlier favourable growth are those of anterior growth rotation (*see* p. 46). Retroclination of the lower incisors may also point to previous dento-alveolar adaptation due to occlusal factors, which could reasonably be reversed in conjunction with a change in the level of the upper incisors relative to the lower lip. The problem is that even when the indications for lower labial segment advancement are favourable, there is no reliable guide to the amount that will be stable. Some clinicians use an anterior bite plane in the hope that the lower incisors will then adopt a position of muscle balance, but the occlusion of the incisors on the bite plane may impede their movement, particularly if they are retroclined. Others rely on the A–Pog line to indicate a position of lower incisor stability, but there is no sound biological basis for this because stability depends on soft tissue, not skeletal balance. Clinical experience does suggest that in Class II cases the lower incisors will not be stable if they are moved forwards further than the A–Pog line, and so it does provide some guide to the reasonable limits of labial advancement.

In this area of uncertainty a reasonable approach is to advance the lower incisors only as far as is necessary to obtain a secure edge–centroid relationship. If this can be done in the mixed or early permanent dentition using a functional appliance there is the opportunity to test the stability of the incisor position by leaving the appliance out for some months prior to detailed finishing with a fixed appliance if this is necessary. Should the lower incisors start to drop back during this period, it is an indication that bodily retraction of the upper incisors with the fixed appliance will be required.

In the older patient, where treatment begins with a fixed appliance, it may be advisable to retain any advancement of the lower incisors with a lingual retainer until facial growth is virtually complete. This ensures that if there is favourable facial growth during the retention period, dento-alveolar adaptation will occur with labial movement of the upper rather than lingual movement of the lower incisors. In all cases where the lower labial segment has been advanced during treatment, there is the risk of some relapse and so there is the increased likelihood of the development of lower incisor crowding after treatment. The patient should be warned of this.

Treatment of Cases with Minimal Space Requirements
Uncrowded cases or those where there is only mild crowding and a moderately

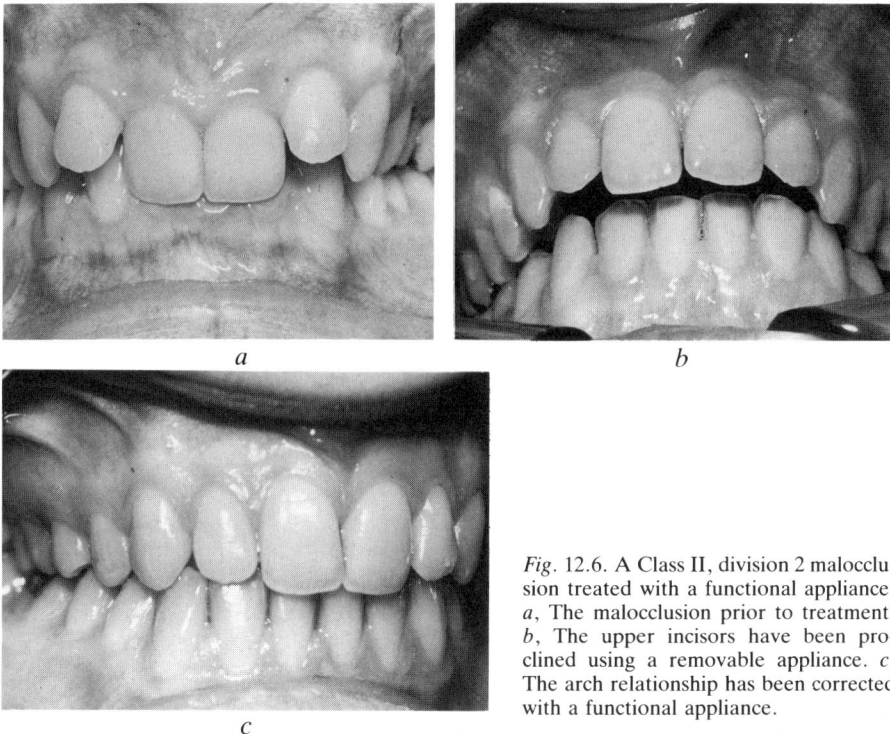

Fig. 12.6. A Class II, division 2 malocclusion treated with a functional appliance. *a*, The malocclusion prior to treatment. *b*, The upper incisors have been proclined using a removable appliance. *c*, The arch relationship has been corrected with a functional appliance.

deep overbite, may be treated without extractions; or possibly with extraction of second or third permanent molars. In some cases a functional appliance fitted after the retroclined upper incisors have been proclined to an average inclination, can give a good result (*Fig.* 12.6). Functional appliances should not be used in mild cases with a degree of lower arch crowding as this may be aggravated due to anterior movement of the entire arch followed by lingual relapse of the labial segment.

Where there is slight lower arch crowding, the lower buccal segments can be retracted. This may be done with a lip bumper (*see* p. 255) or with headgear to the lower arch, either before the second molars have erupted or following their extraction. However, headgear to the lower arch is often not well tolerated. Distal movement of lower first permanent molars is best undertaken just before exfoliation of the second deciduous molars so that the leeway space is not lost by forward drift. The anterior teeth may align spontaneously but if they do not, and certainly if there is an appreciable curve of Spee, a lower fixed appliance is required. Overbite reduction requires space and it is very difficult to reduce a deep overbite in even a mildly crowded lower arch without proclining the lower incisors.

Distal movement of the upper buccal segments can be undertaken using headgear to an 'en masse' appliance or to bands on the upper first permanent molars, either before eruption of the upper second molars or subsequent to their extraction if third molars are favourably positioned.

Following creation of adequate space by buccal segment retraction, the

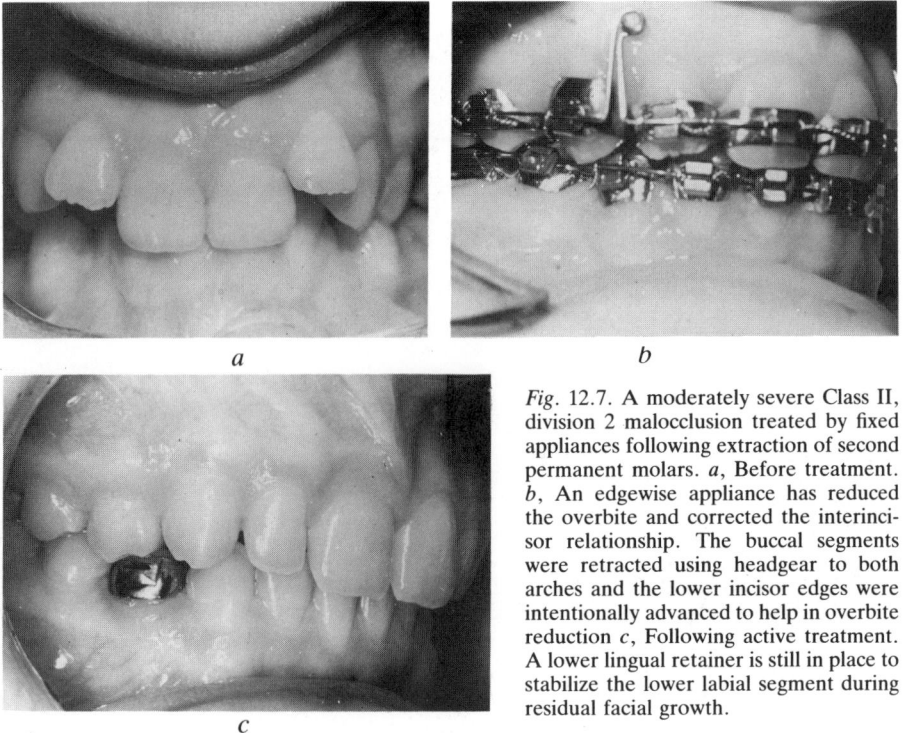

a

b

c

Fig. 12.7. A moderately severe Class II, division 2 malocclusion treated by fixed appliances following extraction of second permanent molars. *a*, Before treatment. *b*, An edgewise appliance has reduced the overbite and corrected the interincisor relationship. The buccal segments were retracted using headgear to both arches and the lower incisor edges were intentionally advanced to help in overbite reduction *c*, Following active treatment. A lower lingual retainer is still in place to stabilize the lower labial segment during residual facial growth.

interincisor relationship must be corrected. This involves overbite reduction and palatal root torque of the upper incisors and will normally require fixed appliances (*Fig.* 12.7). The latter movement in particular requires good anchorage and this is provided most reliably by headgear. High-pull headgear to the upper labial segment helps to control its vertical level as well as supplementing anchorage.

Crowded Cases

Where there is definite crowding, extraction of premolars and treatment with fixed appliances is required (*Fig.* 12.8). With severe crowding, and particularly where the overbite is very deep so that appreciable palatal root torque is required, first premolars are the teeth of choice for extraction from both arches. Care must be taken not to retract the lower labial segment because this would exaggerate the tendency to dental retrusion and would increase the amount of palatal movement of the upper incisor apices that is required for overbite stability.

Ideally the overbite should be reduced as far as possible by intrusion of the upper and lower incisors. This depends on there being sufficient cancellous bone above the incisor apices, and the inclination of the teeth may have to be adjusted (*see Fig.* 11.9) to allow intrusion to occur. Almost invariably some extrusion of premolars and molars will occur as the curve of Spee is flattened, but provided that the anterior intermaxillary height is not opened up excessively, growth in

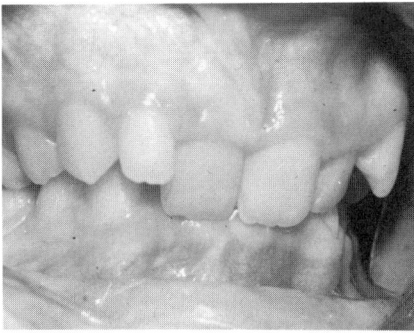

a

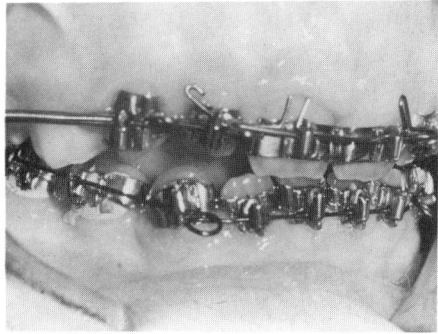

b

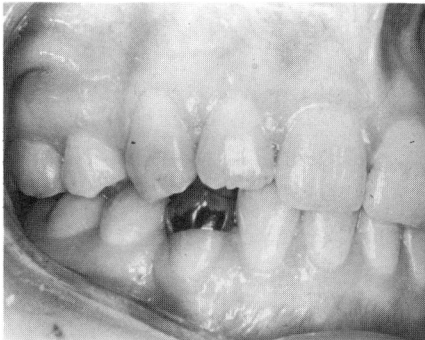

c

Fig. 12.8. A severe Class II, division 2 malocclusion treated by fixed appliances following extraction of first premolars. *a*, Before treatment. *b*, A Begg appliance has been used to reduce the overbite and overjet, align the teeth and close the extraction spaces. This is at the commencement of stage 3, when the tooth inclinations will be corrected. *c*, Completed treatment. A lower lingual arch is being used to stabilize the lower labial segment until growth is nearly completed.

posterior face height should catch up. In patients in whom growth is nearly completed or in adults, overbite reduction is a major problem and any increase in anterior intermaxillary height is very liable to close up with possible overbite deepening. In severe Class II, division 2 cases, intrusion of upper incisors is as important as is depression of the lower incisors, because unless they are elevated relative to the lower lip, the crowns will be held back and it will be almost impossible to obtain a stable incisor edge–centroid relationship.

Where crowding is only moderate, second rather than first premolars may be a better choice for extraction because the anchorage balance favours closure of excess space by mesial movement of the molars rather than by retraction of the labial segments, which can be difficult to avoid following first premolar extractions.

Chapter 13

Class III Malocclusions

In Class III malocclusions, the lower incisor edges lie anterior to the cingulum plateau of the upper incisors (*Fig.* 13.1). Class III malocclusion is found in about 3 per cent of children. Frequently it is the associated skeletal malrelationships and the prominence of the chin as much as the malocclusion itself that is of concern to patients and their families.

OCCLUSAL FEATURES

The severity of the incisor malrelationship varies greatly. In mild cases the incisors meet in an edge-to-edge relationship, when there may be an anterior mandibular displacement to obtain a posterior occlusion (*Fig.* 13.2). This exaggerates the severity of the incisor malrelationship. In more severe cases there is an appreciable reverse overjet. Frequently there is some degree of dento-alveolar compensation for the skeletal malrelationship and so the malocclusion may be less severe than would have been expected from the skeletal pattern (*Fig.* 13.1). The buccal segment relationship may be Class I and it is unusual to find a full premolar width of mesiocclusion.

The upper arch is often narrow as well as being short, and the lower arch is

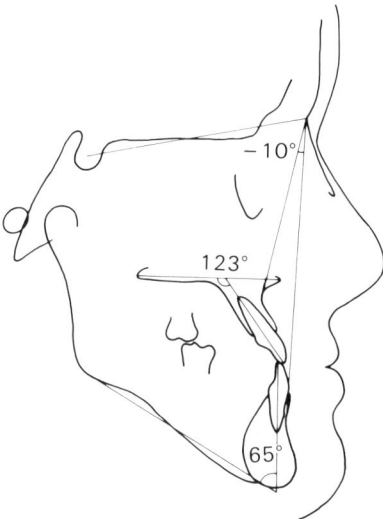

Fig. 13.1. A Class III malocclusion. The incisor malrelationship is milder than would have been expected from the skeletal pattern, due to dento-alveolar compensation.

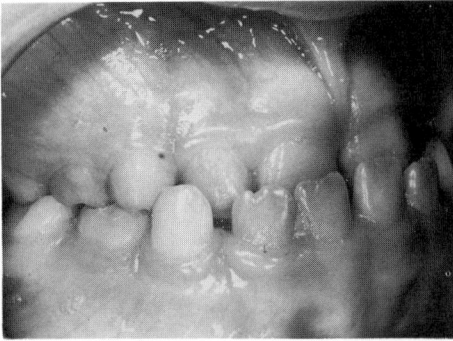

a

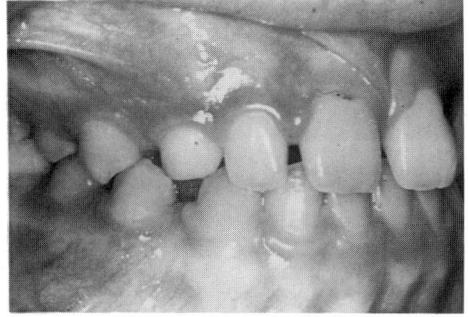

b

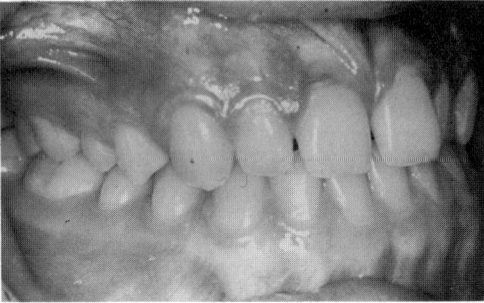

c

Fig. 13.2. a, Although an edge-to-edge incisor contact can be obtained, the mandible is displaced forwards to obtain maximum occlusion. b, Correction of the reverse overjet by proclination of the upper incisors eliminates the mandibular displacement. c, The occlusal correction has been stable due to the good overbite and a favourable pattern of facial growth.

broad; thus crossbites are common. This tendency is exacerbated by the antero-posterior arch malrelationship in that a broader part of the lower arch opposes a narrower part of the upper. Where the arch widths are equal, there is generally a displacement of the mandible to one side, producing a unilateral crossbite. Sometimes, a unilateral crossbite is a reflection of asymmetry of one of the arches. Where there is a more severe discrepancy in arch widths there is a bilateral crossbite (Fig. 13.3).

There are wide variations in intermaxillary height. Quite frequently the anterior intermaxillary height is increased and there is a skeletal open bite (Fig. 13.4a). In moderately severe cases where the lower incisors lie anterior to the

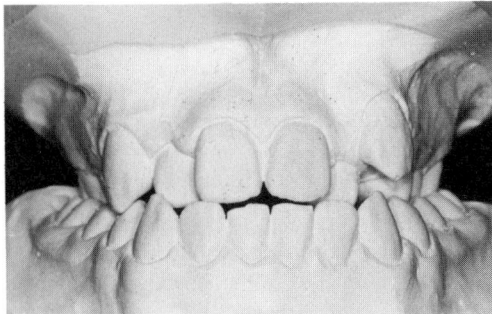

Fig. 13.3. A Class III malocclusion with a bilateral crossbite.

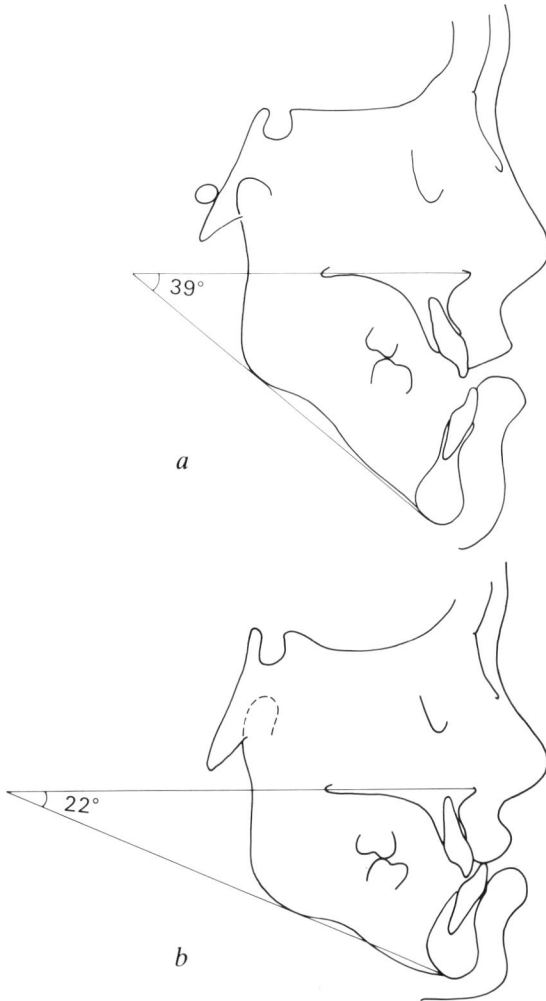

Fig. 13.4. Different facial types associated with Class III malocclusions. *a*, The anterior intermaxillary height is large and there is an associated skeletal open bite. This type of facial pattern can be expected to grow primarily vertically. *b*, The anterior intermaxillary height is reduced and the overbite is deep.

uppers, and the intermaxillary height is reduced, the overbite may be deep (*Fig. 13.4b*). When the incisors meet edge-to-edge, the overbite is of course reduced, regardless of the anterior intermaxillary dimensions.

The upper arch is frequently crowded because it is short and narrow, while the lower arch may well be spaced. Severe lower arch crowding is not common.

SKELETAL RELATIONSHIPS

There is usually a Class III skeletal pattern and its severity is reflected in the arch malrelationship. Particularly when measurements are made from a cepha-lometric radiograph which has been taken with the teeth in maximum occlusion, it is important to check clinically for a mandibular displacement, which would exaggerate the mandibular prognathism.

It is often assumed that in Class III cases it is only the mandible that is at fault. Frequently there is an element of maxillary retrusion; and the mandibular prominence may be due not only to its length but to some shortness of the cranial base. Where surgical correction is planned, it is very important to evaluate the different components of the skeletal malrelationship so that the appropriate surgical procedures are undertaken. In some cases a degree of maxillary advancement, instead of or in conjunction with a mandibular set back, is necessary for the best facial appearance.

FACIAL GROWTH

In Class III cases, facial growth is often unfavourable: the usual tendency for the mandible to become more prognathic relative to the upper face is adverse. Dento-alveolar adaptation may maintain the occlusal relationship, but in many of the more severe cases this is at its limits by the commencement of the pubertal growth spurt and further adaptation is not possible. Thus the reverse overjet tends to become worse.

Vertical facial growth increases any tendency to skeletal open bite, particu-larly where there is a high maxillary–mandibular planes angle and a tendency towards a posterior growth rotation of the mandible (*Fig.* 13.4*a*). In these cases, the vertical growth of the anterior intermaxillary height exceeds the growth potential of the alveolar processes and the open bite may extend to involve the buccal segments so that only the last molars are in occlusion.

SOFT TISSUES

In Class III cases the soft tissues do not generally play any part in the aetiology of the malocclusion. Indeed, they tend to encourage dento-alveolar compensa-tion for skeletal malrelationships, both anteroposterior and transverse, so that the arch malrelationships are less severe than might have been expected from the skeletal pattern. Where there is a severe anterior open bite the lips are usually incompetent and an anterior oral seal may be obtained between the tongue and upper lip or between tongue, alveolar mucosa and lower lip. The upper incisors are in a position of balance between the upper lip and tongue, and the lower lip has little part to play. The lower lip may be rather full and pendulous (*see Fig.* 13.4*b*) and in these cases the lower incisors may even be proclined, exaggerating the reverse overjet.

The different occlusal malrelationships that may be found in Class III cases may necessitate a variety of adaptations in obtaining an anterior oral seal and in swallowing behaviour. These are of little importance in diagnosis and treatment planning because they will modify in response to orthodontic treatment. When surgical treatment is planned, however, it must be remembered that if the oral cavity volume is reduced, the tongue may have to be postured forwards to avoid encroachment on the airway and so dental relapse may occur. In addition, orthognathic surgery will affect the balance of the circumoral musculature and if presurgical decompensation has not been undertaken, this may happen spontaneously under the influence of the soft tissues, and the occlusion may relapse to some extent. This is discussed at greater length in Chapter 19.

MANDIBULAR FUNCTION

The occlusal malrelationships frequently lead to mandibular displacements (*see* Fig. 13.2). If these are left uncorrected, muscle dysfunction and pain are often experienced. Correction of the occlusal malrelationship, which is usually possible with orthodontic appliances in these cases, eliminates the displacement and relieves the pain and dysfunction.

Lateral mandibular displacements are often found where there is a unilateral crossbite. These are not associated with mandibular overclosure, but in the long run may well give rise to muscle dysfunction and pain. Even when the patient does not complain of discomfort, areas of muscle tenderness can frequently be found on palpation, and electromyographic records will demonstrate a disrupted pattern of muscle activity. Correction of a unilateral crossbite in a Class III case is not always simple. The upper teeth are often already inclined buccally and further upper arch expansion is neither very effective nor stable. In some of these cases, rapid maxillary expansion to separate the midpalatal suture may be undertaken, but this may have the undesirable side effect of propping open the occlusion and reducing any overbite. In cases where the anteroposterior skeletal discrepancy is to be corrected surgically, this will at the same time lead to some improvement in the transverse arch relationship.

Occlusal function in Class III cases is often disrupted. Where there is a severe anterior open bite for example, only the last standing molars may meet in occlusion. However, in the absence of mandibular displacements due to premature occlusal contacts, symptoms of pain and dysfunction are surprisingly uncommon.

TREATMENT OBJECTIVES

Correction of the occlusal malrelationships with orthodontic appliances is possible only in the milder malocclusions, although these do form the greater proportion of all Class III cases. In severe cases, surgical intervention is required if the malocclusion is to be corrected (*see* Chapter 19). The greatest diagnostic problems arise in young patients who are already at the limits of orthodontic correction. Even if orthodontic treatment is reasonably successful at that age, further facial growth may produce a relapse, and if surgical treatment is then undertaken, the earlier orthodontic treatment may have been not only inappropriate but may prejudice the quality of the result. For example, if lower first premolars have been extracted to allow retraction of the lower labial segment, which later has to be proclined as part of the decompensation prior to surgery, the extraction spaces may then be very difficult to close.

TREATMENT

Early Mixed Dentition

The patient can often obtain an edge-to-edge incisor occlusion but displaces forwards to obtain occlusion of posterior teeth, thereby creating a reverse overjet. There is often some overclosure of the mandible. Provided that the upper incisors are not already proclined and that there is an adequate overbite, they are proclined with a removable appliance to correct the incisor malrelationship and eliminate the displacement as early as possible (*see Fig.* 13.2). This should take only a few weeks of treatment with a removable appliance. In the more severe cases, or where there would be insufficient overbite to retain the incisor correction, treatment should be delayed until the early permanent dentition stage.

In many Class III cases, the upper arch is narrow and the lateral incisors are trapped palatally (*see Fig.* 13.3). They will then erupt into lingual occlusion, even when the central incisor position has been corrected. In addition, the upper permanent canines may lie labial to their roots, preventing labial movement until the canines have erupted and can be retracted. Where this problem is recognized before eruption of the lateral incisors, extraction of the upper deciduous canines may provide space for the lateral incisors to escape labially and erupt in alignment with the central incisors. This is not always successful, but is worth attempting in suitable cases.

Even when the incisor relationship has been corrected in the early mixed dentition, relapse may occur later because of unfavourable facial growth.

Late Mixed/Early Permanent Dentition

The patient whose incisor malrelationship was corrected earlier may still require treatment to relieve crowding and align the other teeth. The principles of treatment are the same as those for the Class I case with crowding. There may be problems with lateral incisor alignment if these teeth are still positioned palatally. Frequently they are palatally displaced and labial movement may require a fixed appliance; and even when they have been corrected, the overbite may not be sufficient to hold them there. If the overbite is tenuous, some extrusion of all the upper incisors may be attempted using a fixed appliance, but as the face continues to grow vertically, the overbite is liable to reduce again and the upper incisors may slip back into reverse overjet.

Frequently the upper permanent canines erupt rather far forwards, where lateral incisors are positioned palatally, lacking the normal guidance from the lateral incisor roots. Occasionally an acceptable result can be obtained by extracting the lateral incisors themselves, rather than first premolars. As is the case where lateral incisors are absent developmentally, however, the appearance of the canine adjacent to the central incisor may not be ideal.

In deciding whether orthodontic treatment to correct the reverse overjet is advisable, the first step is to assess whether the facial appearance would be acceptable without surgical correction of the skeletal pattern. This evaluation must be undertaken with the mandible in the rest position so that a misleading impression is not given by an anterior displacement or overclosure.

Having decided that the facial appearance would be acceptable, the incisor relationship can be evaluated. If the patient cannot obtain an edge-to-edge occlusion of the incisors, or if there is an anterior open bite, orthodontic correction is probably not feasible. Finally, the incisor inclinations have to be taken into account. Only if the teeth can be tipped to obtain a normal overjet and a secure overbite, without the upper incisors being excessively proclined, is it reasonable to proceed with orthodontic correction of the incisor malrelationship. Where it is decided that orthodontic correction is not practicable, then either the arch malrelationship will have to be accepted, and any orthodontic treatment directed towards alignment of the teeth or surgical correction, possibly in conjunction with orthodontic treatment, will be required. This is usually best delayed until facial growth is nearly complete so that there is no uncertainty about later and possibly unfavourable growth changes.

Treatment of the Class III case with a removable appliance is possible only where a corrected incisor overjet can be achieved with an adequate overbite and without undue proclination of the incisors. The upper arch is often crowded and first premolars are the teeth of choice for extraction, assuming that all other permanent teeth are present, sound and satisfactorily positioned. Distal movement of the upper buccal segments to relieve even mild crowding is generally contraindicated because the molars are often rather distally inclined and because any possible restraint to forward growth of the maxilla and upper arch is to be avoided. Any crowding in the lower arch will usually be dealt with by the extraction of lower first premolars, even though this may leave residual spacing at the extraction site. This encourages the lower labial segment to drop back if there is a worsening of the skeletal pattern with growth, provided that there is an adequate overbite and that the lower incisors are not already very retroclined.

In the more severe case where the overjet cannot be corrected simply by proclining the upper incisors, or where the overbite is tenuous, or where other teeth are positioned unfavourably, fixed appliance treatment will be indicated. It is usually a good policy to aim to obtain as much improvement of the overjet as possible by retroclination of the lower incisors because this does not reduce the overbite. This will usually necessitate the extraction of the lower first premolars, which will also provide space for the relief of any crowding. If the lower incisors are already retroclined, further retraction may not be possible, but this may well indicate that the case is at the limits of orthodontic treatment and surgical correction should at least be considered. Having decided how much retraction of the lower labial segment is feasible, it is clear how much labial movement of the upper incisors will be required.

Chapter 14
Tooth Movement

A tooth is suspended in its socket by the periodontal ligament which, consisting of collagenous connective tissue, cells, blood vessels and tissue fluids, has visco-elastic properties. The periodontal ligament thus cushions the tooth and absorbs the forces of mastication and tooth contacts; it allows the tooth to erupt and to maintain its relation to the alveolar crest in the growing face; its sensory receptors are important in the control of masticatory activity; and it allows tooth movement to take place in response to muscular imbalance or orthodontic forces.

Periodontal ligament and alveolar bone remodelling do not occur in response to the transient imbalance in forces produced by, for example, mastication, speech, swallowing or laughter. Continuous and intermittent forces of sufficient duration and magnitude do prompt a cellular response and, if the loading is consistent in direction, alveolar bone remodelling and tooth movement occur.

The threshold in terms of pressure, duration or periodicity below which bone remodelling will not occur has not yet been quantified. Intermittent and interrupted forces are capable of producing tooth movement: for example, certain

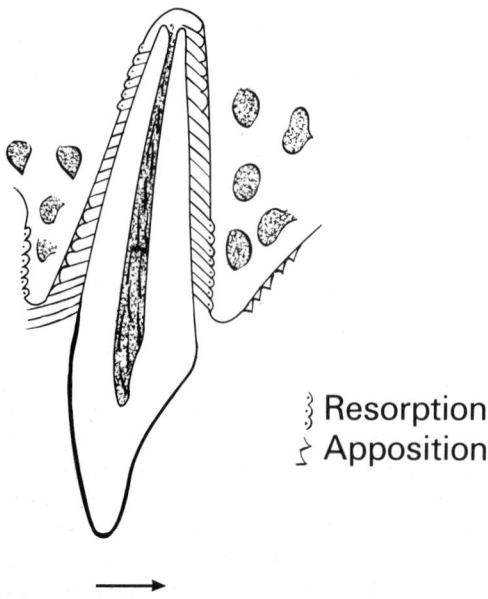

$\}$ Resorption
$\{$ Apposition

Fig. 14.1. The distribution of bone remodelling changes on socket walls and alveolar process when a gentle force tips an upper incisor palatally. The centre of rotation of the tooth is at about 40 per cent of the root length from the apex.

functional appliances generate intermittent forces and are worn only part of the time, yet they are capable of producing extensive tooth movements. The force threshold required to produce tooth movement must be rather low: the slight muscular imbalance produced by labial movement of lower incisors, for example, is often followed by relapse.[1] The question of what constitutes muscular balance is difficult to answer because recordings of the forces applied to the teeth when the orofacial musculature is at rest and during function, indicate that it is rare for all the forces applied to a tooth at a particular moment to cancel one another out. It must be assumed that when the teeth are in a position of muscle balance, the force thresholds are not exceeded in some critical respect.

The nature of the initial tooth movement within the confines of the periodontal ligament depends on the forces applied to the crown and so determines the distribution of pressure changes within the ligament. The centre of resistance to movement lies at about 40 per cent of the root length from the apex and so when a simple force is applied to the crown, it will tip about a fulcrum close to this point.[2] Thus, the pressure within the periodontal ligament varies along the root length (Fig. 14.1), the greatest pressure changes occurring close to the alveolar crest. When a tooth is moved bodily, the pressure distribution is more uniform along the root length, but varies around its circumference.

HISTOLOGICAL CHANGES IN AREAS OF COMPRESSION

The observed changes depend on whether or not capillary blood pressure is exceeded. Where this happens, the blood vessels are crushed, the cells die and the compressed connective tissue has a structureless glassy appearance when viewed in histological sections under the light microscope: this is called hyalinization.[3] This commonly occurs close to the alveolar crest in the area of maximum compression when teeth are tipped, even with quite light continuous orthodontic forces. If excessive forces are used, hyalinization may be extensive. Areas of hyalinization are less common with true bodily tooth movements because of the more uniform pressure distribution along the root; but, of course, even with fixed appliances it may be difficult to avoid some tipping of the tooth and hyalinization is still liable to occur at any irregularities in the socket wall.

Areas of Compression Below Capillary Blood Pressure

Within a few days, cellular proliferation occurs in the fibroblasts and other cells of the periodontal ligament. Osteoclasts, which are believed to be formed by fusion of cells which migrate to these areas from the blood vessels, appear along the socket wall and bone resorption commences. Soon the osteoclasts come to lie within shallow depressions known as Howship's lacunae. Osteoclasts are large complex multinucleated cells, and the one osteoclast may be responsible for resorption at several different locations. Resorption does not take place over a large continuous front, and so while some of the fibres of the periodontal ligament become detached, others remain intact. After some bone has been resorbed, the osteoclasts migrate or are replaced and bone is resorbed at the previously passive sites. Meanwhile, the detached periodontal fibres become re-attached at the former resorption sites[4] and so the integrity of the ligament is maintained.

The factors mediating between the change in pressure and the cellular response are still a matter of speculation. They are probably the same as those that come into play when pressure is applied directly to the periosteum. Suggestions have been made that changes in electrical charge occur at the surface of the bone and these promote the observed cellular response.[5] Experimental work has shown that the application of a direct current to the alveolar process close to a tooth does accelerate its movement in response to orthodontic forces.[6] However, it is not at all clear whether this is a specific effect or whether it merely reflects a general perturbation of cellular activity.[7]

There is some evidence that local hormones, for example prostaglandins, may also have a role.[8] These have been identified in pathological lesions associated with bone resorption; their inhibition reduces but does not prevent resorption in areas of compression of the periodontal ligament and the injection of prostaglandins into the alveolar mucosa has been shown to accelerate orthodontic tooth movement.[9] Although prostaglandins may be important, other chemical factors also have a role in the promotion of osteoclastic activity.

Areas of Compression Exceeding Capillary Blood Pressure

As explained above, where the capillary vessels are crushed, the cells die and the compressed connective tissue appears structureless under the light microscope. If the pressure is reduced, these hyalinized areas rapidly become revascularized and colonized by new cells.[10] Bone resorption cannot take place on the surface of the socket wall beneath a hyalinized area. Peripheral to the hyalinized area, however, the periodontal ligament is compressed slightly and direct surface resorption occurs. This peripheral resorption may completely remove the bone underlying a small area of hyalinization. However, more extensive areas of hyalinization are removed by undermining resorption within the cancellous spaces deep to the affected area; osteoclasts appear and the bone is removed from below so that tooth movement occurs.[10] If the appliance continues to exert an excessive force, a further zone of hyalinization will be produced. When the force is reduced by the tooth movement so that the area is compressed only gently, however, the hyalinized area will be revascularized and direct surface resorption can proceed.

HISTOLOGICAL CHANGES IN AREAS OF TENSION

The periodontal fibres are stretched, and with excessive forces, some may be torn and blood vessels may be ruptured. In contrast to areas of compression, however, there is no fundamental difference in the nature of the tissue response to light and heavy forces. Within a few days cellular proliferation occurs among the fibroblasts of the periodontal ligament and the osteoblasts lining the socket wall. The extension of the principal fibres occurs throughout their length and not specifically at either end. Osteoid is laid down along the socket wall and this becomes calcified and reorganized as woven bone. The irregular and vascular woven bone is very susceptible to resorption, but is progressively remodelled into mature bone.

THE SUPRA-ALVEOLAR CONNECTIVE TISSUES

The transeptal fibres that pass between adjacent teeth also adjust to tooth movement. If two teeth are being moved apart, the fibres stretch, but the residual tension is sufficient to promote tooth movement. Thus, for example, when a first premolar is being retracted, the canine will follow if it is free to do so, although some stretching of the fibres will occur and there will be a space between the teeth. It is good practice to avoid elongating the transeptal fibres because, when teeth are approximated, these fibres do not seem to shorten readily and so the interdental contacts may be less tight than would be desired. This is particularly noticeable at extraction sites, across which the transeptal fibres reform,[11] and may be one reason why extraction spaces are liable to open up following closure if there is any general tendency to spacing.

The free gingival fibres pass from the neck of the tooth into the connective tissue system of the mucoperiosteum. When a tooth is moved orthodontically, it does not pass through the mucoperiosteum but carries it with it; and any adjustment occurs within the mucoperiosteum. This is of particular relevance when teeth are rotated because the free gingival fibres seem to stretch but not to remodel fully.[12] Residual tension within the supra-alveolar connective tissue system is probably an important reason why teeth that have been rotated mechanically are so liable to relapse.[13]

REMODELLING OF THE ALVEOLAR PROCESS

The tissue changes associated with orthodontic tooth movement are not confined to the periodontal ligament and socket wall. Any labiolingual tooth movement is associated with remodelling of the alveolar process: subperiosteal apposition occurs on the bone surface towards which the root is moving, and resorption on the surface from which the tooth is moving. Thus the alveolar process 'drifts' with the tooth (*see Fig.* 14.1). Remodelling is most complete close to the alveolar crest but may be negligible at apical level. Thus, it is possible to move the root apex through the alveolar plate where it is thin. This may provoke root resorption and clearly is undesirable.[14] If the root is moved back again, however, the alveolar bone may reform.[15]

TISSUE CHANGES DURING THE RETENTION PERIOD

If a tooth is released immediately after having been moved with an orthodontic appliance, it will spring back due to residual tension in the periodontal ligament and the force may even be enough to produce some resorption of bone on surfaces that were previously formative. Although this reversal is clearly limited in amount, it is desirable to retain the tooth until the periodontal ligament has adapted fully. More important is the fact that the recently formed bone is very readily resorbed and even slight forces that would not normally provoke a tissue response, may initiate resorption. Thus it seems prudent in most cases to retain the tooth position until more mature bone has been formed. This takes between 3 and 6 months. During this period a new lamina dura forms on previously resorptive surfaces, and some adjustments may take place in the supra-alveolar connective tissue. Adaptation of the supra-alveolar fibres seems to be very slow, however, and may cause relapse of rotations even after quite long periods of retention.

PATHOLOGICAL CHANGES ASSOCIATED WITH TOOTH MOVEMENT

From some points of view it is surprising that there are not more complications of orthodontic tooth movement. Even following extensive hyalinization of the periodontal ligament, recovery is complete. This does not mean that large forces can be used with impunity: other side effects described below are more liable to occur with excessive forces; and there can be problems of anchorage control and appliance management.

Crestal Bone Loss

A slight reduction in crestal bone height occurs with many types of fixed appliance treatment. This may be a direct result of tooth movement, or it may be secondary to a deterioration in plaque control. When treatment is well managed, however, this crestal loss should be less than 1 mm and is of limited clinical relevance;[16] but with poor oral hygiene, it may be more severe and can be a matter of concern. Severe crestal loss and periodontal recession can occur when a tooth is moved labially or buccally with heavy forces where the buccal plate is already very thin. If hyalinization of the periodontal ligament occurs at the alveolar crest, and the plate of bone is thin with few or no cancellous spaces, undermining and peripheral resorption can result in the loss of crestal height. If at the same time oral hygiene is less than ideal, gingival recession will also occur. Labial movement of lower incisors and buccal movement of upper or lower canines is particularly liable to be associated with periodontal recession of this type.

Labial or buccal movement of a root apex may result in fenestration of the alveolar plate. This is not such an immediately serious periodontal problem because bone may reform when the apex is moved lingually again, and it does not predispose to gingival recession in an otherwise healthy mouth.

Root Resorption

Small areas of root resorption are commonly found on teeth that are being moved orthodontically.[17] These may occur laterally or apically, they are repaired by secondary cementum and are of no long-term importance. However, appreciable apical resorption with permanent shortening of the root can occur, particularly where extensive apical movements are undertaken, as with fixed appliances. It has been suggested that 'round tripping', where the apex is moved first in one direction and then in another, is particularly liable to produce root resorption;[18] but this may merely reflect the total distance through which the root is moved. Heavy forces have also been implicated, but again there is no objective evidence that this is so.

The teeth most commonly involved are the upper incisors and the first permanent molars. One-quarter of the root length or even more can be lost from previously healthy teeth and clearly this is a matter of serious concern. The teeth retain their vitality, they do not generally suffer further spontaneous resorption, and after the normal retention period do not demonstrate increased mobility so there are no immediate problems for the patient. However, should periodontal disease with alveolar bone loss become established subsequently, the prognosis for teeth with appreciably shortened roots is poor.

Some teeth are particularly susceptible to root resorption during orthodontic tooth movement and very extensive root loss can occur, even with simple tipping movements. These teeth almost always have signs of idiopathic resorption before orthodontic treatment is commenced and it is very important to examine the root length on radiographs of all teeth that are to be moved. If there are signs of blunting and shortening of the roots, then orthodontic movement of these teeth should be avoided if at all possible. Not only may rapid and extensive resorption occur, but because the centre of resistance to tooth movement is closer to the crown, they tilt more than usual with removable appliances or other simple forces. If it is essential to move teeth that have been affected in this way, the patient (and parent if appropriate) must be warned of the dangers of serious root shortening reducing the life expectancy of the affected teeth, and only if they are prepared to accept the risks, should treatment be commenced. It may be wise to confirm the warning and discussion in writing as a defence against subsequent litigation.

Light forces are mandatory and it is better to use fixed appliances with controlled tipping about the apex in order to minimize apical travel. Root length should be monitored and standardized periapical radiographs taken at 3-monthly intervals and if further root shortening is detected, the tooth should be stabilized with the appliances for a period of 3 months in order to allow as much repair as possible by secondary cementum.[19] This procedure of stabilization should also be followed if root resorption is discovered in previously normal teeth during orthodontic treatment.

The final tooth position should be planned to be as free as possible from occlusal or other stress. It is surprising how firm a tooth that has lost even three-quarters of its root length can be, and it may be functional for many years provided that plaque control and gingival health are maintained scrupulously. However, such teeth are always at risk from even minor trauma and their long-term prognosis is invariably poor.

Damage to the Dental Pulp

When a tooth is moved by an appliance, the apical vessels are under some tension and a minor degree of pulpal hyperaemia commonly occurs. This is normally reversible, with no symptoms or long-term damage. However, if the pulp is already fibrotic with a poor blood supply, for instance following a previous blow to the tooth, orthodontic movement may strangulate the vessels and finally devitalize the already moribund pulp. The tooth will frequently become discoloured and this will be attributed to the orthodontic treatment. The teeth most commonly affected are, of course, the upper incisors, particularly in Class II, division 1 cases in view of their susceptibility to trauma. The patient may volunteer no history of an accident and may not even remember it. This makes it very important to examine the upper incisors carefully at the time of diagnosis. Enamel fractures, cracks or discoloration all indicate that a vitality test should be performed, and the radiograph should be inspected particularly carefully for root fractures, failure of apical closure or periapical radiolucencies. If the tooth is non-vital, it must be satisfactorily root-treated before tooth movement is commenced.

The decision is more difficult in the case of a diminished vitality response. The danger of moving such a tooth is that the pulp may die and the crown may well become discoloured. On the other hand, the patient will be reluctant to have root treatment for a symptomless tooth. Clearly the problem must be discussed with the patient and parent, and if the tooth's vitality response is appreciably diminished, root treatment should be advised.

MECHANISMS OF TOOTH MOVEMENT

All movements can be described in terms of rotations and translations. We shall deal here only with the small initial tooth movements that occur within the periodontal space. Clearly the larger, longer-term movements are the result of a succession of such minor movements, depending on the pattern of socket remodelling; and these too can be described in terms of rotation and translation. However, these may have been achieved by widely different pathways and so any biomechanical description may be more misleading than helpful.

Although for the purposes of illustration, forces and moments are often discussed in quantitative terms, orthodontic appliances cannot be used with this degree of precision. The clinician should be aware of the general range of forces he applies to the teeth, and of the mechanical properties of his appliances, but the effectiveness of a force delivery system is judged by its results; if a tooth is tipping too much as it is retracted with a fixed appliance, the couple will be increased or the force will be reduced at the next visit of the patient. A sound background knowledge is important so that the appliance can be designed and activated in an informed manner and so that if the tooth movement is not as intended, an intelligent correction can be made to the force system.

When a simple force is applied to a single point on a tooth surface, it can be resolved into two components—one perpendicular to the surface at the point of contact and the other tangential to the surface. Unless care is taken in adjusting the spring correctly, unexpected and unwanted tooth movements may occur (*see Fig.* 15.2, p. 205).

The centre of resistance to movement lies at about 40 per cent of the root length from the apex in a single-rooted tooth, and just apical to the furcation of most multi-rooted teeth. When the line of action of the force passes through the centre of resistance, the tooth will be translated in the direction of the force vector, but otherwise it will tip. The further from the centre of resistance the force vector, the greater its tipping moment will be.

The moment is calculated as the product of the force and its distance from the fulcrum. If we look at a tooth in cross-section, it is apparent that rotation can be induced when the force vector does not pass through the long axis. This is not an effective method of producing a controlled rotation but it is a common side-effect when, for example, a palatal canine retractor is adjusted incorrectly (*see Fig.* 15.2).

If translation of the tooth is required and the force vector does not pass through the centre of resistance, a mechanical couple has to be applied to the crown in order to counter the rotational effect of the moment. A controlled couple is very difficult to apply with a removable appliance, but is readily generated by a fixed appliance (*see Fig*. 16.1, p. 225). It is evident intuitively, and can be demonstrated mathematically, that the ratio between the couple and the force determines the nature of the tooth movement. The forces generated by any orthodontic appliance must be in static equilibrium, otherwise the appliance would not be stable. At the simplest level, for example when canines are retracted with a removable appliance, there is an equal and opposite forward force that is resisted by the anchorage. Within even a simple fixed appliance, the force system can be very complex indeed, and as the tooth moves, the forces change. It is neither possible nor is it necessary to analyse the forces within every fixed appliance in detail, however, it is essential to understand the general principles so that appliances can be designed and activated in a way that will produce the intended tooth movements without unexpected side reactions. If treatment does not progress as planned, the reasons must be analysed and corrective action instituted. This can be done only by careful monitoring of tooth movements and with an appreciation of the biomechanical principles of fixed appliances. Horizontal and vertical forces are always balanced by equal and opposite forces of reaction, and couples can be resolved into horizontal and vertical components with corresponding forces of reaction.

FORCES FOR THE MOVEMENT OF TEETH

It is generally agreed that 'light' forces should be used to move teeth. A light force is one which does not produce hyalinized areas in the periodontal ligament for that type of tooth movement. The division between 'light' and 'heavy' forces depends on many factors, including the root length and shape, the characteristics of the periodontal ligament and the nature of the tooth movement. It is neither possible nor necessary to calculate the appropriate force to be applied from first principles. Empirical clinical and histological evidence suggest that a force of 30 g applied to the crown of a single rooted tooth is appropriate for tipping movements, and that more than 100 g can be used for bodily movements.

Although early tooth movement will be delayed by areas of hyalinization, the rapid movement subsequent to their resorption may mean that progress is similar with both levels of force. Clinical experiments have shown that the rate of tooth movement is not consistently greater with light or heavy forces, even on the opposite sides of the same mouth.[20]

The importance of light forces rests not with the rate of tooth movement but with the undesirable side effects of heavy forces:

1   Where large forces are used with intra-oral appliances, anchorage control becomes difficult. It is possible to dissipate all the space required for correction of the malocclusion by unplanned movement of anchor teeth. For example, when a removable appliance is used to retract upper canines following extraction of first premolars, it is only too easy to lose all the space in this way. Where extra-oral anchorage is used, this danger is reduced or eliminated.

2   Control of tooth movement becomes difficult because fixed appliance

archwires are not stiff enough to counter the tipping moment created by large forces. For example, where teeth are moved along an archwire, excessive tipping and 'dumping' may occur, even with wide brackets, due to flexion of the archwire. The mechanical properties of sectional archwires are particularly unsatisfactory when they are activated excessively.

3   Large forces make the teeth tender, and the risks of root resorption and damage to the pulpal vessels are increased.

4   When removable appliance components are activated excessively, the patient may have difficulty in inserting the appliance correctly. For example, canine retraction springs may be positioned distal to, rather than mesial to, the teeth.

REFERENCES

1. Weinstein S., Haack D. C., Morris L. Y. et al. (1963) On an equilibrium theory of tooth position. *Angle Orthodont.* **33**; 1–26.
2. Yettram A. L., Wright K. W. and Houston W. J. B. (1977) Centre of rotation of a maxillary central incisor under orthodontic loading. *Br. J. Orthodont.* **4**; 23–7.
3. Rygh P. (1973) Ultrastructural changes of the periodontal fibres and their attachment in rat molar periodontium incident to orthodontic tooth movement. *Scand. J. Dent. Res.* **81**; 467–80.
4. Kurihara S. and Enlow D. H. (1980) An electron microscopic study of attachments between periodontal fibres and bone during alveolar remodelling. *Am. J. Orthodont.* **77**; 516–31.
5. Bassett C. A. L. and Becker R. O. (1962) Generation of electric potentials by bone in response to mechanical stress. *Science (New York)* **137**; 1063–4.
6. Davidovitch Z., Finkelson M., Steigman S. et al. (1980) Electric currents, bone remodelling and orthodontic tooth movement. I. The effect of electric currents on periodontal cyclic nucleotides. II. Increase in rate of tooth movement and periodontal cyclic nucleotide levels by combined force and electric current. *Am. J. Orthodont.* **77**; I, 14–32; II, 33–47.
7. Norton L. A., Hanley K. J. and Turkewicz J. (1984) Bioelectric perturbations of bone. Research directions and clinical applications. *Angle Orthodont.* **54**; 73–87.
8. Sandy J. R. and Harris M. (1984) Prostaglandins and tooth movement. *Eur. J. Orthodont.* **6**; 175–82.
9. Yamasaki K., Shibata Y., Imai S., et al. (1984) Clinical application of prostaglandin E upon orthodontic tooth movement. *Am. J. Orthodont.* **85**; 508–18.
10. Rygh P. (1974) Elimination of hyalinized periodontal tissues associated with orthodontic tooth movement. *Scand. J. Dent. Res.* **82**; 57–73.
11. Erikson B. E., Kaplan H. and Aisenberg M. (1945) Orthodontics and transeptal fibres. *Am. J. Orthodont. Oral Surg.* **31**; 1–20.
12. Reitan K. (1959) Tissue rearrangement during retention of orthodontically rotated teeth. *Angle Orthodont.* **29**; 105–13.
13. Edwards J. G. (1968) A study of the periodontium during orthodontic rotation of teeth. *Am. J. Orthodont.* **54**; 441–61.
14. Ten Hoeve A. and Mulie R. M. (1976) The effect of anteroposterior incisor repositioning on the palatal cortex as studied with laminography. *J. Clin. Orthodont.* **10**; 804–22.
15. Thilander B., Nyman S., Karring T. et al. (1983) Bone regeneration in alveolar bone dehiscences related to orthodontic tooth movements. *Eur. J. Orthodont.* **5**; 105–14.
16. Zachrisson B. V. and Alnaes L. (1974) Periodontal condition in orthodontically treated and untreated individuals. II. Alveolar bone loss: radiographic findings. *Angle Orthodont.* **44**; 48–55.
17. Linge B. O. and Linge L. (1983) Apical root resorption in upper anterior teeth. *Eur. J. Orthodont.* **5**; 173–83.
18. Goldson L. and Henrikson C. O. (1975) Root resorption during Begg treatment. A longitudinal roentgenologic study. *Am. J. Orthodont.* **68**; 55–66.
19. Rygh P. (1977) Orthodontic root resorption studied by electron microscopy. *Angle Orthodont.* **47**; 1–16.
20. Andreasen G. F. and Zwanziger D. (1980) A clinical evaluation of the differential force concept as applied to the edgewise bracket. *Am. J. Orthodont.* **78**; 25–40.

Chapter 15

Removable Appliances

Removable appliances are well suited to the treatment of simple malocclusions where teeth have to be tipped about a fulcrum close to the middle of the root. Good results can be obtained in suitable cases, but experience and careful case selection are required if they are to be used to maximum advantage. They can be used by the general dental practitioner and they require little surgery time. However, they are not suitable for the treatment of complex cases requiring bodily movement of teeth, and they are not well tolerated in the lower arch, because they encroach on the tongue space. The general practitioner should not become involved in treatment of cases that are beyond the scope of removable appliances, or of his expertise: it is only too easy to maltreat a case so that the malocclusion becomes more complex than previously and the patient is worse off than before.

REMOVABLE APPLIANCE DESIGN

In designing a removable appliance four components should be considered in sequence: active, retentive, anchorage and baseplate. Some components may contribute to more than one function: for example, clasps may be used for both retention and anchorage. A very large number of removable appliance designs have been suggested, and each practitioner will adopt the patterns that suit his approach. The concern of the present text is to illustrate the general principles of design by reference to specific components that have proved to be reliable in clinical practice, while recognizing that alternative methods may be equally satisfactory.

ACTIVE COMPONENTS

These may be grouped broadly as springs and bows, screws and elastics.

Springs and Bows

These are made from hard-drawn stainless steel wire. Removable appliance springs are generally variations of the cantilever spring (*Fig.* 15.1) modified according to local requirements. The force (F) delivered for a given deflection (d) depends upon the wire length (l) and radius (r) and elastic modulus (E) according to the formula:

$$F \alpha \ \frac{Edr^4}{l^3}$$

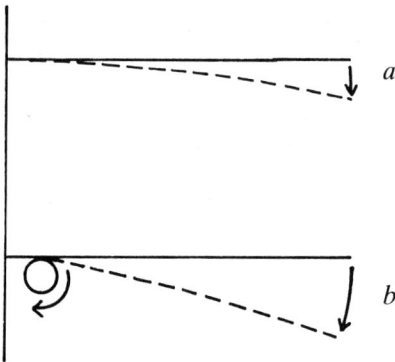

Fig. 15.1. Cantilevered springs. a, A simple cantilever. The deflection for a given load is proportional to the third power of the length of the spring and inversely to the fourth power of its diameter. b, The incorporation of a coil increases the effective length of the spring. For maximum resilience, the coil should be 'wound up' when the appliance is inserted and 'unwound' as the tooth moves.

From this it is apparent that small variations in the length and radius of the wire have a major effect upon its stiffness. Doubling the radius increases the stiffness by a factor of 16, while doubling its length reduces the stiffness by a factor of 8. In most circumstances, the force used to produce a simple tipping movement of a single-rooted tooth should be in the region of 25–50 g (see Chapter 14). It is convenient to have a spring deflection of 2–4 mm so that it is manageable by the patient but the force does not drop off too rapidly as the tooth moves: too large a deflection makes it difficult to insert the appliance correctly, and a very small deflection, of for example only 1 mm, means that by the time the tooth has moved half of that distance, the force has declined by 50 per cent.

The elastic modulus of wires generally used in removable orthodontic appliances varies little and spring length is constrained by the space available in the mouth. The most important factor determining the characteristics of a particular design of spring is thus the diameter of the wire selected. In most circumstances wire 0.5–0.7 mm in diameter will be used for the spring, but it should be noted that the selection of 0.7 mm rather than 0.5 mm wire for a particular spring will increase its stiffness four-fold.

In addition to its load/deflection characteristics, the stability of the spring needs to be taken into account. If the spring is guarded by the baseplate or supported by a stiffer component, this may not be a serious problem, but where the spring has to be self-supporting, as in certain designs of buccal canine retractor (see Fig. 15.5), there may have to be a compromise between stability and stiffness and so the properties of the spring are not entirely satisfactory in either respect. For optimal load/deflection characteristics the spring would be made in 0.5 mm diameter wire, but it would then be so unstable vertically that it would not function satisfactorily. Accordingly, it is made from 0.7 mm wire, which improves the stability to a limited extent but makes the spring so stiff that for a buccal spring of average dimensions, a deflection of just 1 mm will generate a force of 75 g! This is not entirely satisfactory.

Stability Ratio

These problems highlight the necessity of taking account of spring stability when designing an appliance. The stability ratio is *the stiffness in the direction* of *unwanted displacement* divided by *the stiffness in the intended direction of tooth movement*. This ratio should be as high as possible, and at least 1. A simple cantilever spring is equally flexible in all directions of bending and so has a stability ratio of 1 when unsupported, but generally this will be increased by support from the baseplate. The typical unsupported buccal canine retraction spring has a stability ratio of less than 1 and it is very liable to be displaced by lips or cheeks, or by its action on a sloping surface. This design is rather unsatisfactory and alternative patterns (*see Fig.* 15.5) will be found to be preferable in terms of both stiffness and stability ratio.

Coils

Most removable appliances incorporate coils. These increase the effective length of the spring, reducing its stiffness. For the maximal effect, they should be made reasonably large (a diameter of about 2.5 mm is satisfactory) and be placed close to the attachment point of the spring (*see Fig.* 15.1). For small deflections, the direction in which the coil is loaded does not affect its stiffness, but it is important in its resilience: a coil spring loaded in the direction of its formation (*see Fig.* 15.1) has an enhanced resistance to permanent deformation.

Point of Contact

When a tooth is contacted by a spring at a single point, it will move in the direction of the resultant force, which is perpendicular to the tangent at the point of contact with the tooth (*Fig.* 15.2). Thus, great care must be taken to ensure that the spring is positioned and adjusted to move the tooth in the direction required: this should be considered at design stage. For example, when a

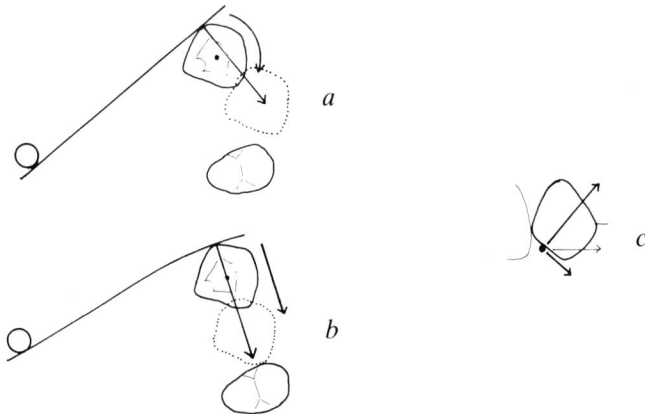

Fig. 15.2. The design of a cantilever spring. The force applied to the tooth is perpendicular to the tangent at the point of contact. *a*, It is a common mistake to have the contact of the spring on the tooth too far palatally. This means that the tooth will not move along the line of the arch but will be deflected bucally. Particularly with an upper canine, the force may also pass laterally to the centre of resistance of the tooth, setting up a mechanical couple which will rotate the tooth. *b*, The coil of the spring should be centred on the line through the midpoint of the tooth and perpendicular to its intended path. Generally the spring should be cranked so that the point of contact with the tooth is positioned sufficiently bucally. *c*, If the spring acts on a sloping surface, an intrusive component may interfere with the eruption of the tooth; and the component along the tooth surface will make the spring unstable.

buccally positioned canine is to be moved distopalatally into the line of the arch, a palatal spring is not suitable and will tend to move the tooth further buccally and perhaps even to rotate it (*Fig*. 15.2). Even if the canine is in the line of the arch, it is very easy to produce unwanted tooth movements if the spring is designed or adjusted carelessly.

Spring Design

SPRINGS FOR MESIAL AND DISTAL TOOTH MOVEMENTS

Palatal springs: Where the tooth is in the line of the arch a palatal cantilever spring is indicated: design principles are shown in *Fig*. 15.2. If the tooth is to be moved over an appreciable distance, the spring should be cranked to ensure the correct point of contact with the tooth. The coil is positioned so that it is 'wound up' when the appliance is inserted. The spring will usually be made from 0.5 mm diameter wire, giving a stiffness of about $15\,g\,mm^{-1}$ for a spring 1.75 cm long. Stability of the spring is helped by boxing in by the baseplate (*Fig*. 15.3). The incorporation of a guard wire on the palatal aspect of the spring (*Fig*. 15.4), so that it acts in a slot between guard and baseplate, enhances the stability further; but care must be taken to ensure that it can still move freely.

Detailed adjustment to ensure a correct contact between spring and tooth is undertaken first. The spring is then activated, typically by 2–3 mm. This is done in the free arm of the spring, not at its point of emergence from the baseplate

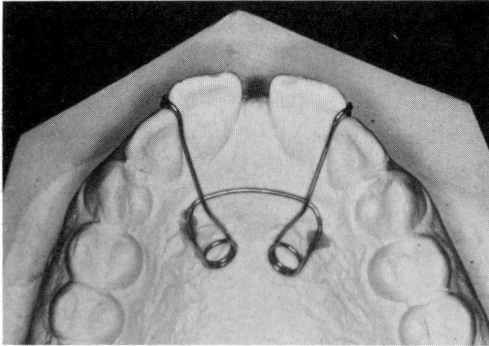

Fig. 15.3. Springs to move central incisors mesially.

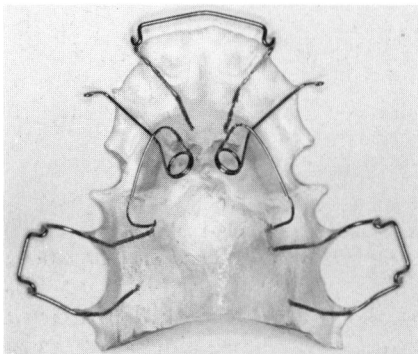

Fig. 15.4. Palatal springs to retract upper canines. A guard wire lies between the springs and the palate. This helps to protect them from distortion when the appliance is inserted and removed. The 'boxing' by the baseplate and the guard wire both stabilize the spring. It is important that the spring acts freely in the slot between the guard wire and base plate.

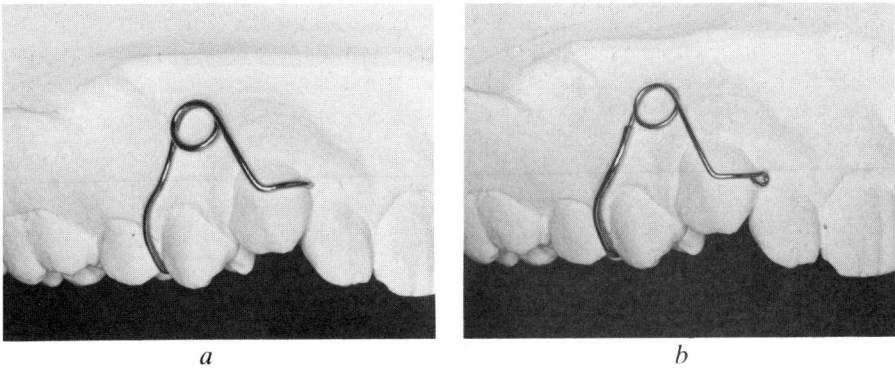

a   *b*

Fig. 15.5. Buccal canine retraction springs. *a*, A self-supporting buccal spring in 0·7 mm wire. Note that this design controls the position of the tooth buccolingually as well as mesiodistally. This type of spring is very stiff and has a poor stability ratio (it is more flexible vertically than anteroposteriorly). *b*, A supported buccal spring of 0·5 mm wire supported in tubing. This has a better stability ratio and is at the same time more flexible than the spring in (*a*).

where it is more liable to fracture due to work-hardening and stress concentration.

Buccal springs: These have to be used where a tooth is to be moved palatally as well as distally. They are often uncomfortable for the patient, their stability tends to be poor and they can be difficult to adjust. The classic design made from 0.7 mm wire (*Fig.* 15.5*a*) is unsatisfactory in all these respects. The supported design (*Fig.* 15.5*b*) is more stable, less stiff and is easier to adjust. All these designs are liable to be uncomfortable for the patient and to cause traumatic ulceration if they are extended too far into the buccal sulcus. The problem is that if they are not high enough, they are excessively stiff and have a very limited range of adjustment. However, other designs of buccal spring, of which there are many, tend to be even less satisfactory.

It will be noted that in these springs the coil is the wrong way round for maximal resilience. This is a minor disadvantage, but a coil made the 'correct' way round is more liable to be uncomfortable for the patient.

Self-supporting springs in particular are very stiff and should be adjusted by only a small amount (about 1 mm). Buccal springs are activated by inserting the round beak of a pair of spring-forming pliers into the coil and bending the anterior limb further round the beak. Palatal activation is in the anterior limb. Supported springs must *not* be adjusted where they emerge from the tubing, as they are most liable to fracture at this point.

SPRINGS FOR MOVING TEETH BUCCALLY

Incisors: Cranked (*Fig.* 15.6) or double cantilever springs (*Fig.* 15.7) are used most commonly. The spring is designed to be clear of other teeth throughout its action. Cranked springs have the point of attachment as far forwards as possible so that they remain in contact with the tooth for the entire movement. Even

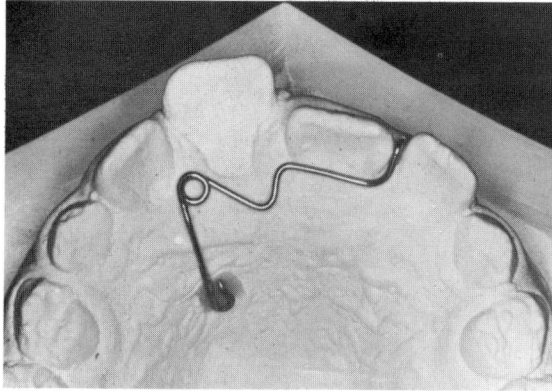

Fig. 15.6. A cranked palatal finger spring. The crank keeps the spring clear of the correctly positioned central incisor. If the teeth were not spaced, the free end of the spring would be recurved palatally. Note that the coil is positioned as far anteriorly as possible.

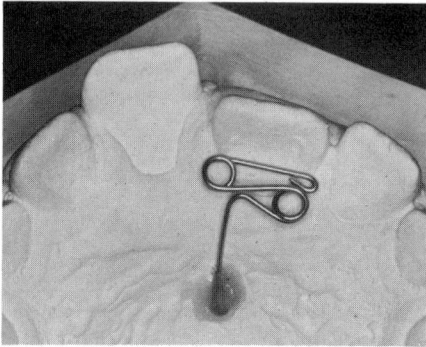
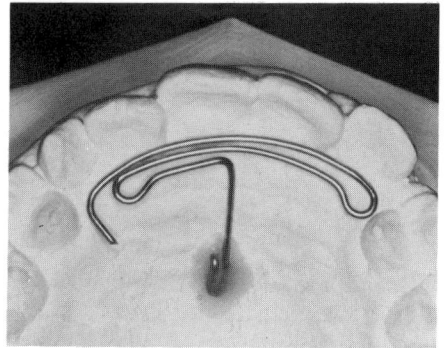

a   *b*

Fig. 15.7. Double cantilever or Z springs. *a*, On a single tooth. On a narrower tooth such as a lateral incisor, the springs are stiff and have a rather poor stability ratio. *b*, A double cantilever spring on four teeth. It is not necessary to incorporate coils as there is already a sufficient length of wire in the spring.

when the tooth has moved away from the baseplate, the spring is still supported by it and so stability is not a problem. The double cantilever spring is satisfactory if it can be made of sufficient width—as when two or more teeth are to be moved labially. When used on a single, narrow tooth, it tends to be rather stiff and if the tooth has to be moved an appreciable distance from the baseplate, it tends to be unstable. For moving several incisor teeth labially, crossed cantilever springs (*Fig.* 15.8) can be useful.

Buccal teeth: A cantilever spring can be difficult for the patient to insert correctly and so, while a cranked finger spring can be used, a self-positioning T spring (*Fig.* 15.9) is often more satisfactory. This works most effectively on a tooth such as a premolar or molar with a rather vertical palatal surface.

The spring is constructed from 0.5 mm wire and care should be taken that it

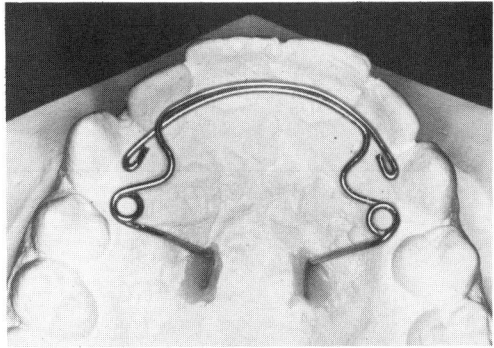

Fig. 15.8. Crossed cantilever springs are an effective way of proclining all four upper incisor teeth.

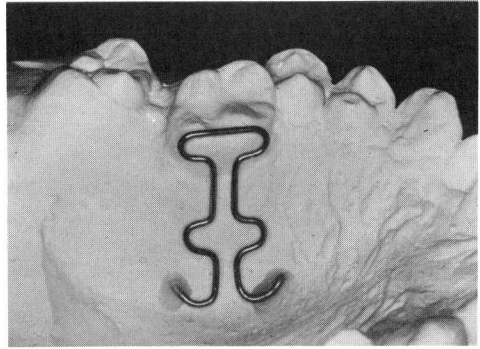

Fig. 15.9. A T spring to move a molar bucally. These are also effective on premolars and canines. The adjustment loops allow the spring to be extended as the tooth moves. Note that the spring is constructed to lie well clear of the palatal mucosa.

stands clear of the palatal mucosa so that it does not dig in as the tooth moves. If appreciable tooth movement is required, adjustment loops should be incorporated to allow the spring to be lengthened (*Fig.* 15.9). It is activated by pulling it away from the baseplate, though not too far as it is difficult to bend it back again.

Where a canine needs to be extruded as well as moved buccally, as is often the case following surgical exposure, it is best to bond an attachment to the tooth, into which a removable appliance spring can fit (*see Fig.* 16.20).

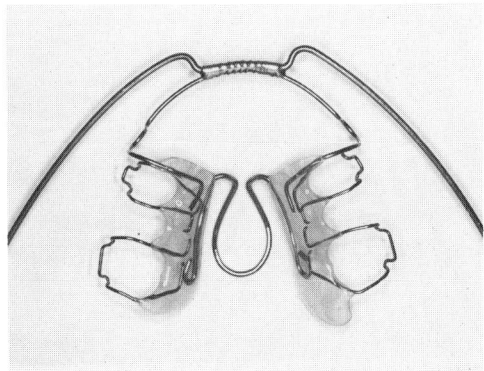

Fig. 15.10. A Coffin spring in an 'en masse' appliance designed to retract the upper buccal segments. Small pits in the acrylic allow the amount of expansion of the appliance to be checked with dividers.

Transverse expansion: As an alternative to a screw plate (*see Fig.* 15.17), a Coffin spring may be used (*Fig.* 15.10). This is constructed from 1.25 mm wire and has the advantage that differential expansion of the arch, anteriorly and posteriorly, is possible. These springs are cheaper and less bulky than screws but, unless they are well made and correctly adjusted, the appliance may be rather unstable.

Pits drilled into the baseplate allow the initial width of the appliance to be checked with callipers. The spring is expanded anteriorly first, then posteriorly by pulling it apart, care being taken not to twist the appliance. This is easier and quicker than adjustment with pliers. An expansion of 2–3 mm will generally be appropriate.

SPRINGS TO MOVE INDIVIDUAL TEETH PALATALLY The amount of movement is generally quite small and self-supporting buccal springs in 0.7 mm wire are satisfactory (*Fig.* 15.11).

BOWS FOR INCISOR RETRACTION As with buccal canine springs, the problem is

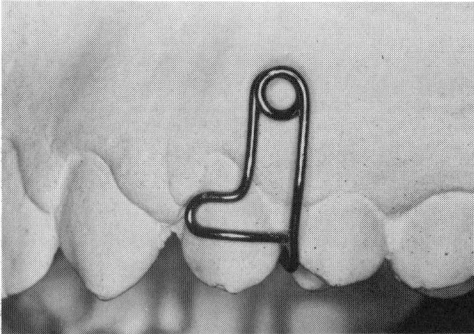

a

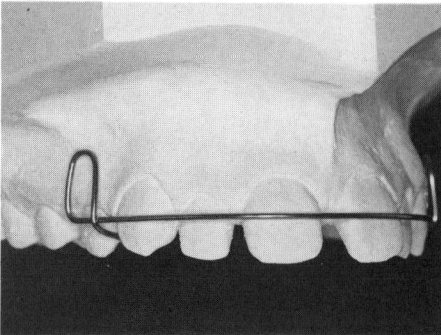

Fig. 15.11. A self-supporting spring to move a tooth palatally.

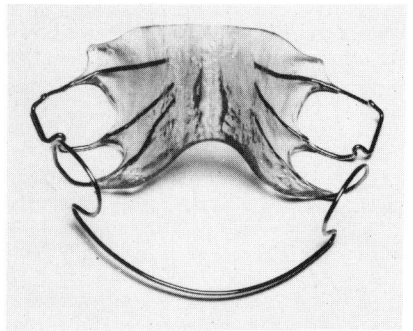

a   *b*

Fig. 15.12. *a*, A labial bow with reverse loops. This is too stiff for effective incisor retraction and the stability ratio is poor (it tends to slide up proclined incisors). It can be used for retaining tooth positions and for minor tooth movements. *b*, A labial bow with large C loops is more flexible but still has a poor stability ratio.

a   *b*

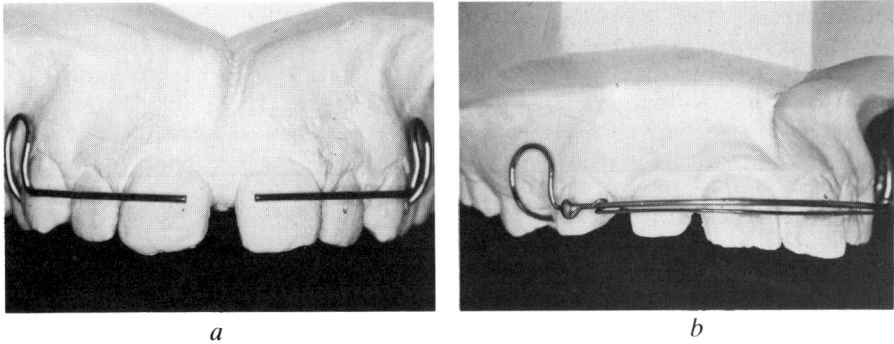

Fig. 15.13. Modifications to a labial bow for incisors retraction. *a*, Splitting the bow reduces the stiffness. *b*, A 0·4 mm wire can be attached to the bow. It tends to spring back to its passive straight form and so exerts a force on the teeth.

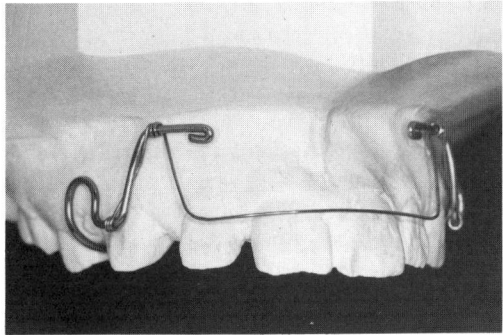

Fig. 15.14. A high labial bow with apron spring.

to design a retractor that will be flexible yet stable, and which will not be uncomfortable for the patient. Many bows in 0.7 mm wire have been devised but these have a poor stability ratio and are very stiff. They can be useful for minor adjustments to irregular teeth (*Fig.* 15.12) but are not really suitable for the reduction of large overjets. A 0.7 mm bow can be modified by splitting it (*Fig.* 15.13*a*) or by the addition of self-straightening wires (*Fig.* 15.13*b*). Both of these are light and flexible but it is very easy to flatten the labial segment too much,

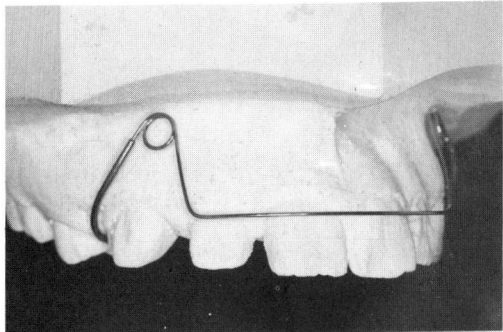

Fig. 15.15. A Roberts retractor.

and they have to be adjusted with care.

The supported incisor retraction bows are stable and flexible but are liable to break if they are adjusted incorrectly. The high labial bow with apron spring (*Fig.* 15.14) consists of a base arch in 1.0 mm wire with a 0.4 or 0.5 mm apron spring wound on. If the apron spring fractures, it can be rewound, although this requires some skill if it is to be done neatly. The Roberts retractor (*Fig.* 15.15) is an excellent retraction bow but is difficult to repair. However, provided care has been taken in its construction not to damage the wire, and provided that it is not adjusted where it emerges from the tubing support, fracture is not common.

Screws

The principle of the orthodontic screw (*Fig.* 15.16) is that its two ends are threaded in opposite directions so that when it is turned, the metal end plates move apart (or towards one another if a closing screw is to be used). Guide pins prevent the end plates from rotating and enhance appliance stability. Because the basic orthodontic screw is rigid, it can be adjusted by only a small amount at any one time, otherwise the appliance cannot be inserted. The teeth are displaced within the limits of the periodontal ligaments and bone remodelling allows them to move. The screw can then be adjusted again.

Typically one-quarter of a turn of the screw will separate the parts of the baseplate by 0.2 mm and the patient will be instructed to turn the screws by one-quarter turn each week. More frequent adjustment, of up to one-quarter of a turn every 3 days, is sometimes possible with children, but care must be taken not to adjust the appliance too frequently or it will not seat fully and will become progressively more ill fitting.

Many different designs of screw are available. Some are spring-loaded, but it is questionable whether these are more effective than the conventional type. Others can hinge, allowing differential expansion anteriorly and posteriorly, which can be useful in the treatment of cleft palate patients (*see* Chapter 20). Heavy duty screws are used for rapid maxillary expansion (p. 162). Spring pin screws are available for the labial movement of individual teeth.

Although screw plates can be designed to undertake many of the tooth movements that can be achieved with springs, the latter are generally cheaper,

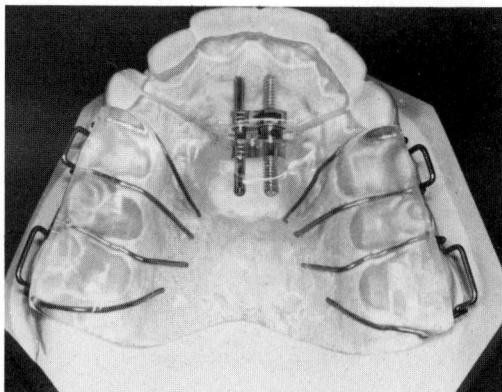

Fig. 15.16. Screw plate to correct a Class III incisor relationship. If retention is a problem, a clasp on the central incisors can be incorporated on the anterior segment. Posterior bite planes free the occlusion.

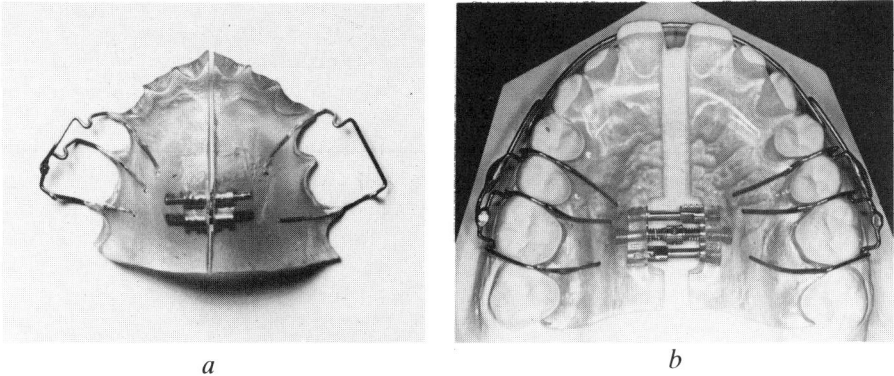

a   *b*

Fig. 15.17. *a*, A screw plate to expand the upper arch. It is usually advisable to incorporate posterior bite planes to clear the occlusion so that the lower arch is not expanded at the same time. Note the different patterns of clasping that can be used to ensure adequate retention where the first permanent molars alone do not give adequate retention. These avoid bringing wires from clasps on adjacent teeth across the same embrasure. *b*, A screw plate to contract the upper arch. The appliance is made with the screw expanded. Buccal wires must contact all the teeth to be moved palatally otherwise they will be left behind.

less bulky and more adaptable. Screws are useful in anteroposterior (*Fig.* 15.16) and transverse arch expansion (*Fig.* 15.17*a*) and in contracting a wide maxillary arch (*Fig.* 15.17*b*) because they enhance appliance stability, but even for these purposes many orthodontists prefer to use springs of suitable design.

Elastics

Rubber or latex rings are used with extra-oral traction (*see Fig.* 15.21) and to provide intra- and intermaxillary traction with fixed appliances (*see Fig.* 16.18). They are occasionally used as the intra-oral active component of a removable appliance, usually to retract upper or lower incisors (*Fig.* 15.18). They have the advantage of being inconspicuous and comfortable for the patient to wear. However, they tend to ride up the crown of the tooth and can cause serious gingival damage. If they are to be used for this purpose, it is desirable to bond

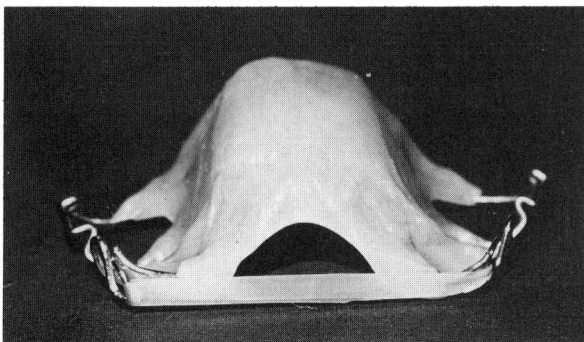

Fig. 15.18. An appliance with an elastic to retract upper incisors.

plastic brackets or composite 'blobs' on to the labial surfaces of the central incisors so that the elastic cannot slide gingivally. These should be at the same level on both central incisors, so that any intrusive effect acts on both teeth to the same extent. Ordinary 'rubber bands' obtainable from a stationery supplier are satisfactory for use with extra-oral traction, but latex elastics are preferred for intra-oral use. All elastics under tension exhibit some stress relaxation, and this is greater in the mouth due to water absorption. However, it is not great enough to be a serious problem with orthodontic appliances.

Elastics are available in various sizes and one should be selected which gives an appropriate loading. Fine adjustments can be made by altering the positions of the hooks to which they are attached. The patient is instructed to renew the elastics every few days or sooner if they break. More frequent change is unnecessary.

RETENTION

Adequate retention is essential because if the appliance is loose, the patient may have difficulty in wearing it. Adhesion between baseplate and oral mucosa contributes little to the retention of an orthodontic appliance, and this depends on clasps and bows.

The most successful clasp for retention of removable appliances is the Adams clasp (*Fig.* 15.19). The most useful undercuts for orthodontic appliances are at the mesiobuccal and distobuccal aspects of the teeth. In children the gingival margin may still cover these and it is necessary to trim the model before making the clasp (*Fig.* 15.19), so that it will slip into the gingival crevice and lie in the undercut when the appliance is fitted. In adults, the gingival margin may have receded so far that the undercut is excessively deep (*Fig.* 15.19). If the clasp is made to engage this fully, it will be too difficult for the patient to insert and remove the appliance, the clasp will have to be loosened and retention will then be poor. Thus, the clasp must be designed to lie just far enough into the undercut to give adequate retention.

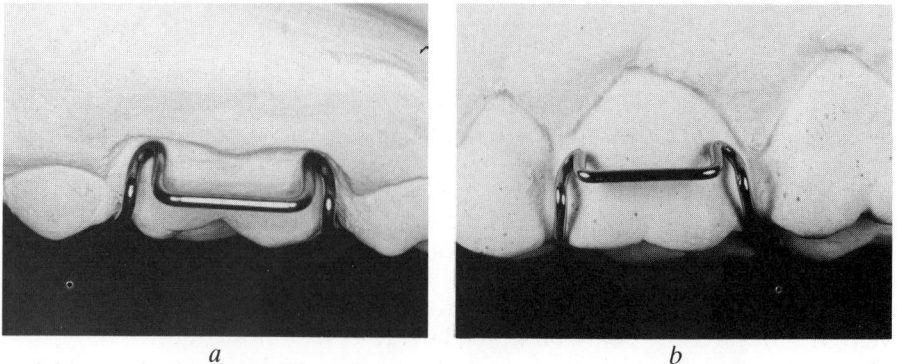

a   *b*

Fig. 15.19. Location of undercuts utilized by the Adams clasp. *a,* In a child, the undercuts may be beneath the gingival margin and so the model must be trimmed carefully to expose them. *b,* In an adult, the undercuts may be quite deep and the arrowhead of the clasp must be located at the correct level as shown.

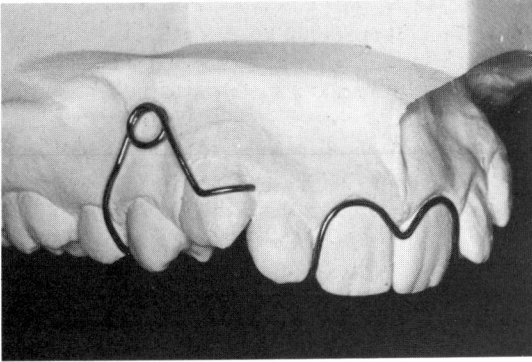

Fig. 15.20. A Southend clasp. This is tightened by pushing it in at the interdental crest.

The number of teeth clasped will depend on the factors tending to displace the appliance, and on the retention potential of the teeth. Where extra-oral traction is used, particularly with a neckstrap that exerts a downward component of force on the appliance (*see Fig.* 15.22), retention has to be excellent and more teeth should be clasped than would otherwise be necessary. If the teeth are rather conical in shape, with few undercuts, then more teeth may have to be used; excessive clasping should be avoided, and the retention should be distributed sensibly.

First permanent molars will usually be clasped and they alone will provide adequate retention for many appliances. If there is a tendency for the appliance to be displaced anteriorly, a clasp on the central incisors is very effective, although this cannot usually be used if these teeth are to be moved by the appliance.

The Southend clasp (*Fig.* 15.20) is preferred where incisors are to be used for retention. Stiff labial bows assist retention anteriorly, but unless they are also to serve another purpose, a Southend clasp will usually be found to be more effective and less obtrusive.

Clasps should be adjusted only when necessary, not as a matter of routine at every visit. When the appliance is seated, the clasp should be passive otherwise it can move the tooth palatally under the baseplate. This is most liable to occur when retention is poor due to lack of undercuts or poorly constructed clasps and the retention potential of the tooth will be diminished still further as it is tipped palatally. If retention is inadequate, attempts should be made to improve it by adjusting the clasp to lie correctly within the undercut; if this fails the appliance may have to be remade clasping other teeth. In some cases where no suitable undercuts are available, retention can be enhanced by fitting a band with a buccal attachment to the tooth, or by directly bonding a buccal attachment, or even just a composite 'blob', on to the buccal surface of the tooth.

Retention problems may be caused by springs, which tend to unseat the appliance—for example, a spring acting on a sloping surface. Extra-oral traction to a cervical strap tends to displace an appliance and if retention is in doubt, it is wiser to use headgear with an upward force vector (*see Fig.* 15.21).

ANCHORAGE

Anchorage is the source of resistance to the reaction from the active components. For example, if canines are to be retracted by springs, there is an equal and opposite force on the appliance which has to be resisted by the anchorage. This will tend to move the anchorage teeth by an amount which will depend on the forces used, the number of teeth incorporated in the anchorage and their resistance to movement.

In some circumstances movement of anchorage teeth is desirable. For example, when the upper arch is to be expanded bilaterally to correct a crossbite, each side acts as anchorage for the other. This is called reciprocal anchorage, In other cases, limited movement of the anchor teeth is acceptable, as when extraction of premolars has provided excess space for retraction of canines and some forward movement of the posterior teeth is to be encouraged. Where space is at a premium, no movement of the anchor teeth is permissible. In these circumstances as many teeth as possible should be included in the anchorage and only a few teeth should be moved at any one time.

The greater the root area of the anchor teeth relative to the teeth to be moved, the more secure the anchorage. If teeth can be prevented from tipping, their anchorage value is increased. This is a measure commonly used with fixed appliances but is difficult to obtain with removable appliances. The forces applied to the teeth are very important. Light forces in the active components (25–50 g per single-rooted tooth) are sufficient, but when distributed over a larger number of anchor teeth they should fall below the threshold that appears to be necessary for rapid movement. Heavier forces generated by the active components will not move these teeth faster but, when distributed over the anchor teeth, may well be high enough to ensure their rapid movement. Where unacceptable movement of the anchorage teeth is occurring, or where it is decided that it would be unwise to risk even a small amount of movement of the anchor teeth, reinforcement with extra-oral traction is necessary.

Extra-oral Anchorage

Extra-oral anchorage can be used either as the sole anchorage to retract buccal segments with an 'en masse' appliance (see Fig. 15.10), or to reinforce intra-oral anchorage. Where buccal segments are to be retracted, appreciable forces have to be used (250–500 g per side depending upon what the patient will tolerate) and it is desirable to use headgear with a slightly upward directed force (Fig. 15.21) rather than a neckstrap (Fig. 15.22), which tends to displace the appliance. The headgear and appliance should be worn for 12–14 hours per 24 hour day. It is helpful in monitoring the response to treatment, and it encourages patient motivation, if they are asked to keep a record of wear and to produce it at each visit.

Where the extra-oral anchorage is used to supplement intra-oral anchorage, it should be adjusted to at least double the force generated by the active components and the headgear should be worn for 10 hours in 24. If anchorage control is not achieved, patient cooperation is suspect; the need for conscientious wear should be emphasized and the amount of wear is increased to 14 hours per day at least until control is reestablished.

While neck straps and headcaps can be made up from plastic or fabric tape, it

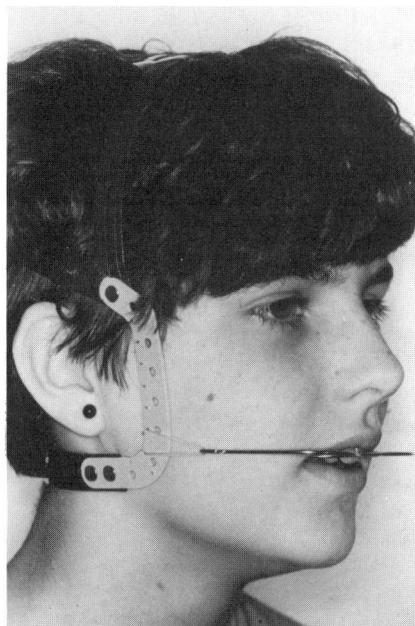

Fig. 15.21. A headcap used to provide anchorage to retract the upper buccal segments with a removable appliance. The direction of pull should be slightly above the occlusal plane so that it does not tend to displace the appliance. This Interlandi design of headcap provides a choice of attachment points for the elastics.

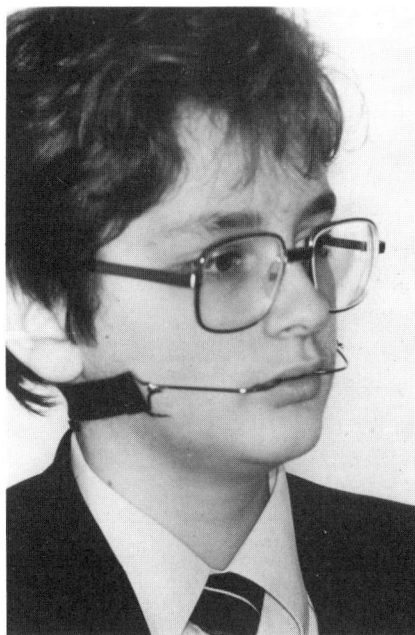

Fig. 15.22. A neckstrap used to reinforce anchorage with a removable appliance. This is less conspicuous than a headcap, but usually delivers a downward direction of traction which tends to displace a re-movable appliance.

is much more convenient to obtain them from an orthodontic supplier. They can be fitted in a few minutes, taking care to ensure that they are comfortable and do not rub on the ears. Many different designs are available and most are suitable for use with removable appliances. Select a type of headcap with a choice of attachment points for the elastics that will be connected to the face bow, so that the correct direction of traction can be assured (*Fig.* 15.21).

Extra-oral traction can be connected to the appliance anteriorly by J hooks which clip on to spurs or other attachments in the incisor or canine region (*Fig.* 15.23); or by a face bow which will usually slide into tubes on the molar clasps (*Fig.* 15.24). J hooks are liable to rub the angles of the mouth if they are not fitted correctly, and face bows are adjusted so that the outer bow stands just clear of the cheeks when the elastics are fitted. The cervical strap or headcap may be elasticated so that the J hooks or face bow can be attached to it directly, but better force control is possible with elastics. Elastics obtained from a stationery supplier are quite satisfactory for this purpose, or high quality latex elastics may be obtained from an orthodontic supplier. The gap to be bridged by the elastic should be about 5 cm. Too small a gap means that a very small elastic with little extensibility has to be used, while a large gap may mean that the elastic rubs the patient's cheeks.

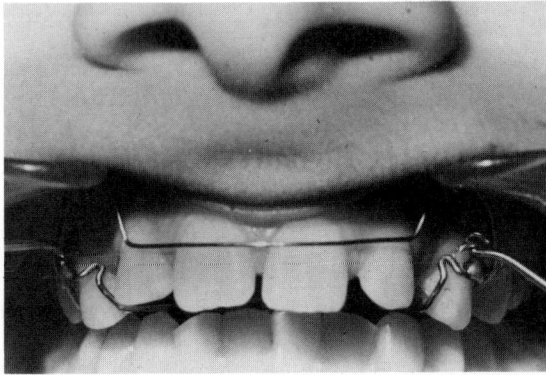

Fig. 15.23. J hooks attached to spurs on a removable appliance.

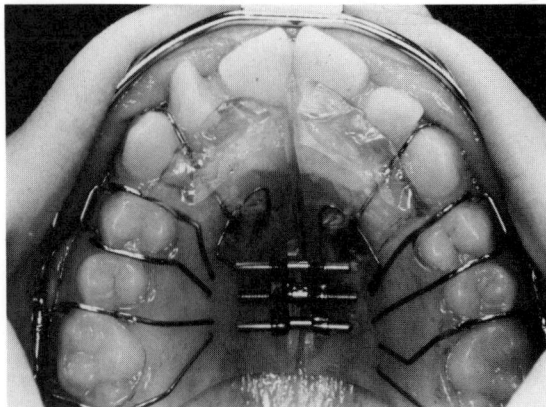

Fig. 15.24. A facebow engages in tubes soldered to clasps on a removable appliance.

J hooks and face bows are potentially dangerous to the patient or another child if they engage in horseplay and it is important that they, and their parents, are warned of this. Another child may be injured by the extra-oral hook and this danger can be minimized by finishing the hook neatly so that the end recurves. The J hook or face bow must never be removed from the mouth while still attached to the headgear, as there is a risk of its being released and lacerating the face or damaging the eyes.

BASEPLATE

The baseplate serves to hold together the other components of the appliance and may be built up into bite planes to clear the occlusal interferences or to help in overbite reduction. It contributes little to anchorage or retention in most appliances.

Scant attention is often paid to baseplate design but it is very important for patient comfort. A baseplate that is unduly bulky will be uncomfortable and may interfere with speech, while if it is incorrectly trimmed, it may allow food packing or hinder tooth movement.

The baseplate is made from acrylic. Clear acrylic is usually preferred by the patient and has the advantage that any areas of undue pressure can be detected by observing blanching of the palatal mucosa when the appliance is in the mouth. Cold-cured acrylic is used most commonly because it is simpler for the technician and there is no risk of thermal distortion. However, heat cured acrylic is appreciably stronger and its use is recommended for appliances with bite planes that will be loaded heavily, and for lower appliances which are weak in the section behind the incisors.

Undercuts are rarely a problem in fitting upper removable appliances for children, but in adults and in lower appliances they may interfere with the insertion and removal of the appliances. It takes only a few moments to survey a model and to block out undercuts that might be a problem, and this should be done as a matter of routine in these cases. Thus it should never be necessary to trim the baseplate in order to allow the appliance to be inserted.

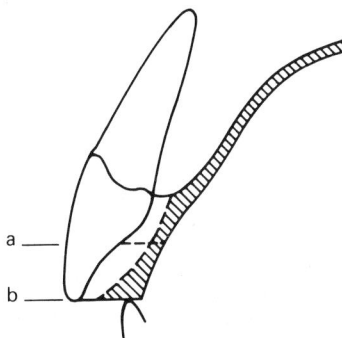

Fig. 15.25. Bite plane design. A bite plane built up to level (*a*) may clear the occlusion and initiate overbite reduction during canine retraction. However, a bite plane, to the level of the incisor edges (*b*) is required during incisor retraction to allow the appliance to be trimmed away from the upper incisors while maintaining control of the lower incisors.

Bite Planes

Bite planes are used to clear possible occlusal interference with tooth movement and to reduce overbites.

Anterior bite planes (*Fig.* 15.25) are used for the purposes mentioned above. Overbite reduction is obtained by accelerated dento-alveolar development of the lower buccal segments; the upper buccal segments are restrained by the appliance and little intrusion of the lower incisors is produced. This is tolerated in children and subsequent facial growth will catch up so that the height of the intermaxillary space is not affected permanently. Attempts to reduce overbites in adults with anterior bite planes are not usually successful because the lower buccal segments may not grow vertically when the appliance is fitted. Even if this does happen, the overbite will often relapse: the orofacial musculature may not adapt to the increased intermaxillary height and so the posterior teeth are intruded while the incisors slide past one another.

The bite plane should be just deep enough to engage the lower incisors: there is no advantage in encroaching further on the oral space. For complete overbite reduction, the bite plane will have to be level with the upper incisor edges (*Fig.* 15.25), but few patients can cope with this level immediately. Initially a bite plane to the mid-height of the upper incisors should be tolerated and either this can be raised progressively by layers of cold-cure acrylic at subsequent visits, or the next appliance can be constructed with a full-height bite plane.

Posterior bite planes (*Fig.* 15.16) are used to clear the occlusion where there is reverse overjet or where the overbite is tenuous and should not be reduced.

FITTING AND ADJUSTING REMOVABLE APPLIANCES

As with all routine tasks, appliance fitting and adjustment is completed more quickly and more reliably if a standard procedure is followed. The procedures for fitting and for subsequent adjustment of appliances are similar.

The Baseplate

First ensure that there are no blebs of acrylic on the fitting surface. These should have been removed by the technician. The thickness of the baseplate is also checked and it is trimmed down if it is too bulky. This will not be necessary if the technician has received clear instructions; the well-constructed appliance should fit immediately.

Difficulties in insertion are due to clasps carried too far into buccal undercuts, or failure to block out palatal or lingual undercuts on the model before the appliance was constructed. If the cause of the difficulty is not apparent immediately, bend the clasps back slightly in order to determine whether they are at fault. If there are undercuts on the baseplate, they are removed judiciously, taking particular care not to remove the edge of the acrylic at the polished surface where contact with the tooth must be maintained in order to avoid food packing and gingival hyperplasia. The clasps are now readapted.

Provided that the bite plane dimensions have been specified in the appliance prescription (*Fig.* 15.26), trimming will be minimal. Posterior bite planes are

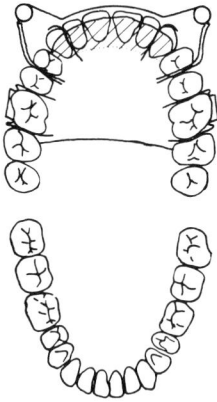

| PATIENT'S NAME | | LAB. No. |
| ORTHO. No. | **ORTHODONTIC DEPT.** | TECHNICIAN |

INSTRUCTIONS TO TECHNICIAN

Upper removable appliance to retract upper incisors.

1. Adams clasps 6|6

2. Stops 3|3

3. Roberts retractor

4. Anterior bite platform – level with lateral incisor edges – (Overjet = 8 mm)

| DATE OF IMPRESSION | DATE FOR FINISH | SURGEON'S SIGNATURE |

Form 304

Fig. 15.26. An appliance prescription must be clear and unambiguous in design specification.

adjusted so that the patient occludes evenly on both sides with just sufficient clearance to allow the required tooth movements. The bite plane may be perforated over molar cusps but this does not matter. Anterior bite planes are trimmed so as not to extend further back than necessary and to a level that the patient can cope with. If the lower incisor edges are at different heights, the bite plane is adjusted to allow at least three contacts and at subsequent visits it is flattened progressively by addition of acrylic.

Now the baseplate is trimmed to allow the teeth to move as intended. Acrylic is cut back as generously as possible so that the teeth will be free to move throughout the period between visits. If the tooth is too close to the baseplate, not only will its movement be impeded, but the gingivae will tend to pile up between tooth and baseplate, and this can be uncomfortable for the patient. Sometimes when one tooth is moved along the line of the arch, it is helpful to allow adjacent teeth to follow, and the baseplate should be trimmed to permit this.

Where incisors are to be retracted and there is an anterior biteplane, this will have to be cut back to allow the teeth to move, while maintaining contact with the lower incisors (*Fig.* 15.25). This is not possible if the bite plane is too low and it may first have to be built up with cold-cure acrylic.

Retention

Retention components should be adjusted only if this is necessary. If retention is still poor after the clasps have been adjusted correctly, it may be necessary to construct a new appliance to an improved design, possibly with extra clasps. It is quite unreasonable to expect a patient to wear an appliance that is unstable.

Anchorage

Anchorage is planned at the stage of appliance design and nothing has to be done when the appliance is fitted, unless extra-oral traction is to be used. The important points have already been mentioned and instructions to patients are discussed below.

Active Components

At the first visit these are adjusted only to a small extent. This is sufficient to initiate the tissue changes in the supporting structures and allows the patient to get used to the appliance. Full activation at the first visit may make the teeth tender and the patient may insert the appliance incorrectly (e.g. canine retraction springs may be incorrectly positioned distal, not mesial to the teeth).

Ensure that buccal springs and bows do not impinge on the gingivae or oral mucosa. Care should be taken not to damage the spring during the adjustment: if the wire is nicked with pliers, or if it is regularly adjusted at the same spot, subsequent fracture is more likely. This is also liable to happen if the spring is adjusted at the point of stress concentration where the wire emerges from the baseplate or from a supporting tube.

INSTRUCTION AND MOTIVATION

The clarity and conviction with which instructions on appliance wear are given can greatly influence subsequent cooperation. It is unreasonable to expect a patient to remember instructions that are given casually and without reinforcement. It is preferable to restrict the number of new instructions given on each visit to two or three, and so advice on oral hygiene and general information on the wear of appliances should be given on visits prior to fitting the appliance. Practical points, such as cleaning the teeth and appliance, and its insertion and removal, should be demonstrated to the patient and then practised under supervision in the surgery. The most effective way of conveying instructions to a child is to explain them simply and clearly, to check that they are understood and then ask the child to repeat them to the parent and demonstrate how the appliance is removed and inserted. This emphasizes that the primary responsibility for appliance care and wear is the patient's, and gives the parent the opportunity of asking for clarification of any points. Ideally, a leaflet containing the same instructions in writing should also be given to the parent.

The conviction and commitment of the dentist has an important effect on patient cooperation in appliance wear, particularly of headgear and functional appliances. Instructions given with confidence that the patient can and will wear the appliance as prescribed are much more effective than if the same information is given in a manner lacking conviction that the treatment is worth while or likely to be successful. Particularly with children wearing headgear and functional appliances, which should be worn for as many hours as possible but not full time, it is effective to give patients a target and ask them to keep a log book or chart of wear. This record of treatment progress is readily appreciated by the patient and can boost their interest and cooperation. At each visit, progress should be compared with the account of wear, and praise or reproach given according to the results. Obviously it is counter-productive to ask the patient to keep a record of wear but take no further interest in it; or to emphasize the need for full-time wear of the appliance but be unable to detect when this is not happening!

FOLLOW-UP VISITS

First chat to the patient, asking whether he or she has had any problems. Do not ask leading questions as to whether the appliance has been worn as instructed because almost inevitably the reply will be affirmative and it may then be difficult for the patient to retract this when clinical evidence suggests that the appliance has in fact not been worn correctly. Observe whether speech is affected by the appliance: most patients adapt to appliances within a few days, and if speech continues to be affected this may be a sign that the appliance is not worn full time.

A thorough inspection of the general oral condition, with the appliance removed, follows. Examine the oral mucosa for trauma or ulceration from the appliance and check the teeth for caries. The standard of oral hygiene is recorded and if it is not satisfactory, a bleeding index is estimated and recorded. Any deficiency in general oral care is discussed with the patient. A persistently poor standard of oral hygiene may necessitate abandonment of orthodontic appliance treatment,

The orthodontic review begins with an assessment of the changes that have occurred since the previous occasion. Whenever possible, measurements are taken and noted so that an objective record of progress can be obtained.

First check anchorage. Anchorage problems generally arise during retraction of teeth when the natural mesial drift tendency of the anchor teeth is increased. Provided that no active lower appliance is being worn, the lower arch can be used as a reasonably reliable reference against which to check the upper anchorage. Care must be taken to ensure that the lower jaw is in true centric relation when this is done: if the upper buccal teeth are coming forward, the patient may posture the mandible, masking a change in occlusal relationships and giving a misleading impression that nothing has altered. Where the upper incisors are not being retracted but the appliance contacts them palatally, a measurement of the overjet provides a simple record of anchorage stability. Where active appliance treatment is being carried out in the lower arch, and particularly if the lower incisors are contacted by the appliance, it is not easy to monitor anchorage and on occasions it may be necessary to obtain a lateral skull radiograph to check it.

Clearly if the anchorage is not stable, measures must be taken to control it. If the spring or bow has been activated too much, this is adjusted but if the problem lies with the anchorage, then reinforcement with headgear (or increased wear if it is already fitted) is necessary. Only when the anchorage has been checked can a reliable record of the intended tooth movements be obtained. If it is known that the anchor teeth are stable, measurements from them can be used to record the tooth movements. The landmarks selected for the measurement must be identifiable readily: cusp tips and buccal fissures are good landmarks, and the margins of fillings may also be used. It is best to obtain the measurement with dividers and then record it directly on the patient's notes by punching holes through the page. A comparison with previous measurements gives an indication of whether or not the teeth are moving at the rate anticipated. If the teeth have moved less than expected a series of points should be checked:

1   Are the teeth free to move? The baseplate, wirework or contact with opposing teeth may impede tooth movement.
2   Is the spring correctly activated? The spring (or bow) may be passive, or may be excessively active, and both faults may impede tooth movement.
3   Is there any reason to expect a slow rate of movement? Buccally placed teeth or 'necking' of the alveolar process may result in very slow movement because of the dense cortical bone surrounding the tooth. Provided that light forces are used, tooth movement will be progressive but slow.
4   Is the appliance being worn as instructed? The patient may position the spring incorrectly or the appliance may be left out. Even short periods of non wear may greatly delay progress.

Appliance Adjustment

Now it is time to adjust the appliance components, following the procedure outlined above.

Chapter 16
Fixed Appliances

Control of tooth movements is enhanced when appliances are fixed to the teeth. While removable appliances can only tip teeth, fixed appliances can produce any type of movement. By applying a mechanical couple of forces to the tooth crown in conjunction with a simple force, apical and bodily movements, as well as rotations, can be obtained (*Fig.* 16.1). Controlled intrusion and extrusion of teeth is also possible.

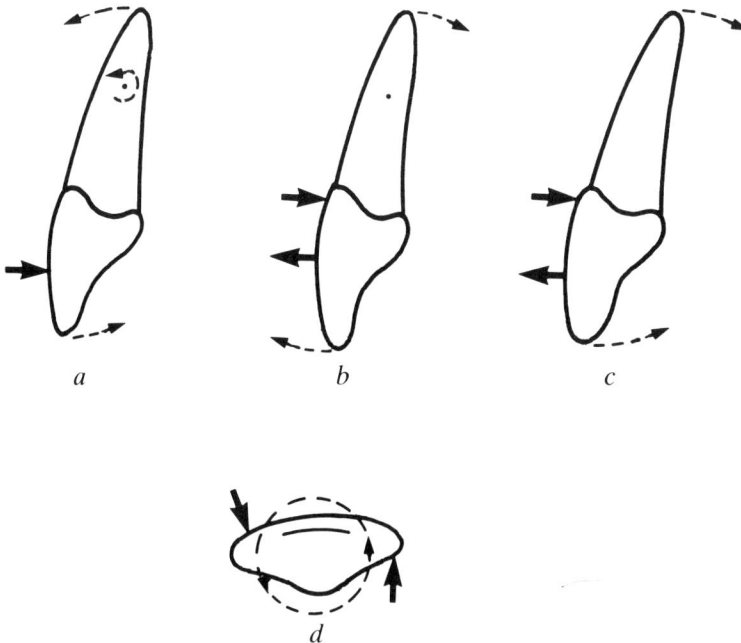

a   *b*   *c*

d

Fig. 16.1. Forces applied to teeth. *a*, A simple force applied to the crown of a single rooted tooth will tip it about a fulcrum within the root. *b*, A pure mechanical couple of equal forces in opposite directions applied to the crown of a tooth will tip it about a fulcrum within the root. *c*, An appropriate combination of a force plus a mechanical couple will move a tooth without rotation. *d*, Rotation of a tooth about its long axis will be produced by a pure couple applied in an appropriate manner to the crown.

COMPONENTS

The principal components of fixed appliances are attachments, archwires and auxiliaries. It is not possible to separate the active and anchorage components in fixed appliances because both these functions are served by the archwires and auxiliaries. However, in planning and monitoring treatment, anchorage and active tooth movements must be evaluated separately.

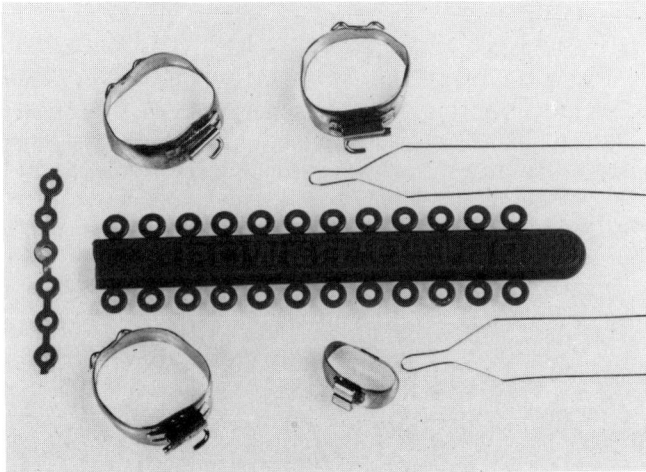

Fig. 16.2. Bands and brackets used in the edgewise technique together with different methods of fixation: wire ligatures, polyurethane rings on a dispenser and a polyurethane chain.

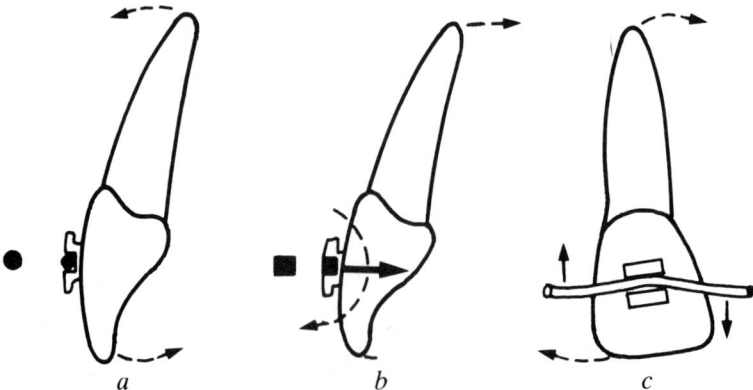

a   *b*   *c*

Fig. 16.3. Force systems used in the edgewise technique. *a*, Retraction of an incisor with a round wire generates no mechanical couple and so the tooth is free to tip. *b*, Retraction of an incisor with a rectangular wire: the fit of the wire in the bracket means that as the tooth tends to tip, this is constrained by the fit of the wire in the bracket. A mechanical couple is generated and so the tooth undergoes a translational movement. Play between wire and bracket or flexure in the archwire may allow some tipping to take place. *c*, If the bracket slot is not parallel to the archwire a mechanical couple will be generated which tends to move crown and root in opposite directions. If a force is applied to the crown so that it cannot move, only the root will move.

Attachments

The main attachments are brackets and tubes. Buttons and cleats may also be used in some situations. The different fixed appliance techniques are characterized by their attachments. For example, the brackets and tubes used in the edgewise technique and its variants have a rectangular channel, and the archwire is secured to the bracket by soft stainless steel ligatures or by plastic rings (*Fig.* 16.2). Round archwires are used in the initial stages of treatment but labiolingual movement of the tooth apices is achieved by rectangular archwires (*Fig.* 16.3).

In contrast, the bracket in the Begg technique is designed to allow free tipping of the teeth, both mesiodistally and labiolingually (*Fig.* 16.4). Round archwires are used and secured to the brackets by metal pins. Control of apical movement

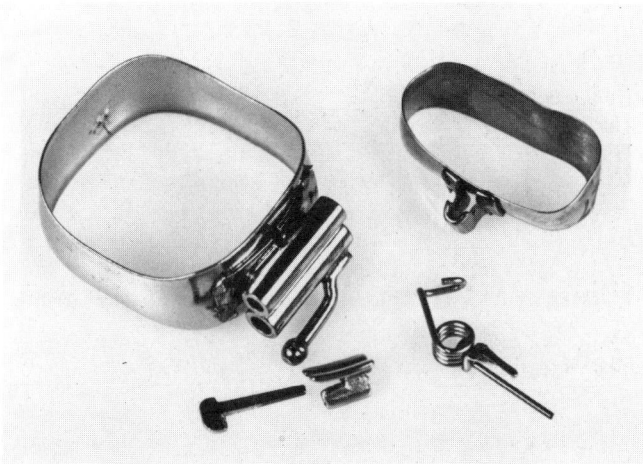

Fig. 16.4. Bands and attachments used in the Begg technique. Brass pins are used to hold the wire in the bracket slot. These can be replaced by uprighting springs in stage 3.

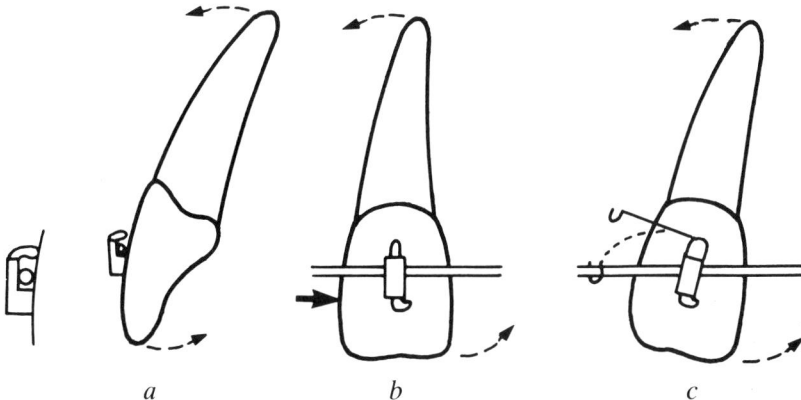

a   *b*   *c*

Fig. 16.5. Force systems in the Begg technique *a, b,* The round archwire fits loosely in the bracket slot allowing the tooth to tip freely. *c,* Auxiliary springs are used to generate mechanical couples so that controlled root movement can be undertaken.

is obtained by auxiliary springs (*Fig.* 16.5) rather than by the fit of the archwire and bracket.

Bonds

Attachments may be fixed to the teeth directly with composite resins following acid etching of the enamel surface (*see Fig.* 16.9). Chemically cured resins are generally used. The fitting surface of the bracket is designed to allow a mechanical locking with the composite resin because there is no chemical adhesion to stainless steel. The tooth surface is etched for about 45 seconds with phosphoric acid gel and is then washed, dried and primed with unfilled resin in order to protect the enamel from subsequent demineralization due to plaque. The attachment is fixed to the tooth with a small amount of the composite resin. It is very important that the attachment is positioned accurately and that excess resin is cleared away before it sets, otherwise it will encourage plaque accumulation and gingival irritation.

In ideal conditions modern filled composite resins are strong enough to withstand all orthodontic forces, including those of headgear. However, bond strength is reduced greatly if the tooth surface is not dry when the attachment is placed. In areas where moisture control is difficult, in particular in the lower buccal segments and upper molar regions, direct bonding may not be satisfactory. Some clinicians administer anti-sialagogues prior to bonding, but these are unpleasant for the patient. Most orthodontists prefer to use metal bands, to which the attachments are welded, in areas where moisture control is difficult (*see Fig.* 16.9).

Plastic brackets are available for direct bonding and these have the great merit of being inconspicuous. However, at the present time they are not rigid or strong enough for most uses: the fit with the archwire is not sufficiently precise and the wings are liable to fracture. For these reasons, most orthodontists continue to use metal brackets, although plastic brackets can be useful on the upper incisors in adults when only simple tooth movements are required.

Bands

The traditional method of fixing attachments is by welding them to metal bands which are then cemented to the teeth with zinc-oxyphosphate or similar cement. The cement not only holds the band in place, but prevents the formation of plaque between band and enamel. It is very important that the integrity of the cement is checked at every visit because if it leaches out, plaque will accumulate and serious enamel demineralization can occur rapidly.

While bands can be made up from stainless steel tape, preformed bands are much more convenient (*Fig.* 16.4). These are available in a wide range of sizes for each tooth and can be supplied with brackets already welded in place. The band must fit the tooth well so that the bracket is at the correct height on the tooth crown and so that the gap that must be filled with cement is minimal. Molar bands and the lingual aspects of premolar bands should fit into the gingival crevice so that there is no unprotected enamel. Elsewhere the bands should be sufficiently clear of the gingival margin to allow plaque control.

So that the bands can be placed accurately, the teeth have to be separated if

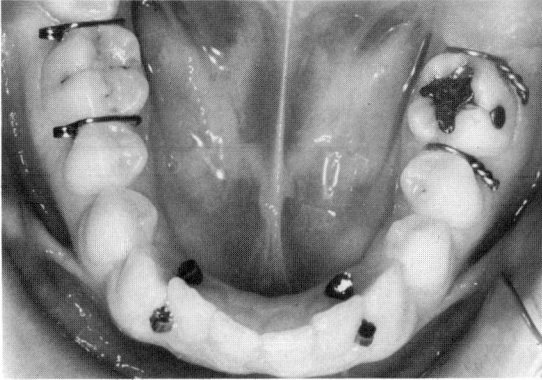

Fig. 16.6. Different methods of separating teeth; on the patient's left, brass ligature wire has been twisted tightly around the contact areas of the molar. Separating springs have been placed mesially and distally to the right molar: a short arm of the spring passes under the contact area and applies a separating force to the teeth. Elastic separating strips have been placed mesially to the lower canine teeth.

the contacts are tight. This can be done by 0.5 mm brass ligature wire tightened around the contact area, or by separating springs (*Fig.* 16.6), left in position for a few days. If it is necessary, incisor contacts can be separated by rubber strips cut from a broad elastic band and placed 1–2 hours before the bands are placed (*Fig.* 16.6). The patient can insert these on the day of the appointment for banding.

Bonds and Bands Compared

Direct bonding has a number of advantages over bands. The attachments can be positioned more precisely and more quickly than when bands are used. Teeth of unusual shape or that have not erupted fully can be bonded readily, whereas banding may be very difficult. Frequently teeth need to be separated prior to banding, which may entail an extra visit; and at the end of treatment band spaces have to be closed. Although the band material is not thick, the band space in each arch can amount to 3–4 mm and this is a disadvantage, particularly in cases where space is at a premium. Bands make the appliance more conspicuous. Thus the bonding of attachments is quicker, more precise and less stressful to the patient.

Bonding of attachments does, however, have some disadvantages. The most important of these is the need for excellent moisture control during bonding, which can sometimes be difficult. Removal of bonds and composite after treatment is tedious and more time-consuming than for bands. If plaque control is less than excellent, the enamel is more liable to be demineralized with bonded attachments: the bands themselves protect the most vulnerable areas of enamel, provided that the cement is intact, while plaque gathering interproximally and around bonded attachments results in rapid demineralization of the tooth surface. The risk can be minimized by ensuring that there is no excess resin around the attachments to encourage plaque accumulation, by sealing the labial surface of the enamel with resin following etching, and by insisting on a high standard of oral hygiene, backed up by fluoride mouth rinses.

Archwires

Elastic recovery (springback) and flexural rigidity (stiffness) are two of the most important physical characteristics of an archwire.

A good elastic recovery is important, otherwise the arch is liable to become distorted in use, which at best will render it inactive, but may result in unwanted tooth movements. Where the archwire is to be used to align irregular teeth, a low flexural rigidity is desirable so that the wire can be deflected through a reasonable distance without generating an excessive force. With a stiff archwire, even a small deflection will produce a large force and either the teeth will be subjected to undue loads or the arch will have to be activated very frequently. While a low flexural rigidity is desirable for the alignment of irregular teeth, the archwire may also have to resist external forces such as those generated by elastics (*Fig.* 16.7). In this case, too flexible a wire may allow unwanted tooth movements.

There are a number of other situations where a rather high flexural rigidity is desirable to maintain control—for example, when retracting a canine into a premolar extraction space, too flexible a wire will allow the tooth to tip. These conflicting demands may be met in one of two ways. A relatively stiff wire (e.g. 0.016 in diameter round wire) may be used and its flexibility can be increased locally by the incorporation of loops (*Fig.* 16.8). Alternatively, the initial alignment of irregular teeth can be achieved with a thin flexible arch, and the use of elastics or other operations requiring a higher flexural rigidity can be delayed until stiffer arches are placed.

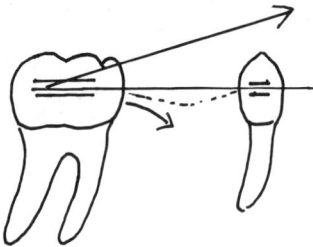

Fig. 16.7. When elastic traction is applied to a lower molar, the unsupported span of the archwire tends to flex. If this happens to an appreciable extent, the tooth will tip. In order to prevent this, the wire must be stiff enough and a tip back bend should be incorporated to counter the effect of the elastic.

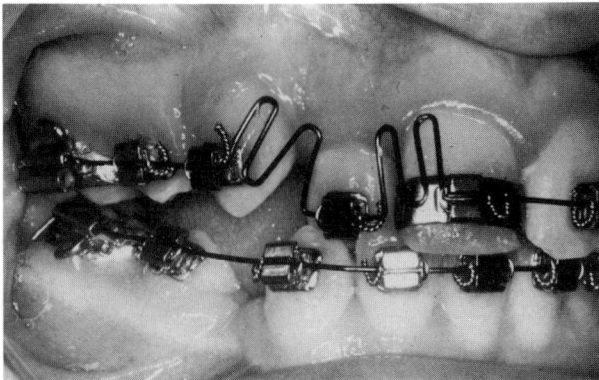

Fig. 16.8. Vertical loops are incorporated in an archwire to increase its flexibility locally.

Originally archwires were made from gold alloys, but these were very expensive and stainless steel became the material of choice. Recently a number of titanium alloys have been introduced. These have a lower modulus of elasticity and so are more flexible than a stainless steel wire of the same dimensions. This is useful in some situations. The elastic recovery is also superior to that of stainless steel, and while this makes a titanium alloy archwire more difficult to form, its resistance to permanent deformation in use is clearly advantageous. Braided multiple strand stainless steel archwires are also available. These have a much higher elastic recovery and a lower flexural rigidity than solid stainless steel wires of the same nominal diameter, and are useful for the alignment of irregular teeth. For most stages of orthodontic treatment, however, high tensile stainless steel wires are used.

Archwires have to satisfy many different requirements, some of which may be mutually contradictory: non-toxicity, resistance to corrosion, fatigue and fracture, ease of formation and economy, are all important considerations. Suitability for welding and soldering are advantages.

ACTIVE TOOTH MOVEMENT WITH FIXED APPLIANCES

In most appliance systems, the archwire itself is the major active component in the alignment of irregular teeth, both vertically and radially. Because the span between adjacent brackets is short, the archwire segments tend to be stiff, and if a full-size archwire (e.g. 0.018 in diameter, or more) is used, a straight span would be almost rigid and quite unsuitable for tooth alignment. This problem can be circumvented by using very thin wires initially and then working up through progressively thicker wires until a full size arch can be engaged. Alternatively, a relatively heavy wire (0.016 in) can be used and its flexibility can be increased at irregular contacts by the incorporation of loops (*Fig.* 16.8). Looped segments are very much more flexible radial to the arch than vertically,

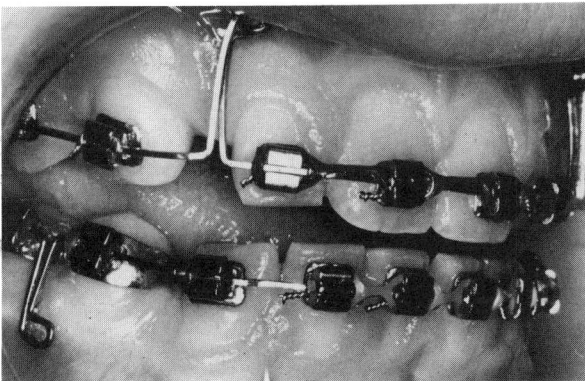

Fig. 16.9. Loops incorporated in an upper arch in order to retract the incisors and in a lower arch to close extraction spaces. The loops are activated by pulling the distal ends of the archwires through the brackets and tying them back or bending them up behind the molar tubes.

but this is generally advantageous because the major tooth irregularities are usually labiolingual. The force systems generated by looped arches are very complex and adverse side reactions can occur, and so it is desirable to progress to a plain archwire at as early a stage as possible.

Loops may also be used to retract incisors or to bring forward buccal segments to close spaces (*Fig.* 16.9). These are activated by pulling a small amount of the archwire through the molar tubes and holding it either by a ligature or by turning up the end.

Archwires must be made accurately because the teeth are generally drawn to the form of the archwire and any faults will be difficult to correct. Arch form and symmetry must be preserved.

Movements of teeth along the archwire may be accomplished by auxiliary coil springs or elastics (*Figs.* 16.10, 16.11). Appreciable binding may occur between brackets and archwire but care has to be taken to avoid the use of excessive forces otherwise the archwire may be deformed, allowing unwanted tooth movements and prejudicing the stability of the anchorage.

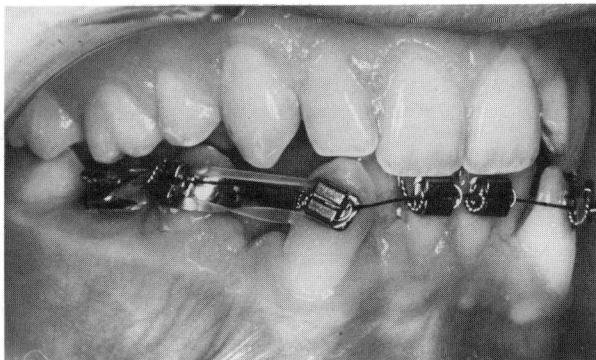

Fig. 16.10. A latex elastic used to retract a lower canine along an archwire.

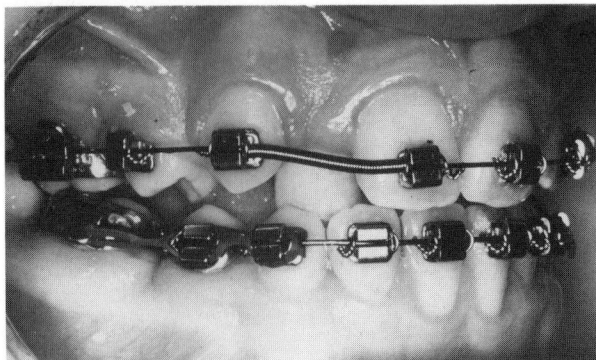

Fig. 16.11. In the upper arch, a coil spring has been threaded on to the arch and compressed between the canine and central incisor to open up space for the lateral. In the lower arch, a polyurethane chain is being used to close the space at the site of extraction of the lower second premolar.

Adjustment of arch relationships is often achieved by the use of intermaxillary elastics (*see Fig*. 16.18*b*). Anchorage balance is very important here and the arch malrelationship must not be corrected at the expense of the stability. For example, in the correction of a Class II malocclusion with intermaxillary elastics, it is only too easy to advance the lower incisors unintentionally, particularly when lower premolars have not been extracted.

Headgear is commonly used to reinforce anchorage or to achieve active tooth movement. Retraction of the upper buccal segments and of upper and lower canines are the tooth movements most commonly undertaken with extra-oral traction (*Fig*. 16.12). High-pull headgear can be valuable in intruding the upper incisors in certain Class II cases (*Fig*. 16.13). In conjunction with a rectangular archwire, high-pull headgear is also very effective in achieving bodily retraction of the upper incisors.

Palatal and lingual arches (*Fig*. 16.14) may be used for anchorage reinforcement. They may also be used for arch expansion and in some techniques they

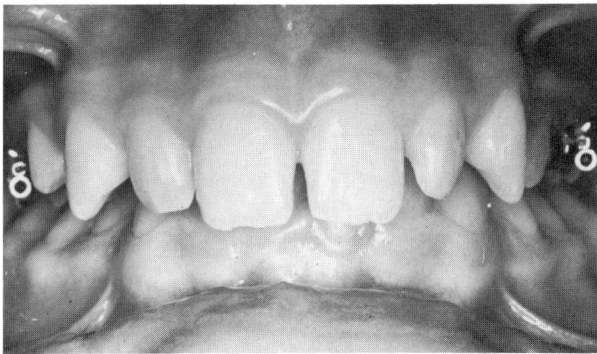

a

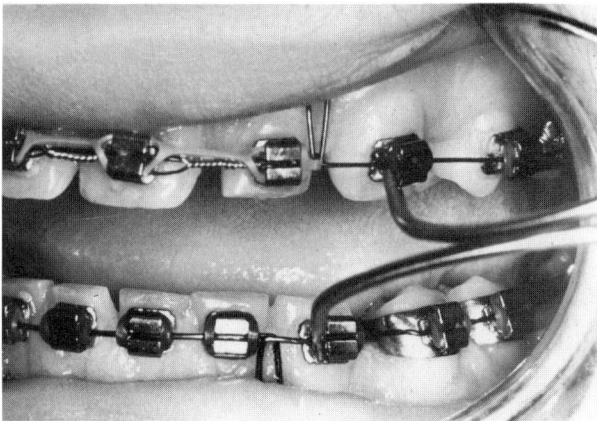

b

Fig. 16.12. *a*, Molar bands with double tubes. The upper rectangular tubes will carry an archwire while the lower tubes will house the facebow for extra-oral traction. *b*, J hooks being used to retract upper and lower canines along an archwire. The J hooks are attached to a headcap by elastics.

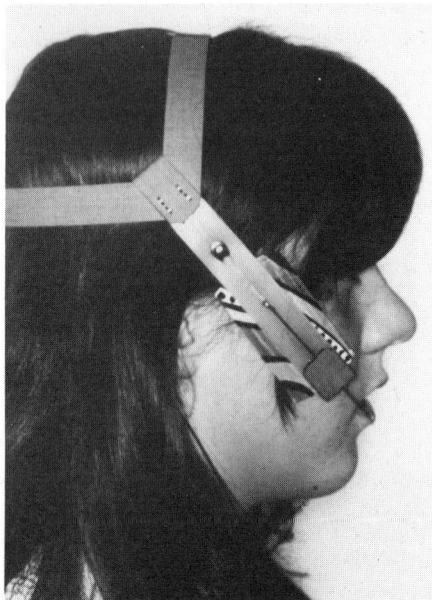

Fig. 16.13. High-pull headgear. This is being used to apply an intrusive and retraction force to the incisor segment of the upper archwire.

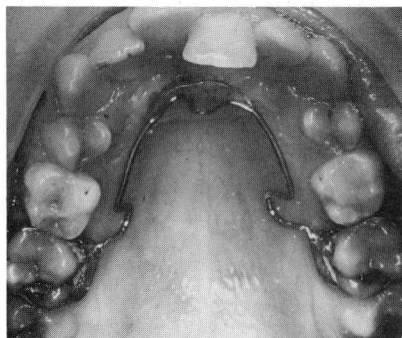

a

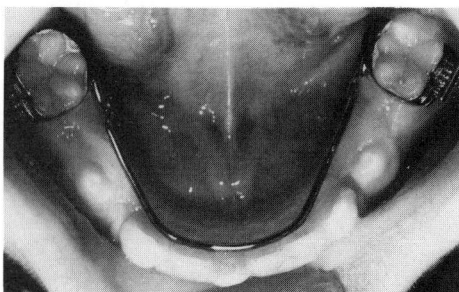

b

Fig. 16.14. *a*, An upper palatal arch attached to bands on the upper first permanent molars. This increases their anchorage value by preventing them from rotating or tipping. Note the button of acrylic anteriorly which prevents the archwire from becoming buried in the palatal mucosa if the teeth do tend to tip, so reinforcing anchorage. *b*, A lower lingual arch to enhance the anchorage of the lower molars.

may carry auxiliary springs, which tip teeth in the same manner as removable appliance springs.

ANCHORAGE CONTROL WITH FIXED APPLIANCES

As with removable appliances, anchorage control is fundamental to successful treatment. Loss of anchorage can mean that essential space is dissipated and this can be very difficult to regain.

The anchorage value of a tooth or group of teeth depends in part on root areas and in part on the type of movement that is allowed. With fixed appliances it is possible to prevent anchor teeth from tipping or rotating and their anchorage value is increased greatly by ensuring that only bodily movement can occur. Equally, this means that when a tooth does have to be moved bodily, substantial demands are made upon the anchorage.

Anchorage balance must be taken account of when treatment is planned. For example, if substantial space is required for the relief of incisor crowding and correction of a large overjet, and particularly if the tooth inclinations are unfavourable so that they cannot be tipped simply into the correct positions, the demands on anchorage will be considerable. It will usually be appropriate to extract first premolars so that the maximum number of teeth can be included in the anchorage (*Fig.* 16.15*a*), and to ensure that the maximum anchorage is obtained by preventing the tipping or rotation of anchor teeth, and by using headgear where appropriate,

On the other hand, if only a small amount of space is required for the correction of labial segment irregularities, the extraction of first premolars is undesirable because active closure of excess space can easily result in too much retraction of the labial segments. In these circumstances a better anchorage balance would be given by the extraction of second premolars, which encourages a greater amount of space closure by forward movement of the molars during correction of the labial segments (*Fig.* 16.15*b*). If, by the time the labial segment irregularity has been corrected, substantial space remains at the extraction site, the anchorage value of the anterior teeth should be maximized by ensuring that they are not allowed to tip.

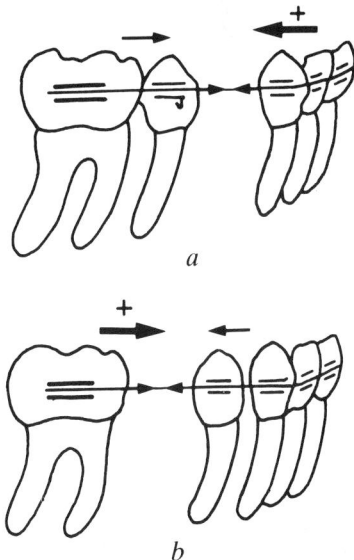

Fig. 16.15. The concept of anchorage balance. *a*, When the lower first premolars have been extracted and intramaxillary traction is applied to close the space, the labial segment tends to move more than the buccal teeth. The anchorage value of the labial segment can be enhanced by using an archwire that will prevent it from tipping. *b*, When second premolars have been extracted, anchorage balance encourages closure of the space by forward movement of the molars.

One of the major benefits of fixed compared with removable appliances is that excess space at extraction sites can be closed by forward movement of buccal teeth in a controlled manner, but if full advantage is to be taken of this, attention needs to be given to anchorage balance during planning and treatment.

Monitoring Anchorage with Fixed Appliances

One of the major problems in evaluating treatment progress with fixed appliances is in monitoring anchorage. In fully banded appliances there are no assured stable reference points within the dentition. Cephalometric radiographs can be used to check the stability of the lower incisor position relative to the A–Pog line, for example, and then other tooth movements can be related to the lower incisors. Cephalometric control of this sort, however, can be used only very occasionally—not more than once or twice during a course of treatment. This means that anchorage management depends greatly on the clinician's acumen and ability to control the force systems that are used, with few opportunities to check objectively that unwanted anchorage loss is not occurring. This is one of the reasons why prolonged training in the use of fixed appliances is required.

FIXED APPLIANCE TECHNIQUES

A large number of different fixed appliance techniques have been developed and there would be little value even in enumerating these. Many are variants of the edgewise technique, while others attempt to combine the best features of several different systems but rarely succeed in doing so. Continual development of materials and refinement of techniques has resulted in a number of powerful appliance systems that are capable of achieving good results for most malocclusions. For the orthodontic specialist, the limitations to what can be achieved should be biological rather than technical. The orthodontist will usually confine his practice to one or at the most two fixed appliance techniques in the interests of practice efficiency. Although the proponents of each appliance system extol its virtues, the expert will be able to obtain excellent results whatever system he uses. Advances in one appliance technique are soon matched by developments in its competitors.

Edgewise Technique (Fig. 16.16)

This technique was introduced in 1928 by Edward Angle but has evolved radically since that time. It is based on the use of brackets with a rectangular slot. In some versions of the technique the slot is 0.018 in wide and in others it is 0.022 in. It is a very versatile system with many variants, only one of which will be outlined here.

The brackets are placed on the tooth surfaces so that when the teeth are in ideal positions, the bracket slots will be level. Initial bracket levelling and tooth alignment is obtained by first using a flexible archwire (Fig. 16.16a) (0.012 in stainless steel or 0.015 in multiple strand wire) and then progressively heavier arches (0.014 and 0.016 in). The 0.016 in archwire is suitable for achieving bodily movements of teeth around the arch and labiolingual tipping movements as well as overbite control. Many simpler malocclusions can be treated completely with round archwires and can be finished with a 0.018 in archwire. The heavier archwires (0.016 and 0.018 in) should incorporate offsets to allow for the differing thickness of the teeth. These offsets are usually required mesial to the canines and to the first permanent molars. The upper and lower archwires must be coordinated in form so that the dental arch malrelationships are corrected in all dimensions.

Where buccolingual root movements are required, a rectangular arch is used after either an 0.016 or 0.018 in round wire (*Fig.* 16.16*d*). By incorporating torque in the rectangular archwire, controlled buccolingual root movements and bodily tooth movements can be obtained. The rectangular arch must be formed very carefully so as not to produce unwanted torque and adverse buccolingual movements in teeth that were originally correct.

Techniques Using Pre-torqued Brackets

Archwire fabrication is simplified if each bracket slot is inclined in such a way that when the teeth are positioned ideally, the bracket slots lie on the one plane (*Fig.* 16.17). Thus, the final rectangular archwire would not require the incorporation of any torque. The bracket slot orientation for each tooth is different and thus separate bracket specifications are required for each tooth. The base thickness of each bracket can also be designed to allow for the different thickness of the teeth and so the need for offsets in the archwires can be eliminated. The pre-torqued systems work well on teeth of 'average' form but, of course, in most patients at least some of the teeth vary from this and so some individualization of archwires is required.

Pre-torqued bracket systems do offer a number of advantages over the conventional edgewise systems in ease of archwire fabrication, but with the variety of brackets, inventory control is more complex and they tend to be more expensive than conventional brackets.

Begg Technique (*Fig.* 16.18)

With edgewise appliance systems very large forces can be generated when heavy arches are used. Dr Raymond Begg, an Australian orthodontist, introduced a technique based upon tipping teeth with light forces, followed by root movements with auxiliary springs. The Begg technique[1] has developed greatly since it was introduced in 1956, but although it has won widespread acceptance, it is used by a minority of orthodontists.

The Begg bracket (*see Fig.* 16.4) is designed to allow free tipping of teeth in all directions. Treatment is divided into three stages (*Fig.* 16.18). The objectives of stage 1 are to align the teeth and to correct incisor malrelationships. This is done using 0.016 in round arches with vertical loops at interdental contact irregularities. overjet and overbite are corrected with the aid of intermaxillary elastics. At the end of stage 1, the teeth should be well aligned and the incisors should meet edge to edge.

In stage 2 the extraction spaces are closed using plain 0.016 in arches and intra- and intermaxillary elastics. The edge-to-edge incisor relationship is maintained while the incisors are tipped further back. At the end of stage 2, the upper and lower incisors are often very retroclined (*Fig.* 16.18*c*).

In stage 3 the inclination of the incisors and of teeth adjacent to extraction spaces is corrected by the use of auxiliary springs (*see Fig.* 16.18*d*). The objectives at the end of stage 3 are to have the teeth well aligned with correct

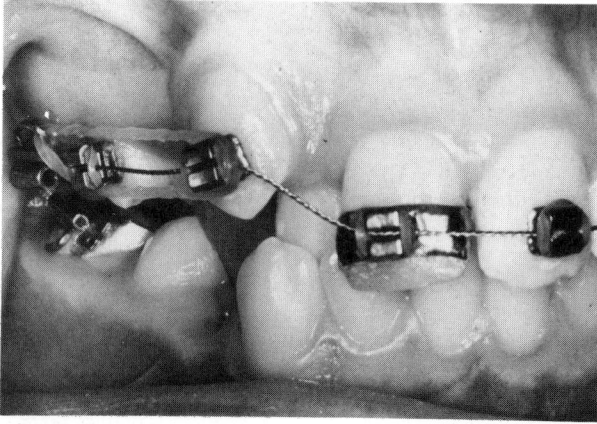

a

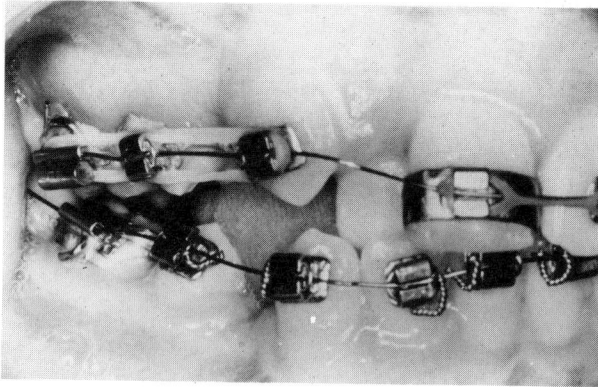

b

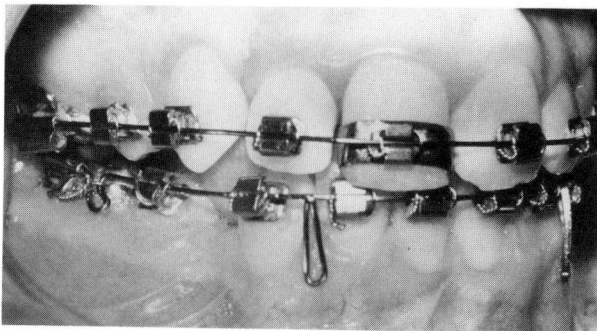

c

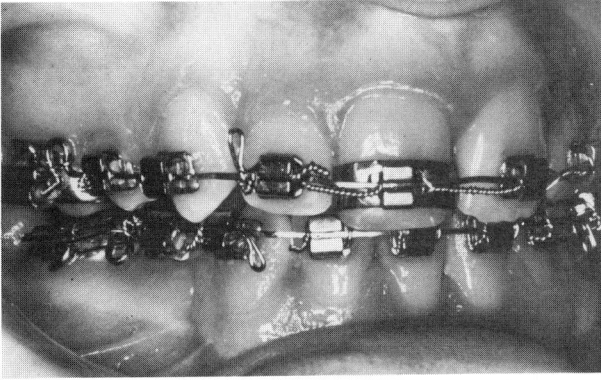

d

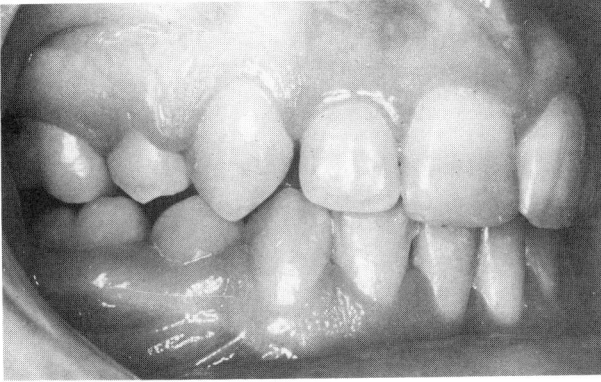

e

Fig. 16.16. A case treated by an edgewise technique. Note that a band has been used on the upper right central incisor because it has been crowned. *a*, Light multiple strand arches are used to align the brackets. *b*, Alignment is progressing and a heavier round wire arch is now in place. *c*, Most of the alignment is now complete, and a still heavier round wire arch is used. *d*, A rectangular arch is being used for detailed tooth positions and control of labiolingual root positions. *e*, The appliances have just been removed, but the occlusion has still to settle in fully.

Fig. 16.17. *a*, With conventional edge-wise brackets, the slot is not horizontal when the tooth is in the correct position and so the wire must be torqued. *b*, This is not necessary with pre-torqued brackets.

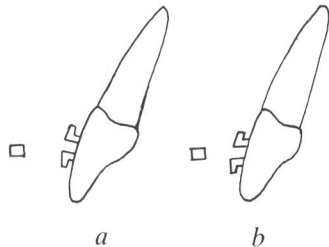

a   *b*

axial inclinations but with arch relationships somewhat overcorrected (*Fig. 16.18e*). Occlusal guidance will then carry the teeth into the correct relationships during the retention and settling in phase. This may seem a little haphazard, but it is what happens during the normal development of the occlusion and excellent results can be obtained with the Begg technique.

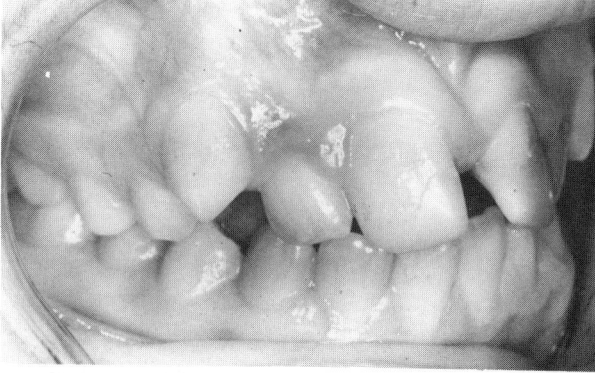

a

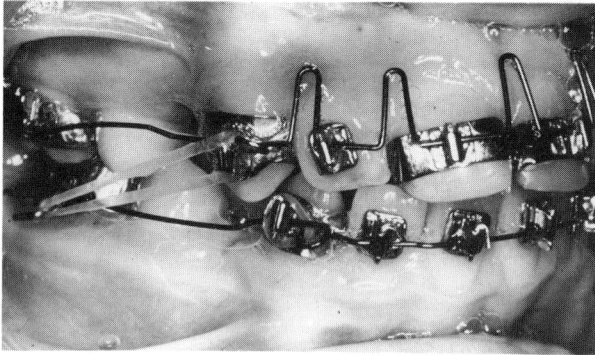

b

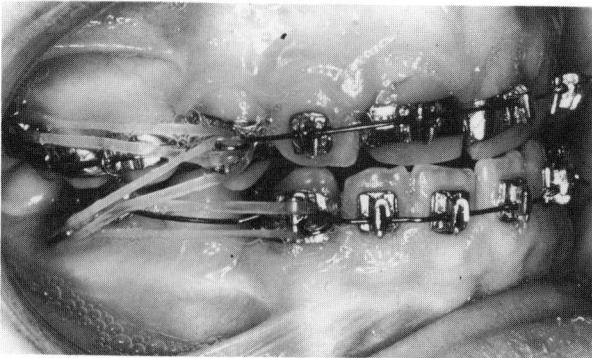

c

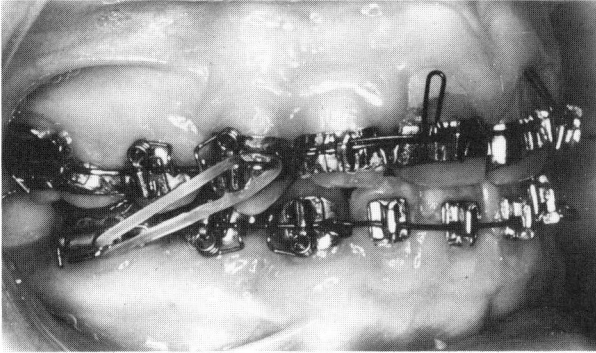

d

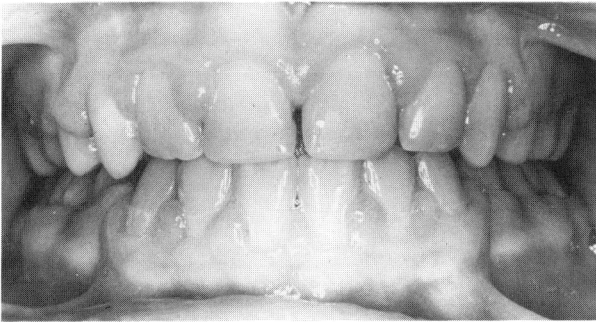

e

Fig. 16.18. A Class I malocclusion treated with the Begg technique. Note that both upper central incisors have been fractured and restored with etch retained composite. Because of this, bands rather than directly bonded attachments have been used on these teeth. *a*, The malocclusion before treatment. *b*, Stage 1. The round wire arches are quite stiff, but their flexibility has been increased locally by incorporation of vertical loops. The overbite is being reduced by the archwires and the overjet is being reduced by the intermaxillary elastics. *c*, The commencement of stage 2. Note that the incisors are in an edge-to-edge relationship. Spaces are being closed by intramaxillary elastics. *d*, Stage 3. the incisors are being uprighted by a torquing auxiliary. Uprighting springs are used to correct the mesiodistal inclinations of the teeth, particularly those adjacent to extraction sites. *e*, The corrected occlusion on removal of the appliances and before any settling in of the teeth.

Lingual Techniques

This recently introduced approach involves brackets and other attachments bonded to the lingual surfaces of the teeth. The advantage is that the appliance does not show and this is more acceptable, particularly to adults who might otherwise be unwilling to undergo fixed appliance treatment. However, this approach has a number of disadvantages and limitations.

It is more awkward to attach brackets to the lingual surfaces of teeth because of their small height and irregular surfaces. Access is much more difficult for the orthodontist and complex archwire adjustments are very exacting and time-consuming. Moreover, the appliance systems cannot control tooth movements as effectively as conventional appliances. Thus treatment with these appliances is expensive and limited in scope. It will be interesting to see whether these techniques evolve and become more readily manageable, or whether tooth-coloured attachments will be developed that will undermine the demand for lingual appliance systems.

Finishing Procedures

At the completion of treatment, bands and bonded attachments have to be removed. This is a somewhat tedious task that is accomplished with special pliers. Band cement can be removed with scalers but residual composite from bonds has to be removed carefully with fluted tungsten carbide burs and composite finishing stones. It is obviously very important that the enamel is not damaged by these instruments.

Removable retainers are then fitted, as with cases treated by removable appliances (*see* Chapter 18).

Fixed-Removable Appliances

In some cases treatment could be undertaken successfully with a removable appliance, except for a specific malposition of one or two teeth. In these circumstances the best solution may be to use a removable appliance with fixed attachments only to the teeth in question. Rotations and traction of teeth (for example of a palatally positioned canine that has been exposed surgically) are the operations most successfully undertaken with this approach. This treatment can be undertaken by the general practitioner who is skilled in the use of removable appliances. It is important to obtain brackets designed for direct bonding.

Derotation of teeth

An edgewise bracket is bonded to the labial surface of the tooth and a whip engages in a bow (*Fig.* 16.19). It is important that the whip is free to slide along the bow as the tooth derotates, and that it is constructed so the patient can take out the removable appliance for oral hygiene.

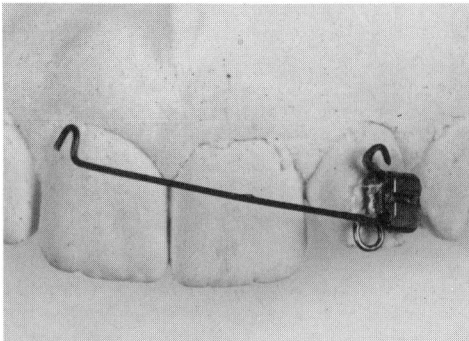

Fig. 16.19. A whip spring and edgewise bracket to derotate a tooth. A wire ligature between the loops in the whip spring holds it in place. The free end engages on the labial bow of a removable appliance.

Traction

Fixed–removable appliances are particularly useful for this purpose because with a conventional fixed appliance there is the danger of intruding and tipping adjacent teeth due to reciprocal effects on the archwires. In some circumstances composite material can be used to build up a ledge which a spring or buccal arm can engage. More frequently, a bracket is required. A Begg bracket lends itself particularly well to this purpose but an edgewise bracket can also be used (*Fig.* 16.20).

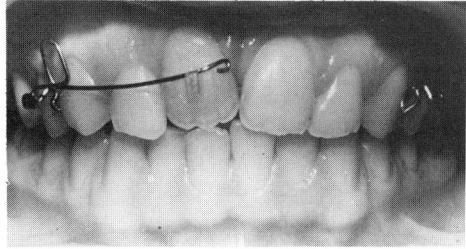

Fig. 16.20. A removable appliance being used to extrude a tooth by the action of a buccal arm on a plastic edgewise bracket bonded to the crown.

INDICATIONS FOR AND DISADVANTAGES OF FIXED APPLIANCES

The main advantage of fixed over removable appliances is in the possibility of precise control of all tooth movements. Thus they are indicated in malocclusions where rotations, bodily tooth movements and controlled root movements are required and for controlled closure of extraction spaces.

The principal disadvantages are that they are unsightly, oral hygiene requires special care and treatment is expensive. With direct bonding and relatively narrow brackets, modern fixed appliances are less unsightly than when bands were used on incisors. Plastic brackets and lingual appliance systems both have serious limitations, despite their superior appearance.

Provided that the patient maintains oral hygiene carefully, using a suitable toothbrush with disclosing tablets as necessary, and supplemented with fluoride mouth rinses, plaque control should be good and oral health should not deteriorate during appliance treatment. The adult patient with periodontal recession may need to use extra aids such as flossing, using a floss threader to feed the floss over the archwire. Thus plaque control can be difficult and time-consuming.

Fixed appliance treatment is more costly than removable appliance treatment. The materials themselves are expensive and surgery time is appreciable. Fixed appliances are not suitable for use by practitioners without special training and specialist treatment may not be available locally to patients in some communities.

REFERENCE

1. Begg P. R. (1956) Differential force in orthodontic treatment. *Am. J. Orthodont.* **42**; 481–510.

Chapter 17
Functional Appliances

Functional appliances depend for their action upon the activity of the orofacial musculature. Many designs of functional appliance have been proposed, and special claims have been made for each type. However, they can all be allocated to one of two groups, depending on the degree of displacement of the mandible: some displace the mandible only to a moderate extent and are intended to stimulate muscle activity; others induce a more extreme displacement and rely on the elastic properties of the muscles and fascia for their action. Graber[1] has called them myodynamic and myotonic appliances, respectively.

Functional appliances are most effective in the correction of Class II arch malrelationships in children in the mixed dentition. They have limited application in the permanent dentition, particularly when facial growth is more or less complete. Many ingenious variations have been proposed to deal with individual tooth malpositions, but these are seldom very useful. Major dental irregularities are best dealt with by a preliminary removable appliance and, if detailed tooth alignment is required, a short course of fixed appliance treatment should follow the functional appliance.

Although crossbites, anterior open bites and Class III malocclusions can be treated with certain functional appliances, they are generally dealt with more effectively and more rapidly in other ways. For example, many of the cases of anterior open bite for which successful treatment is claimed could have been expected to resolve spontaneously had the appliance been withheld: some are the results of a digit-sucking habit and others are normally developing dentitions in which an overbite has not yet been established by full eruption of the incisors. The Class III cases that can be treated with a functional appliance are mild and these could often be corrected equally well with a simple upper removable appliance.

The main effect of a functional appliance is to apply traction between the arches (intermaxillary traction) which results in tooth movement by the usual processes of bone remodelling (see Chapter 14). Some appliances produce arch expansion by mechanical devices such as screws, by guidance of eruption of buccal teeth or, as in the Frankel appliance, by holding the lips and cheeks away from the teeth so that their muscular balance is disturbed. As with any other orthodontic appliance, stability of expansion depends upon a permanent change in muscle balance. Claims have been made that this does occur, but they have not been substantiated by long-term controlled clinical trials or by other scientific evidence.

Proponents of functional appliances maintain that part of the correction in arch relationships is due to a change in jaw relationships produced by the appliance. Case reports have been published, showing the improvement in facial pattern that can accompany functional appliance treatment. However, these are usually specially selected, and there are few comparisons with matched control groups treated with other appliances. Many children with Class II malocclusions experience favourable growth changes, whether or not they are receiving orthodontic treatment, and controlled studies that have been published have found little or no effect on facial growth.

Experimental work in monkeys has shown that the forward displacement of the mandible by splints, in a manner comparable to that of certain functional appliances, can promote growth of the condylar cartilage as well as remodelling of the glenoid fossa. It is interesting that the effect seems to be limited in duration and that further displacement of the mandible seems to be necessary to maintain the condylar response.[2]

On balance, it seems probable that certain functional appliances may have a favourable effect on mandibular growth in some children; and they may also restrain maxillary growth to a small extent. However, these effects are limited in amount and most of the correction occurs by dento-alveolar change. Indeed, it is very easy to procline lower incisors and to produce other tooth movements that will not be stable. Claims of the correction of severe Class II malocclusions in a matter of weeks by 'jumping the bite' must be regarded with scepticism. This happens when the patient adopts a forward mandibular posture, which may be difficult to disclose but which will not be stable in the long term, and which cannot be regarded as an acceptable outcome of orthodontic treatment.

In a number of functional appliance techniques, great emphasis is laid on retraining the orofacial musculature by means of the appliance and by exercises.[3] It is certainly true that the activities of lips, cheeks and tongue may be atypical in the presence of a malocclusion, but these are very frequently adaptations to the malocclusion (see Chapter 3) and improve spontaneously as the malocclusion is corrected, whatever type of appliance is used. There is little evidence that training of the orofacial musculature by a functional appliance produces any extra modification that enhances occlusal stability or facial appearance.

Patient motivation is very important with functional appliances. They are bulky and inconvenient and the patient is tempted to wear them for less time than is necessary: treatment does not progress well and motivation deteriorates still further. In addition to the usual techniques of motivation, it is particularly valuable to set patients a target and to ask them to record truthfully their appliance wear each day. If the appliance has to be left out, for example for a social occasion, the time should be made up. Some appliances cannot be worn during the day because the patient cannot speak with them in the mouth, but others can be worn full time except for eating and sports.

A considerable degree of expertise is required in the management of functional appliances, and they are not suitable for use in general practice, except perhaps for the treatment of rather mild, uncrowded Class II, division 1 malocclusions. In most other cases a period of fixed appliance treatment is required following correction of the arch relationships in order to obtain optimal alignment and tooth relationships.

The following discussion refers only to the treatment of Class II malocclusions, because it is in these cases that functional appliances are most successful.

The reader who is interested in the treatment of other types of case is referred to Graber's text.[1]

PRELIMINARY TREATMENT

When a Class II malocclusion is to be corrected, the upper arch has to be expanded transversely to a minor extent in order to conform to the lower. Some expansion can often be incorporated in the functional appliance, but it may be simpler to do this with a removable appliance. If the upper incisors are very proclined and spaced, they can be retracted to some extent using a labial bow on the same appliance; and in a Class II, division 2 case, the retroclined upper incisors can be proclined to average inclinations with a palatal spring. Where the overbite is deep, an anterior bite plane can be incorporated to initiate overbite reduction. It is often noted that some improvement in arch relationship takes place during this preliminary phase of treatment.

REGISTERING THE CONSTRUCTION BITE

Although functional appliances differ greatly in design, this important stage is similar for all of them. Variations in the amount of protrusion or opening are described with each appliance. The amounts of vertical and anterior displacement of the mandible must be coordinated: the greater the anterior displacement, the less the vertical opening and vice versa. The total amount of mandibular displacement depends on the type of appliance and on the features of the malocclusion. For myodynamic appliances, the bite is opened within the normal working range of the muscles of mastication so that their activity is stimulated, while the opening is greater for myotonic appliances, so that the muscles and other soft tissues are stretched. If only a small forward posture is required to correct the buccal segment relationship, a greater degree of bite opening will be required than if there is a more severe arch malrelationship.

The intended mandibular displacement is registered with a wax squash bite. It is helpful to get the patient to practise posturing the mandible by the required amount, with guidance from the clinician. A roll of softened wax is made up, its thickness depending on the degree of bite opening, and is formed to the shape of the lower arch, keeping it clear of the incisors. The wax is settled on the lower arch and the mandible is then guided forwards by the required amount, taking care not to displace it laterally. The patient is then asked to close gently, maintaining the anterior displacement, until the required amount of opening at the incisors is obtained. The patient should be sitting upright when this is done. It is important that the correct registration is obtained and that the occlusal surfaces of the teeth are clearly reproduced in the wax so that the models can unequivocally be registered and articulated.

Several attempts may be required to obtain the correct registration. The squash bite is then chilled and trimmed so that it does not extend beyond the last erupted molars or beyond the buccal cusps of the lower teeth. The bite is now rechecked in the mouth to ensure that it has not warped and that the mandible is displaced symmetrically and the bite is opened as intended. The models are then mounted on an articulator, care being taken that the bite registration is not altered in any way.

THE ANDRESEN APPLIANCE (OR ACTIVATOR)

The activator (*Fig.* 17.1) was popularized by the publication of Andresen and Häupl's text on functional jaw orthopaedics in 1936. The Andresen appliance is loosely fitting and moderately displaces the mandible forwards with limited bite opening. It is thus a myodynamic appliance, designed to stimulate the activity of the muscles of mastication, although it has been found that this does not happen to any great extent during sleep when the appliance is mostly worn.

The Andresen appliance is useful in mild to moderately severe Class II cases with no crowding in either arch. Preliminary treatment with a removable appliance to expand the upper arch to match the lower and to correct upper incisor inclinations simplifies subsequent management, although these changes can be obtained with suitable adjustment of the activator.

The Construction Bite

If it is possible to do so without undue strain, the construction bite is taken with the mandible displaced forwards to obtain an edge-to-edge incisor relationship, with a vertical opening of 2–3 mm at the incisor edges (*Fig.* 17.1). With a large overjet, the advancement has to be done in two stages. It is possible to reactivate the first appliance by trimming it away from the lower teeth so that wax can be added to register the more advanced position of the mandible. The appliance

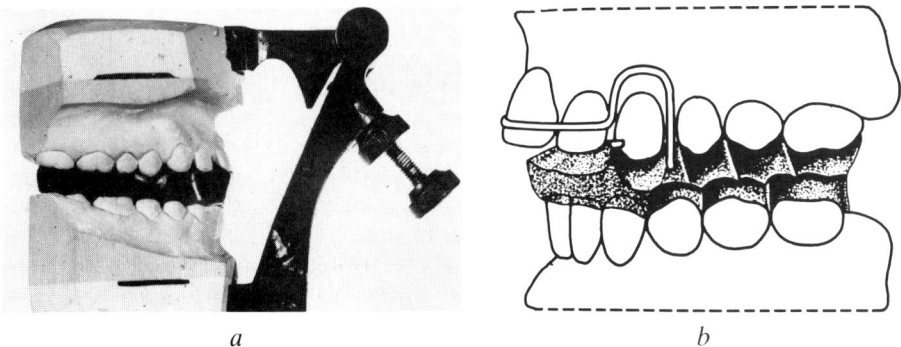

a   *b*

Fig. 17.1. An Andresen appliance. *a*, Using the construction bite, the models are mounted on a plane line articulator. *b*, Channels are trimmed in the finished appliance to guide the eruption of the upper buccal teeth buccally and distally; and to guide the lower buccal teeth mesially. If the upper incisors are spaced, the acrylic may be trimmed away from their palatal aspects to allow their retraction with the labial bow. The capping of the lower incisors must be left intact so that the overbite is controlled.

can then be 'relined' with cold-cure acrylic. However, it is often more convenient to make a new appliance.

The Appliance

In essence, the Andresen appliance consists of upper and lower baseplates sealed together. The acrylic caps the lower incisor edges to prevent them from overerupting and in an attempt to splint them to resist their proclination, although this may still occur. The acrylic is carried across the occlusal surfaces of the buccal teeth and there is an upper labial bow. If the upper incisors are spaced, this bow may be used to retract them, after clearing the palatal acrylic, but this makes the appliance more difficult for the patient to manage. Other springs can be incorporated but these are often troublesome and rather ineffective, and are not recommended.

Clinical Management

When the appliance is inserted initially, check that it fits well and that the mandible is displaced as intended. If the bite registration has been altered in the laboratory, the appliance will usually have to be discarded. In order to reduce a deep overbite, which will usually be present, channels are cut over the occlusal surfaces of the buccal teeth (*Fig.* 17.1). In the upper arch these slope slightly distally and buccally, leaving interdental spurs to contact the mesiopalatal aspects of the teeth so that they are guided distally and buccally as they erupt. In the lower arch the channels slope occlusally and the interdental spurs contact the distolingual tooth surfaces.

Trimming is facilitated by marking on the appliance with a wax pencil the areas of acrylic that are to be left in contact with the teeth. If the upper incisors are to be retracted with the labial bow the acrylic is trimmed away from their palatal aspects and the adjacent alveolar mucosa, but this is often better delayed until a subsequent visit because the appliance becomes rather unstable.

The patient is instructed to wear the appliance for 10–12 hours in every 24: this will be at night with 2–4 hours' wear in the evening. Evening wear is particularly important when the patient is getting used to the appliance: it will often come out during the first few nights, but patients should be reassured that this is normal and that they will soon cope with it easily.

The appliance requires little routine adjustment but the patient should be seen every 4–6 weeks. There should be definite progress at each visit. If there is no obvious change within 3 months the appliance is not being worn as instructed and it may be best to discontinue treatment if full cooperation cannot be obtained.

Unless treatment is monitored carefully it may be allowed to run on for years with little improvement in the occlusion. This wastes everyone's time and undermines the possibility of future cooperation when treatment with a different type of appliance may be indicated.

A problem with the activator is that it is liable to procline the lower incisors while the lower buccal teeth are moved mesially. This may appear to be perfectly satisfactory while the appliance is being worn, but when it is discontinued the lower incisors may drop back to their original position and become crowded. This is one advantage of the lower incisors being spaced initially.

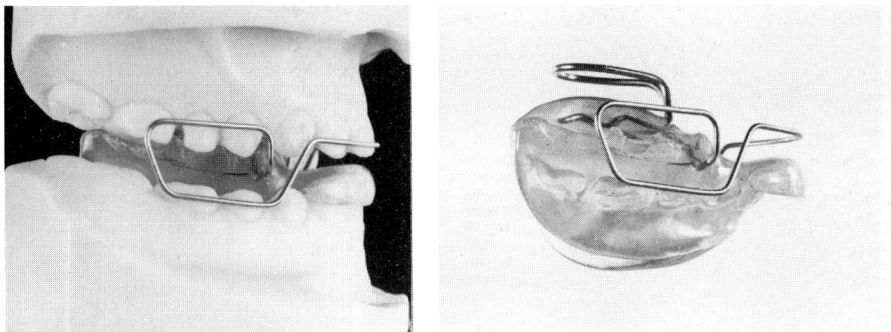

a b

Fig. 17.2. A bionator. *a*, The appliance showing the construction bite. *b*, The finished appliance.

THE BIONATOR

This appliance is derived from Andresen's activator but is greatly reduced in bulk (*Fig.* 17.2) so that it can be worn during the day as well as at night. It is left out for eating and during sports. The increased wear means that treatment results can be obtained more rapidly. The intermittent relapse, which can occur with part time wear because of occlusal contacts or because the lower lip lies behind the upper incisors, is avoided. Therefore, the appliance is effective in correcting certain Class II malocclusions and its lack of bulk, and its simplicity, make it one of the easier functional appliances to use,[5] although it has generally been neglected outside Germany. The effects of the appliance are primarily upon tooth position with questionable influence upon skeletal growth and muscular patterns.

Construction Bite

In Class II cases, an edge-to-edge relationship of the incisors is aimed at, and the bite is opened just sufficiently to allow this. If the overjet is too large for an edge-to-edge incisor occlusion to be obtained readily, the mandible will have to be advanced in more than one stage and a corresponding number of appliances are required,

The Appliance

In the lower arch the acrylic extends as far as the distal surface of the first permanent molar, contacting the mandibular teeth and the lingual alveolar mucosa. It does not extend far into the lingual sulcus. The base is clear of the upper incisors and extends over the occlusal surfaces of the premolars or deciduous molars, leaving the first permanent molars free to erupt. The occlusal platform is ground flat so that the teeth contacting it are free to move buccally. This platform stabilizes the appliance and allows the molars to erupt so that the overbite is reduced. When this has been achieved, the platform can be removed, although this makes the appliance rather unstable. When the mandible is displaced far enough to obtain an edge-to-edge incisor occlusion, the lower incisor edges are left free; but otherwise they are capped to prevent them from overerupting.

The buccal bow contacts the upper incisors but is clear of the buccal teeth by 2–3 mm. Its function is to restrain the upper labial segment and at the same time to keep the cheeks away from the buccal teeth to allow some arch expansion. The palatal loop was introduced by Balters to encourage a forward posture of the tongue and mandible.

Variations of the basic bionator have been designed to deal with different malocclusions but usually there are simpler and more effective ways of treating them.

Clinical Management

For the first few weeks the appliance is worn for 2 hours each evening and at night. Daytime wear is then introduced and within the first month the patient should be wearing the appliance full time apart from during meals and sports.

HARVOLD APPLIANCE

The Harvold[6] appliance (*Fig*. 17.3) is derived from the activator of Andresen, but differs from it in the degree of bite opening and in the trimming of the appliance. This is a myotonic appliance that depends for its action on the elastic properties of stretched muscles and other soft tissues, rather than on muscular contraction.

Impressions must reproduce the full depth of the lingual sulcus, into which flanges extend deeply so that it is difficult for the patient to dislodge the appliance unintentionally when asleep.

Construction Bite

The mandible is advanced a few millimetres less than the maximum the patient can attain and it is opened to give an interocclusal clearance of 10–20 mm measured at the premolars. The principles of taking the bite are discussed on p. 246.

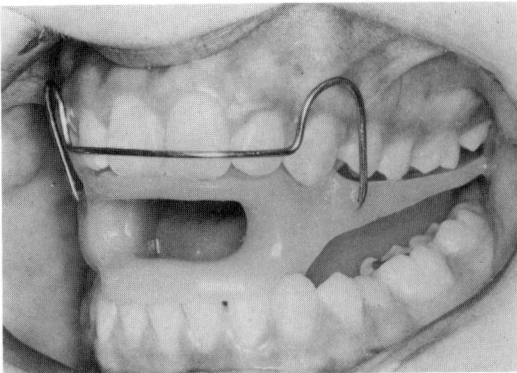

Fig. 17.3. A Harvold appliance.

The Appliance

The upper labial bow (0.9 mm) contacts the upper incisors but it is not activated: it merely restrains the upper incisors and ensures that they are not left behind as the arch relationship is corrected. Palatal springs (0.9 mm) which may be incorporated mesial to the upper first permanent molars are intended to unseat the appliance rather than retract them. They will be activated by about 1 mm. This means that the patient is encouraged to bite into the appliance and this muscular activity complements the soft tissue stretch.

The baseplate extends deeply into the lingual sulci. The acrylic caps both the upper and lower incisors and passes between the occlusal surfaces of the buccal teeth to form a shelf which will contact the upper but not the lower teeth. To obviate very extensive trimming at the chairside, certain areas should be relieved before the baseplate is formed. These are plastered out if heat-cured acrylic is to be used, but can be waxed out for cold-cure acrylic.

The acrylic should be well clear of the upper and lower incisors except incisally and labially. On the upper model the palatal surfaces of the incisors and canines, and the anterior portion of the palate, are waxed out. This allows distal tipping of the incisors and alveolar bone remodelling as the upper arch is retracted. The displacing springs are also waxed out. The lower model is relieved over the lingual surface of the labial segment and immediately adjacent alveolar process. This means that the appliance should not exert any protrusive effect on the lower incisors and that the anterior displacement of the mandible is procured by contact with the lingual mucosa below the relieved area. The occlusal surfaces of the lower buccal teeth are relieved with quite a thick layer of wax which is carried over on to the lingual surfaces as a thin layer, leaving these teeth free to erupt and to aid overbite reduction. Depending on the degree of bite opening, 5–10 mm of clearance may be appropriate. According to Woodside,[7] the undercuts in the lower lingual sulcus should not be relieved because contact with the appliance encourages the patient to bite into it. However, if the undercuts are deep they should certainly be reduced with wax and the acrylic in this region must be thick enough to allow it to be trimmed away from the undercut area if the patient develops ulcers. As the bite has been opened appreciably, a gap can be left in the incisor region which allows the adept patient to speak with the appliance in place.

Clinical Management

Provided that the models have been correctly relieved as described above, trimming is minimized, However, it is important to ensure that the acrylic is adequately clear of the lingual surfaces of the incisors and of the occlusal surfaces of the lower buccal teeth.

The acrylic is trimmed away from the distopalatal aspects of the upper buccal teeth, leaving spurs in contact with their mesiopalatal surfaces, very much as is done with the Andresen appliance except that the acrylic there is left in contact with their occlusal surfaces.

The patient is instructed to wear the appliance in the evenings and at night with a target of 100 hours per week. The appliance needs very little regular attention, other than easing in any areas of persistent ulceration.

Action of the Appliance

As with most functional appliances, claims are made that the growth of the mandibular condyle is stimulated, and that maxillary growth is restrained. The major effects are dento-alveolar. Harvold[6] demonstrated that by manipulating the cant of the occlusal plane a Class II buccal segment relationship could be corrected, and the appliance is effective in doing this. Bite opening occurs by eruption of the lower buccal teeth while the incisors are restrained. The upper labial segment is tipped lingually, particularly when the appliance opens the bite to a major extent.

THE FRÄNKEL APPLIANCE

This appliance, named after its originator, Dr Rolf Fränkel of East Germany, is one of the more recent functional appliances and it has led to a resurgence of interest in functional appliance treatment. Fränkel termed it a function regulator (FR) because it is intended to correct functional anomalies in the circumoral musculature, which he holds responsible for crowding and other aspects of malocclusion. The theoretical justification of the appliance may be questionable, but impressive occlusal changes can be obtained in suitable patients.

There are four variants of the function regulator: FR 1 for Class I and mild Class 2 cases; FR 2 for Class II malocclusions of both divisions; FR 3 for Class III cases; and FR 4 for open bite and bimaxillary proclination.

The Fränkel appliance can be useful in the correction of Class II arch malrelationships but other malocclusions are generally treated more efficiently by other methods. The description here is confined to the FR 2 (*Fig.* 17.4). Details of the other types can be found in the text of Graber,[1] who has done much to popularize the appliance.

Some preliminary treatment, for example correction of incisor inclinations, may be carried out with removable appliances, but detailed tooth alignment is best left until the arch relationships have been corrected, because a short period of fixed appliance treatment will be required in many cases if an ideal result is to be obtained.

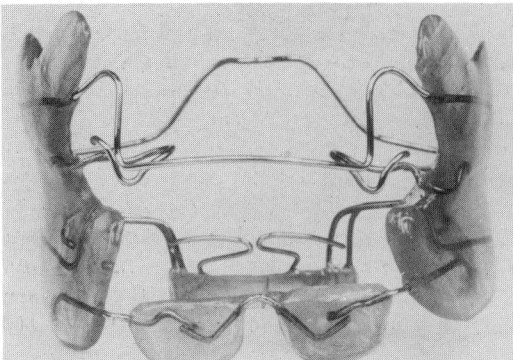

Fig. 17.4. A Fränkel appliance.

The Appliance (FR2) (Fig. 17.4)

The buccal shields extend to the full depth of the buccal sulcus, and indeed the models are trimmed to allow this. Fränkel claims that this produces 'periosteal stretch', which promotes subperiosteal apposition of bone, but the validity of this is questionable. The buccal shields lie clear of the teeth and so the arches are expanded: the teeth are free of muscular pressures on the buccal but not on the lingual surfaces. While this expansion is undoubted, adequately controlled long-term studies of its stability are still awaited. The lip pads are also intended to produce periosteal stretch and to control lower lip activity: in conjunction with the forward posture of the mandible induced by the appliance, the lip pads eliminate any trapping of the lower lip behind the upper incisors.

The lingual pad contacts the alveolar mucosa on the lingual surface of the mandibular alveolar process, but it is clear of the teeth. Thus a forward mandibular posture is induced without any protrusive force on the lower incisors. The labial and lingual pads both create stimuli which result in a controlled forward posture of the mandible, and it is claimed that this is more effective than the anterior displacement produced by some other functional appliances.

The wire components are designed to connect the different parts and to stabilize the appliance. The upper labial bow, upper palatal bow and canine loops (in 0.9 mm wire) and the palatal arch (1.0 mm), with its occlusal rests, stabilize the appliance against the upper arch. The palatal arch passes interdentally, mesial to the first permanent molars. The teeth should be substantially separated with elastic separators before the impressions are taken, or the model can be trimmed so that the teeth are separated as the appliance gradually settles into place.

The lower lingual arch (1.15 mm) supports the lingual pad and this in turn carries the lingual springs. These are designed to prevent eruption of the lower incisors and so to control the overbite. They should not be activated labially unless it is intended to procline the lower incisors. All the wire components must be 2 or 3 mm clear of the alveolar mucosa to avoid trauma or ulceration. The tags of all wire components, except for the lingual springs, are embedded in the buccal shields. The tags of the lower lingual and labial arches are disposed in a way that allows reactivation of the appliance—by sectioning the buccal shields and advancing the mandibular part of the appliance.

Appliance Construction

The impression must extend to the full depth of the buccal and labial sulcus, clearly reproducing muscle reflections. Even the well-taken impression will not generally reproduce the full sulcus depth, because the cheeks and lips are displaced outwards by the tray and impression material. To allow for this, and to ensure some 'periosteal stretch', the sulcus should be deepened carefully by trimming the model. After the wire components have been fabricated, the models are mounted on a plane line articulator using the construction bite. Now wax relief is applied in the areas that will be covered by buccal shields so that they stand clear of the teeth and buccal mucosa. The clearance is greatest at the top (2–3 mm) and tapers to about 1 mm at the lower buccal sulcus. The wires are then fixed to the models with sticky wax and the acrylic shields and pads are made up in cold-cure acrylic resin.

Clinical Management

Wear of the appliance is extended progressively. For the first 2 or 3 weeks it should be worn only in the evenings for about 2 hours. When the patient is confident in its management, night time wear is introduced and then, as soon as possible, the patient should wear it full time, except for meals and sport. The strongly motivated patient will cope with the appliance well. Fränkel lays great emphasis on obtaining a habitual lip seal and recommends that the child should be reminded to do this whenever the parents observe that the lips are parted. He also suggests that the child should practise holding a piece of paper between the lips when doing homework to focus attention on this.

If the buccal shields have been overextended, ulcers may develop in the buccal sulcus and the shields will have to be trimmed very conservatively and polished. The lip pads may also cause trouble, but there is little scope for trimming them. These problems arise most commonly when the lip pads are not sufficiently upright, and so this needs attention during appliance construction.

Within 3 months of the commencement of treatment, progress should be obvious. If this is not the case, the appliance is probably not being worn as instructed. Where there is initially good progress but this declines after 3–6 months, it is probably time to reactivate the appliance by advancing the lower labial and lingual pads.

Although lower incisor proclination should not happen unless the lingual springs have been activated intentionally, this is sometimes a problem. It is most liable to occur if the appliance is not adequately stabilized against the upper arch, or if the lower labial pads have been positioned incorrectly so that the lip is held away from the incisors.

THE ORAL SCREEN (Fig. 17.5)

This very simple functional appliance lies in the labial vestibule. It has been used to discourage thumb-sucking and to correct the associated malocclusion. It has also been used for lip training in patients with incompetent lips. The oral screen has no place in modern orthodontics: it is inefficient and limited in scope as an orthodontic appliance and there is no evidence that its use as a lip training device is of any benefit to the patient.

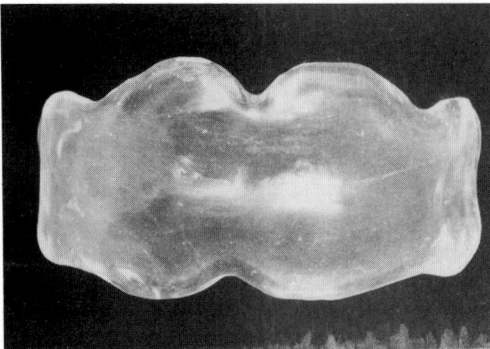

Fig. 17.5. An oral screen.

LIP BUMPER (Fig. 17.6)

This is a functional component, occasionally used in conjunction with a lower fixed appliance. The labial arch fits into tubes on lower molar bands and an acrylic pad, which stands clear of the alveolar process and lower incisors, holds the lower lip forwards. The force of reaction from the lower lip can move the lower molars distally, or can be used to reinforce anchorage. The lip bumper can occasionally be useful in Class II, division 1 cases where there is strong lower lip contraction behind the upper incisors which may interfere with their retraction: by holding the lip clear, overjet reduction is expedited.

If the lower incisors are not included in the appliance, they are liable to be proclined because of the change in muscle balance.

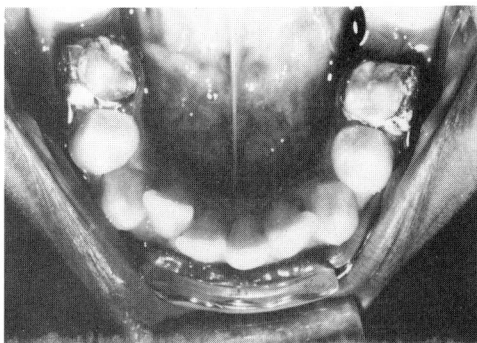

Fig. 17.6. A lip bumper to retract the lower first permanent molars following removal of the second permanent molars,

HEADGEAR AND FUNCTIONAL APPLIANCES

In many Class II cases some retraction of the upper arch is required and treatment will progress more rapidly if headgear is worn in conjunction with the appliance.[8] Spurs to which J hooks can be attached are incorporated readily in a number of activators or headgear can be applied through tubes on upper molar bands. Particularly where the extra-oral traction is applied directly to the functional appliance, the pull should be directed slightly upwards so that the appliance is not displaced, making it excessively difficult to wear.

FIXED APPLIANCE TREATMENT IN CONJUNCTION WITH FUNCTIONAL APPLIANCES

In some cases the results of functional appliance treatment will be entirely satisfactory and no further intervention is indicated. However, where there are dental irregularities or crowding necessitating extraction of teeth, a fixed appliance may be required for an optimal result. This should follow correction of the arch malrelationships with the functional appliance.

It is usually very desirable to allow a period of settling in without retention before the fixed appliance is fitted. This is particularly true where the lower incisors have been proclined, either deliberately or unintentionally, and their stability is in question. An adequate settling period of 12–18 months allows the orthodontist to begin fixed appliance treatment in the knowledge that the teeth are in stable positions; and if there has been any relapse this can be corrected. For example, if the lower incisors had been proclined but have dropped back, the increase in overjet may be treated by upper incisor retraction; and any increase in lower incisor crowding can be dealt with as appropriate. If there is no intervening period, instability will be revealed only at the conclusion of retention following the fixed appliance phase of treatment, and it is then very difficult to cope with.

A settling period may be objected to on the grounds that the risk of relapse is increased: the orofacial musculature might have matured, or the tooth movements during the fixed appliance phase might have enhanced stability. In most cases, however, it will be found that these reservations are outweighed by the advantage of commencing the fixed appliance treatment on an occlusion that is known to be stable.

Interruption of treatment is particularly valuable when the functional appliance has been used in the early mixed dentition. The patient may not be ready to proceed with fixed appliances for several years and it is an undue burden on the patient's cooperation if the functional appliance has to be worn as a retainer during this period.

The orthodontist is faced with a dilemma if the occlusion does start to relapse by lingual movement of lower incisors when the functional appliance is discontinued. Not only may the patient's confidence be undermined, but adverse secondary changes may occur. The overbite may deepen and the upper incisors may start to procline if the lower lip drops behind them. In these circumstances it is probably best to fit an upper removable retainer with a labial bow and a flat anterior biteplane. This allows the lower labial segment to adopt a position of stability while preventing the side effects of this relapse. The retainer may be worn only part-time.

It is important to warn patients who are to have functional appliance treatment as a prelude to a fixed appliance that it may not deal fully with the arch malrelationships and that interim stabilization may be required.

THE ROLE OF FUNCTIONAL APPLIANCES

Functional appliances can be useful in the treatment of mild, uncrowded Class II malocclusions with well-aligned teeth. In these circumstances an entirely satisfactory result may be obtained without any other appliances.

There is no advantage in using functional appliances for mild Class II malocclusions with crowding or dental irregularities. These can be treated more efficiently by using conventional removable or fixed appliances.

Functional appliances do have a place in the treatment of some more severe Class II malocclusions, particularly when these present in the mixed dentition. Advantage can be taken of facial growth in helping overbite reduction and correction of arch malrelationships.

Preliminary functional appliance treatment followed by a period without appliances is a good way of allowing the stability of lower incisor advancement to be verified before definitive fixed appliance treatment is commenced.

Although the effects of functional appliances on facial growth are still questionable, any changes that do occur can only be favourable. Scientific evidence and clinical anecdote do suggest that full-time wear of functional appliances in the mixed dentition period may enhance facial growth in Class II cases, to at least a minor extent.

REFERENCES

1. Graber T. M. and Neumann B. (1984) *Removable Orthodontic Appliances*, 2nd ed. Philadelphia, W. B. Saunders.
2. McNamara J. A. jun. (1980) Functional determinants of craniofacial size and shape. *Eur. J. Orthodont.* **2**; 131–59.
3. Fränkel R. (1980) A functional approach to orofacial orthopaedics. *Br. J. Orthodont.* **7**; 41–51.
4. Andresen V. and Häupl K. (1936) *Funktions–Kieferorthopaedie*. Berlin, Hermann Meusser.
5. Eirew H. L. (1981) The bionator. *Br. J. Orthodont.* **8**; 33–6.
6. Harvold E. P. (1974) *The Activator in Interceptive Orthodontics*. St Louis, Mosby, pp. 92–4.
7. Woodside D. G. (1984) The Harvold–Woodside activator. In: Graber T. M. and Neumann B. *Removable Orthodontic Appliances*, 2nd ed. Philadelphia, W. B. Saunders, pp. 244–309.
8. Pfeiffer J. P. and Grobèty D. (1975) the class II malocclusion: differential diagnosis and clinical application of activators, extraoral traction and fixed appliances. *Am. J. Orthodont.* **68**; 499–544.

Chapter 18
Stability and Retention

The position of teeth in the dental arch is dictated primarily by the shape and relationship of the jaws and by forces from the surrounding soft tissues (*see* Chapter 3).

Following a course of orthodontic treatment, the teeth should be in a position of balance, but a period of retention is still usually necessary to allow the supporting tissues to adapt (*see* p. 197). In rare cases, permanent retention is required.

A distinction should be made between relapse of orthodontic treatment and changes that are a result of facial growth and occlusal maturation. For example, in a Class III case where upper incisors have been proclined but the overbite is inadequate to hold them, they will relapse. Similar changes in incisor relationship can occur in the longer term due to unfavourable facial growth. Another situation where relapse can be mimicked by natural occlusal change is the development of lower incisor crowding: injudicious proclination of lower incisors may be followed by relapse and crowding; but similar lower incisor crowding may develop in the longer term due to late facial growth (*see* p 46). For the patient these changes are undesirable whatever the cause, but the clinician should recognize their different aetiologies. Relapse should be anticipated and avoided, but the prediction of facial growth changes is much more uncertain. The clinician should be aware of the possibility of unfavourable occlusal change and should warn the patient accordingly.

STABILITY

Soft Tissue Factors

An occlusion before orthodontic treatment is in balance between occlusal and soft tissue forces, and unless a new position of balance can be found, changes will not be stable. As a general rule the size and form of the lower arch has to be accepted. Lower arch width is particularly difficult to alter with the assurance of stability and so this should not be done without good cause. Cases can be found where transverse lower arch expansion has been stable, but this is unpredictable and is not a sound basis for treatment.

Labiolingual movement of lower incisors is also liable to be unstable unless other factors are changed at the same time. For example, retraction of lower incisors may be stable in a Class III case if an adequate overbite is established. In a few Class II cases the lower incisors have been restrained by contact with the palate or upper labial segment, or by a thumb-sucking habit, and so proclination to a position of true soft tissue balance will be stable. However, these changes in lower incisor position are problematic and have to be managed skillfully.

Retraction of upper incisors in a Class II, division 1 case will be stable provided their relationship to the lower lip is changed.

Concomitant changes in the upper and lower arches have poorer prospects of stability because occlusal factors cannot help. Thus transverse expansion of both upper and lower arches to relieve incisor crowding is very liable to relapse and was discredited many years ago. It is still claimed that with some functional appliances, such as the Fränkel appliance, the muscle balance can be changed so that transverse expansion is stable but this is a matter of controversy.

Simultaneous proclination or retraction of both upper and lower labial segments is equally problematic. Proclination of upper and lower incisors in cases of bimaxillary retroclination would provide a simple solution to the deep overbite, but would not be stable. In many cases of bimaxillary proclination retraction of upper and lower incisors would be advantageous, but this will be stable only if the soft tissue balance can be changed (*see* p. 157).

Cases can be demonstrated that seem to disprove these general guidelines, but they are exceptions. The experienced orthodontist may be able to recognize these unusual cases where the general rules can be broken, but this is always at the risk of long-term relapse. Stability should not be claimed for such cases until all retention appliances have been abandoned for at least 2, or preferably 5, years.

Occlusal Factors

Teeth that are retained by the occlusion will be stable without retention appliances. For example, instanding upper incisors that have been moved over the bite will be stable provided the overbite is adequate. Similarly, a unilateral crossbite corrected by upper arch expansion should be stable if there is a good intercuspation of the teeth.

The occlusion is also important in maintaining a corrected anteroposterior arch relationships—following retraction of upper buccal segments in a Class II case, for example. Stability of overbite reduction depends on a change in the interincisor relationship; the edge-centroid relationship must be secure (*see* p. 77).

Facial Growth and Occlusal Development

Dento-alveolar adaptation tends to maintain occlusal relationships even when skeletal relationships change with growth. However, if the intercuspation of the teeth is poor, or if dento-alveolar compensation is already at its limits, occlusal changes can occur, particularly where skeletal growth changes are marked. For example, a Class III occlusion will often deteriorate if the underlying Class III skeletal relationship becomes more severe; and a skeletal open bite often becomes worse with growth in lower face height.

Although the arch relationships remain stable in most cases, increase in labial segment crowding is often associated with dento-alveolar adaptation. Mesial drift of buccal teeth contributes to the development of labial segment crowding. Many causes of mesial drift have been postulated, including the anterior component of force, tensions in the supra-alveolar connective tissues and impaction of third permanent molars. It is possible that all these factors can play a part, but the evidence is not clear cut, and certainly the early removal of third permanent molars cannot be justified on these grounds alone.

Supporting Tissues

In normal circumstances, transient variations in occlusal and muscular forces will not result in tooth movement. However, when a tooth has been moved by an orthodontic appliance, the recently deposited bone is particularly susceptible to resorption. Thus relapse can occur due to minor imbalances that would normally have no effect. For this reason it is prudent to retain most tooth movements for a period of months until the supporting tissues have adapted fully. The supporting bone and principal fibres of the periodontal ligament will be reorganized within 3–6 months, but the supra-alveolar connective tissue takes very much longer. This can produce partial relapse of rotations and of labial movement of instanding lateral incisor teeth unless they are held by an overbite (*Fig.* 18.1). Pericision of the free gingival and transeptal fibres following rotation (*Fig.* 18.1)

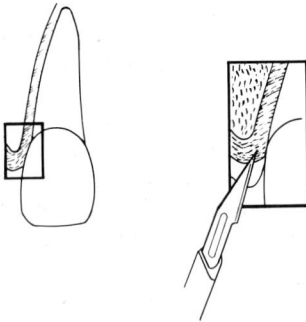

Fig. 18.1. Pericision. A fine pointed scalpel blade is inserted through the gingival margin as far as the alveolar crest and the incision is carried circumferentially around the tooth. Care must be taken that all the free gingival and transeptal fibres are severed.

helps to stabilize the correction, although it does not eliminate the risk of relapse. Overcorrection and prolonged retention also help to deal with this problem, although there are no precise quantitative guidelines because individual response varies so much.

In the adult patient with periodontal disease appreciable drifting of teeth, particularly the upper incisors, may occur. This is in part due to pocket formation producing an imbalance in periodontal support, but to a large extent can be attributed to disruption of the transeptal and other supra-alveolar connective tissue fibres which undoubtedly have an important role in stabilizing tooth positions against minor imbalance in occlusal and soft tissue forces. Particularly where the control of upper incisors by the lower lip is marginal, they may drift labially and space, while the lower incisors overerupt. Stabilization of these teeth following orthodontic treatment can be very difficult. Control of the periodontal condition is mandatory, and if there has been appreciable loss of periodontal support, some form of permanent retention will be required.

RETENTION

Following orthodontic treatment, the occlusion may be self-retentive, as when an upper incisor is moved over the bite, and no retention appliance will be required. Unless there is positive occlusal retention of the treatment result, it is usual to fit a retainer at least until the supporting tissues have reorganized fully.

Retention can be short term, medium term or permanent.

Short-term Retention

This extends from 3 to 6 months while the supporting tissues are reorganized. A removable appliance is most useful because it can be worn only part-time towards the end of the retention period. A typical regime would be full-time wear for the first 3 months, followed by nights-only wear for a similar period. Some operators then ask the patient to wear the appliance only on alternate nights to taper off the retention gradually. The advantage of concluding retention with part-time wear is that if the teeth become more mobile, or if the appliance is difficult to insert after it has been left out, this indicates that the tooth positions may not be stable. There is little merit in then extending the retention period in the hope that things will improve. A decision has to be made either to proceed with further orthodontic treatment or to leave out the appliance to find out how much relapse will occur.

Where active treatment has been completed with a removable appliance, this may be rendered passive and used as a retainer. On some occasions it is better to make a new retainer, and this is generally required following fixed appliance treatment.

For most purposes a Hawley type of retainer (*Fig.* 18.2) is adequate in the upper arch. A similar appliance can be used in the lower arch but the patient may find this difficult to manage, and it is often best to remove attachments of a lower fixed appliance progressively, so that the fixed appliance is used as a retainer. Premolar attachments are removed first and then molar bands, so that a sectional arch is used to retain the labial segment.

Some orthodontists like to use a positioner for retention. This is a flexible splint (*Fig.* 18.3) made from hard rubber or plastic material, into which the

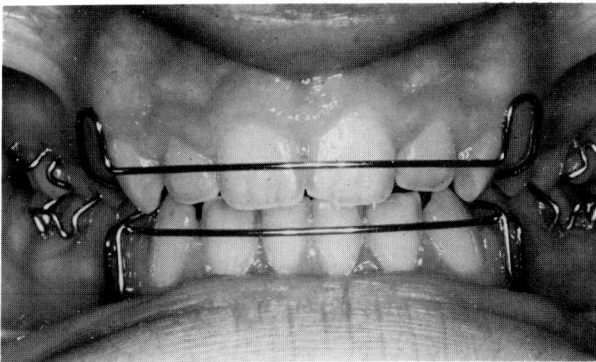

Fig. 18.2. Upper and lower removable retainers.

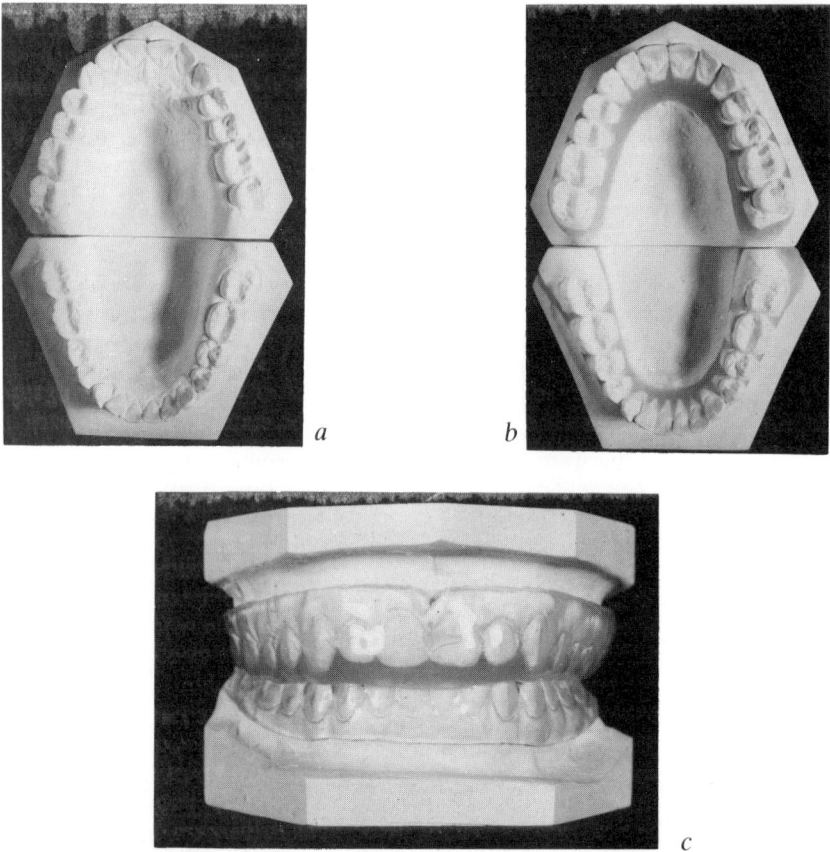

Fig. 18.3. A positioner. *a*, At the completion of appliance treatment, minor irregularities remain. *b*, These teeth are removed from the model and repositioned to correct any minor irregularities. The adjustments to the tooth positions are small and the arch size and form are not changed. *c*, The positioner is made on the adjusted models from a plastic or rubber material.

patient bites. It is intended to adjust any minor dental irregularities, although this should have been done with the active appliance. Preformed positioners are available but these have the serious limitations that unless one can be found that fits the occlusion precisely, they may be ineffective as retainers and may even introduce unwanted tooth movements. Individually prepared positioners are made on models that have been adjusted to correct any minor irregularities (*Fig.* 18.3).

Medium-term Retention

This is appropriate where the supporting tissues will take a longer time to adapt, or where it is decided to stabilize the occlusion during the later stages of facial growth so that dento-alveolar adaptation does not result in adverse occlusal changes, and, in particular, in lower incisor crowding.

Medium-term retention may extend from 1 to 5 years. A fixed retainer will generally be used, and although some orthodontists use positioners in this capacity, this is of questionable benefit.

Medium-term retention should be used only where there are clear indications that it will be beneficial and not merely to postpone the inevitable relapse of an unstable treatment result.

Bonded Flexible Retainers

Where a rotated tooth is to be retained for an extended period a multiple strand wire can be bonded to the lingual surfaces of the tooth in question and its neighbours. With multiple rotations in the upper labial segment for example, the retainer may extend from canine to canine.

The retainer must be clear of the occlusion. The flexibility of the wire allows a small amount of individual tooth movement in response to occlusal forces. Attempts to bond adjacent teeth together directly usually fail because of these minor tooth movements. Retainers of this type will generally be used for between 1 year and 18 months.

Lower Lingual Retainers (Fig. 18.4)

These are particularly useful where the lower incisors were crowded or where the lower labial segment has been proclined and it is considered that relapse could be produced by late facial growth and associated dento-alveolar adaptation. A retainer of this type ensures that dento-alveolar adaptation has to occur

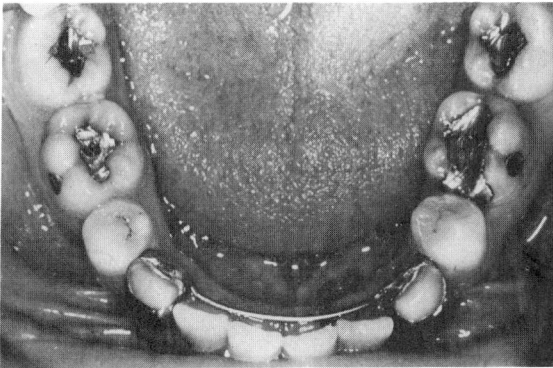

Fig. 18.4. A lower lingual retainer attached to bands on the lower canine teeth.

in other ways, for example by some proclination of the upper incisor teeth. Also, mesial drift of the lower buccal segments is prevented from encroaching on the labial segment. This does not ensure, of course, that adverse occlusal changes will not occur following the eventual removal of the retainer.

The retainer is made from 0.7 mm wire, attached to bands or gauze that will be bonded to the supporting teeth, usually the canines. The retainer may be attached to the canines or premolars.

In many situations the retainer will be in place for 12–18 months; however, if they are to be effective in controlling dento-alveolar adaptation, lower lingual retainers have to be worn until growth is nearly complete. This may mean that the retainer must be left in place until 16–19 years of age in boys, and until 14-17 years of age in girls. Prolonged retention should not be embarked upon lightly. Regular inspection is required to ensure that the appliance is satisfactory, and careful oral hygiene is necessary to prevent plaque accumulation.

Permanent Retention

Permanent retention can be justified only in exceptional circumstances: for example, in the patient with a cleft of the lip and palate where a prosthesis can act as retainer, and in adult patients with periodontal problems where there is no alternative but to stabilize the teeth permanently.

Chapter 19

Oral Surgery for Orthodontic Patients

David Poswillo and Murray Foster

CRANIOMAXILLOFACIAL SURGERY

Techniques developed in Europe in the early 1950s, particularly those of Obwegeser and Trauner,[1] provided the basis for surgical movements of the jaws which would alter, in a stable fashion, the alveolar and basal bones. These techniques now provide the opportunity for orthodontist and oral surgeon to treat, in collaboration, severe orofacial disproportion which was not previously amenable to orthodontic therapy. In this section the guidelines for the planning and execution of orthognathic surgery of the maxilla and mandible will be discussed, with special emphasis on the aspects with which the orthodontist should be familiar.

Case Assessment

Early in treatment planning the consultant responsible for overall case control should discuss, with the patient, the principal complaint and the motives for seeking treatment. At this interview possible treatment options should be outlined and good written records initiated. If it appears likely that the patient will proceed with treatment, or wish further information, additional records such as photographs, study models and radiographs should be obtained. The initial radiographic views required are a lateral cephalogram, plus pan-oral and appropriate intra-oral films. A facebow recording may assist with accurate mounting of the study models.

Early in the assessment phase attention should be given to psychological and behavioural matters, career prospects, educational commitments, marriage plans and other personal matters. Family attitudes to facial appearance should be evaluated, signs of personal embarrassment should be sought (for example, covering the mouth with the hand while conversing) and the expectations of treatment should be compared with the likely results of surgery. An early meeting with parents, spouses or other important members of the family will help to provide a picture of home support and attitudes to treatment. These preliminary observations are essential if the true measure of the patient's concern with facial or dental appearance is to be appreciated.

At an appropriate stage of assessment the patient should be informed of all realistic treatment options, including the masking of deformity by less demanding camouflage or compromise procedures. The advantages, disadvantages and likely complications of the various options should be explained. Special attention should be given to obtaining an accurate history of the general medical status of the patient and the presence or absence of genetic disease in the immediate family. While eliciting all this essential detail the clinician can assemble information related to the specific facial problem. It should be remembered that many factors that affect assessment and the outcome of treatment are outside surgical control; factors such as skin quality, general health, hair, and the shape, size and position of the ears can rarely be changed. Ethnic factors should be considered when planning the 'ideal' facial form: cultural attitudes may not coincide with those that motivate the surgeon.

If treatment is to proceed, it must satisfy the patient's concern with respect to the presenting problem. There is an overriding need, at this stage, to define this area from the point of view of both surgeon and patient. Where the aspirations of the patient can be matched by the technical skills of the surgeon there exists a realistic basis for a successful outcome.

Clinical Inspection

When examining, first inspect critically and then gently palpate to confirm your findings. Note if the face and occlusion are symmetrical, for the ensuing discourse assumes this. If *asymmetry* exists define the main area affected, think hard about which side is at fault and calculate which sites need to be corrected. Is the asymmetry limited to the lower face or are the orbits and temporomandibular joints included? Assuming it is lower facial, does the maxillary plane require lateral levelling and if so would it be best to raise one side or lower the other? Generally the former is felt to be more stable but the decision clearly depends on lip/incisor relationships, the need to alter the anteroposterior occlusal plane angle, existing nasal airway patency and what mandibular procedure is anticipated.

The initial emphasis should be on general impressions, the balance, then proportions of the face, both in profile and full face. Look at the chin, nose and lip balance, both vertical and anteroposterior. Use the labiomental/nasolabial angles for this, and supplement them with the frontonasal and chin–neck angles. Is the nasal profile alone a likely source of complaint by the patient (the size, width, symmetry, shape, humping), are the nostrils flared or pinched, is the columella particularly noticeable? Note the relative facial prominence of the zygomata, orbital rims and orbital globes in relation to the jaws and chin. A higher facial convexity is generally more acceptable in Caucasian females than males. Look at the vertical proportions of the face; are they within an acceptable range or are the upper and lower face too long or short or is the fault a combination of both? As a general rule the distances from glabella to subnasale and from subnasale to the base of chin should be about equal.

When viewing the patient's profile, remember that the patient himself cannot see this. Try to determine clinically whether any anteroposterior discrepancy between the jaws is mainly maxillary or mandibular in origin, or both. Relate this to the earlier assessment of upper and lower facial heights, and palpate the nasolabial areas to determine the underlying bony level. Likewise, palpate the infra-orbital rims and glabella and check the masseteric muscle bulk during clenching, and the symmetry of mandibular opening.

Circumoral assessment must include the relative prominence of the lips and the ratio of the upper/lower vermilion exposure. The degree of lip competence and lip tone is worth noting. What relationship has the upper lip to the upper incisors at rest? Usually 1–4 mm shows in adults. Note this especially when the patient is smiling, and whether there is excessive or deficient upper gingival exposure. How are the lateral facial proportions in the full face view? It is most common to see the inner canthus line up with the lateral alar margins, and the pupils with the oral commissures. Does the intercanthal distance look right (men 34 mm, women 33 mm)? Normal values of soft tissue proportion in the full face view have been published, as have those of soft tissue profile proportion in the predominant ethnic groups.[2]

Radiological Examination

The assessment can now move on to a more exact analysis (but no more or less important) of the hard tissues, best done with radiographs in the light of clinical findings. In the United Kingdom it is unusual to analyse postero-anterior cephalograms for anything other than the site and broad degrees of asymmetry. Most emphasis is put on the proportional and absolute linear, vertical and anteroposterior measurements, in addition to angular assessments. The importance of having standardized lateral cephalograms cannot be overemphasized when comparing patient data.

When inspecting such a film, ensure that appropriate soft tissue outlines can be seen easily and that there is good quality and exposure, including the entire skull, nose, chin and hyoid, and that it is appropriately labelled with the patient's name, date and hospital of origin. Any of the currently accepted methods of cephalometric analysis may be used (*see* Chapter 6). The importance is that the clinical impression and diagnosis of the main source of skeletal and occlusal defects is sharpened or adjusted, and that possible solutions to the basic defect(s) or, alternatively, less complex masking procedures, are generated during the analysis.

Special Tests

At the conclusion of clinical and radiographic analysis a clear impression should exist in the clinician's mind as to the sites of the main anteroposterior, vertical and transverse discrepancies. In addition, an assessment should be made of the compensations that have taken place naturally, and those corrections which it may be reasonable to offer, bearing in mind the patient's complaints and aspirations.

The principles of orthodontic assessment have already been covered in Chapter 7. The differences specific to surgical assessment include the following additional examinations: it is important to have periapical films of the teeth adjacent to a planned osteotomy within the dental arch, and vitality test results must be recorded where teeth are at risk during segmental surgery.

It is a good plan to retake preoperative radiographs after the completion of orthodontic treatment to reassess root and apical positions and any changes that may have followed appliance therapy. While with modern appliance orthodontics and techniques of arch levelling many feel that the place for segmental surgery is receding, there are still instances where the patient and problem merit this type of solution to adjust the occlusal plane or level and achieve better occlusion, e.g. in open bites, both anterior and lateral. The most likely category will be where the patient's age or commitments or dental condition preclude protracted, visible appliance therapy and a surgical alternative can be offered. It is, of course, possible to create space orthodontically to enable easier and safer segmental osteotomy to be performed. Surgical correction of deep overbite and anterior open bite may still be preferred when long term orthodontic stability is uncertain.

Extra study models should be requested and if necessary articulated on an articulator machine, but remember that the patient's own jaw provides the best guide to articulation. Using a fine plaster cutting jig-saw blade, segmental surgery can be tried out by sectioning the model at the sites that would appear most suitable for arch expansion, realignment of anterior segments, or their vertical or anteroposterior repositioning, usually in the canine–premolar region. Beware of removing aproximal tooth substance with a saw: and if small cuspal interferences arise, consider cusp grinding. If a stable final occlusion will result, mark where this has been done, recalling that extreme grinding will produce dentine sensitivity needing treatment. Remove segments of base plaster and keep them as a guide to the necessary bone removal, and make a note of what has been planned.

The mobilized segment may be held in the neutral position, initially with soft pink carding wax, and later by 'sticky yellow wax' or by dual pins in each segment joined by elastics. Test the new occlusion in protrusive and lateral excursive movements. Depending on the method of fixation to be used, a new occlusal impression may be needed to construct a wafer to tie the mobilized segments together. Alternatively, if splints are to be used, an accurate impression should be taken immediately preoperatively and the procedure outlined to the technician, enabling the necessary segmental splints to be prepared with appropriate locking plates and openings to allow the planned cuspal grinding at operation.

Templates

When osteotomies are to be carried out, templates are used by some surgeons. These must be prepared with great care. The template must locate firmly into position in such a way that it relates positively to the teeth, otherwise inadequate or excessive quantities of bone may be removed and require bone grafting or prejudice the stability of the result.

For certain complex and poorly predictable osteotomies, it is often desirable to make up full scale models to facilitate mock surgery and pre-empt operative difficulties and unforeseen rotations. This may be particularly applicable to body ostectomies of the mandible, anterior mandibular osteotomies and certain bimaxillary and midfacial procedures.

Final treatment planning

This is best undertaken at a joint orthodontic and oral surgery clinic, with the patient present and after each clinician has had an opportunity to see the patient or study the records. Having reached an agreed diagnosis and assessed the patient's needs and suitabilities, and thought out varying treatment options, these can be discussed with the patient, their merits compared and a plan of action evolved. Most treatment planning will be performed in this fashion. The emphasis is commonly towards predominantly orthodontic or predominantly surgical solutions and a variety of aids to the processes are used. These include the dental model and jaw model mock surgery, discussed already.

In instances where facial morphology will alter, it has become accepted practice for a number of clinicians to 'profile plan' the changes. Some clinicians point to the value of conducting this process in the presence of the patient, as the planning exercise forms a method of communication with the patient, whose comprehension of the likely change can only be enhanced by seeing the predicted profile and a suitable explanation of its meaning and accuracy. In addition, the method can be used as a valuable teaching and thought-provoking procedure.

While the 'eye-balling' system that comes from experience is the more popular tool, profile planning should be outlined at this point. The method described by Henderson[3] requires a transparent (celluloid) lateral facial photograph to be enlarged to a precise profile fit with the most recent lateral cephalogram. The points S, N, A, B, menton, gnathion, gonion, pogonion, ANS, PNS, are pricked through both the lateral cephalogram and the superimposed profile photograph and the incisor and first molar of each jaw is traced on to the photograph, This is then separated from the cephalogram and checked. The photograph is sectioned and re-positioned to simulate the planned osteotomy movements. The soft tissue profile consequences are then calculated and the chin, nose and lip re-positioned accordingly. Overlaps and defects are eliminated and the result represents a reasonable guide to the likely profile alterations; and it may also serve to reveal unfavourable effects of certain osteotomy plans (*Fig.* 19.1).

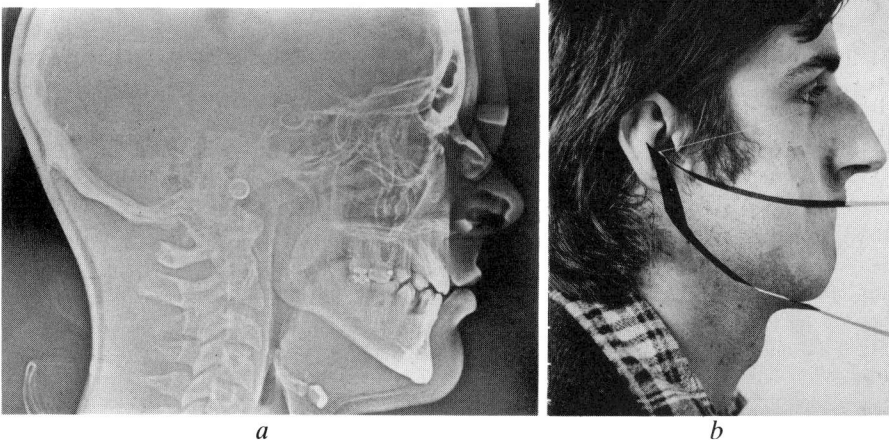

a   *b*

Fig. 19.1. *a*, Soft tissue profile with underlying skeleton and teeth shown on xeroradio-graph prior to profile planning. *b*, Paste up of profile segments on planning photographic print. (From David D. J., Poswillo D. and Simpson D. (1983) *The Craniosynostoses.* Berlin, Springer-Verlag.)

Mandibular Prognathism and Retrognathism

Osteotomy Techniques

In recent years there has been a proliferation of procedures used for the correction of dentofacial anomalies in which the collaboration of the orthodontist and the oral surgeon is paramount. The very fact that diverse techniques exist for the correction of almost every type of orthognathic problem means that no specific operative method is universally applicable to a given type of jaw deformity. Surgeons may prefer to operate by the intra-oral route or by other approaches from the skin surface; and the choice between maxillary, mandibular, intra-oral, extra-oral, segmental and interradicular techniques allows the surgeon numerous options. Every effort should be made to avoid obviously inappropriate procedures, and generally, when the guiding principles of assessment and case planning are applied, an optimal solution is available for each individual problem of orofacial deformity. Clearly the plethora of technical modifications cannot be encompassed in a single chapter. Opportunity will be taken, in this section, to describe in broad outline those basic technical procedures that are frequently used in one modified form or another for the correction of most orthodontic/orthognathic problems.

Body Ostectomy

This method is valuable for closure of gaps in the dental arch, reduction of the abnormally long body of the mandible and the restoration of symmetry (*Fig. 19.2*). It can be used to close an anterior open bite, in conjunction with a reduction in lower facial height. The area of bone contact achieved is often less than adequate, however, and union is not always achieved in the expected time.

This method requires meticulous model planning on a plaster or acrylic mandible. Templates showing the precise amount of bone to be removed are

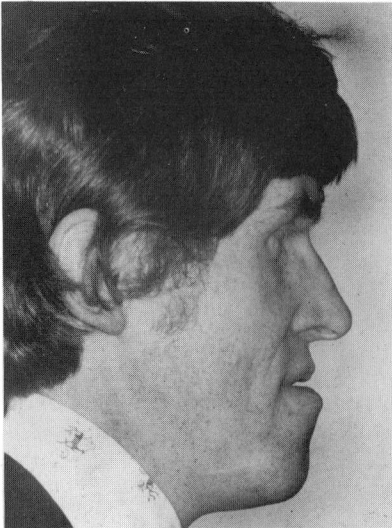

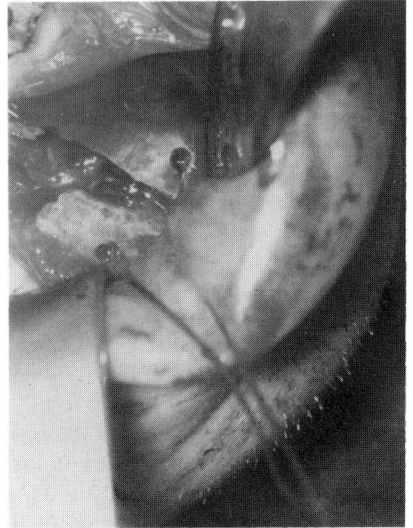

a   *b*

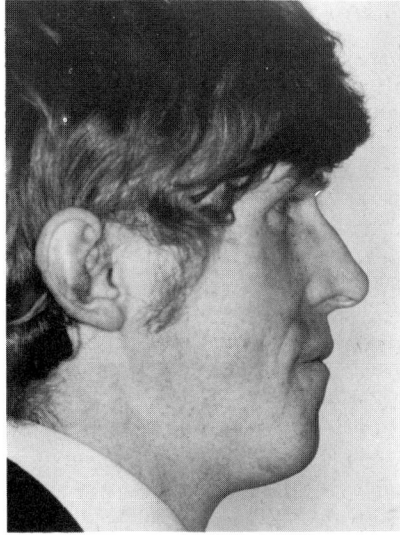

Fig. 19.2. *a*, Profile view showing prognathism with abnormally long body of mandible. *b*, Gap in premolar region of body of mandible after body ostectomy and prior to tightening of fixation wires: mental nerve is protected in 'bone cave' at superior aspect of cut. *c*, Profile following bilateral intra-oral body ostectomy.

c

constructed, due consideration being paid to the sites of teeth and roots adjacent to the bone cuts. The surgical approach is generally intra-oral and bone grafts are useful additions to promote early union. While intermaxillary fixation is not always essential, great care must be taken with the method of splinting, especially where the crowns of the teeth are malposed or small.

The principal disadvantages of this procedure are those connected with the necessity to avoid injury to the mental nerve and the difficulty in fixing a small anterior semilunar segment on widely flared posterior bone cuts. Union is impaired in these circumstances, even when grafting with iliac crest bone mush is employed. When large movements are undertaken, relapse is prone to occur, vertical steps may remain on the lower border of the mandible and excessive submental soft tissue may produce an unacceptable 'double chin' appearance. The procedure does nothing to overcome the poor aesthetics of an obtuse mandibular angle in cases of mandibular prognathism.

C and L Osteotomies

These geometrically designed ramal bone cut procedures permit repositioning of the body and tooth-bearing segment of the mandible in relation to the rami within the pterygomasseteric sling. While the range of movement of the resected parts is somewhat limited, there is some advantage from the minimal positional disturbances of the muscles of mastication. The methods are particularly favoured for the closure of anterior open bite, provided that pure rotation is avoided, for this leads to instability. Bone grafts are usually incorporated in the area of the resection to promote union and stability (*Fig.* 19.3).

The surgical approach is usually extra-oral. Care must be taken to match arch widths and levels, and attention should be given to good final cuspal interdigitation. Intermaxillary fixation is generally required for 6–8 weeks postoperatively. These procedures have the advantage of interfering only minimally with the

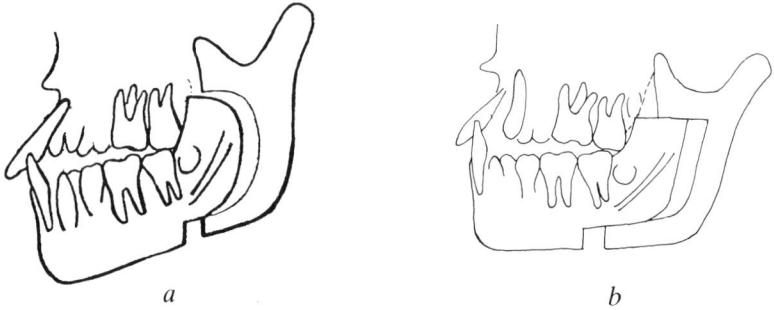

Fig. 19.3. *a*, Diagram of bone cuts in conventional C osteotomy. *b*, Diagrammatic view of modified Trauner L osteotomy in mandible.

coronoid process and temporal muscle. The chief limitation is that of relapse: when considerable mandibular advancement is attempted, relapse may be dramatic. While paraesthesia of the lips is usually avoided, trismus may persist for a long period, especially when the coronoid process is inadvertently fractured during operation. The use of iliac bone grafts may leave an unacceptable external scar at the donor site.

Mandibular Ramus Osteotomies

The aim of these procedures is to reposition the entire body of the mandible in relation to the maxillary teeth, while operating within the pterygomasseteric sling which envelops the site of surgery. While the procedures usually permit great flexibility in the repositioning of segments, there are limits to the degree of retrusion and/or advancement that can be achieved without loss of stability. Attempts to reduce or elongate much beyond 1 cm are often compromised by relapse.

In choosing these procedures, attention should be given to the adequacy of the final occlusion and arch fit; and spot grinding may need to be done at operation to facilitate these aims. The use of forms of fixation which do not cover the crowns of the teeth is essential if occlusal adjustment is to be carried out. It should be ensured that the condyles are correctly repositioned in the fossa prior to establishing intermaxillary fixation. These procedures usually produce large areas of cancellous bone for optimum healing of the fixed segments. Relapse is minimized by periods of fixation extending to 8 weeks and beyond.

In experienced hands there are usually few complications from these procedures. Postoperative swelling can be greatly reduced by the use of steroids, peri- and postoperatively; bleeding is usually slight, especially when local anaesthetic infiltration is employed and incisions are made with a cutting diathermy. Adequate drainage of the wound prevents haematoma formation. Often there is some alteration in sensation of the lips and tongue for variable periods after operation. Rarely, prolonged paraesthesia may occur. Relapse, in well-planned cases, is seldom severe and the patient acceptance of these procedures is uniformly high.

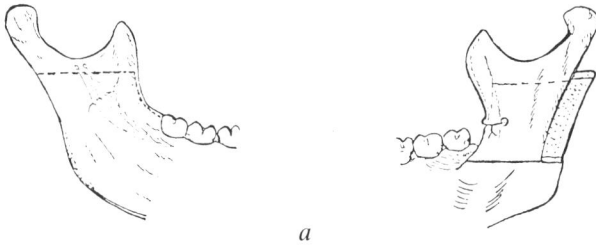

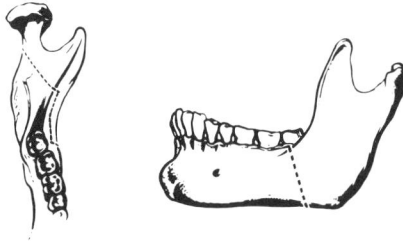

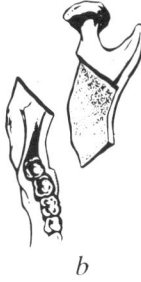

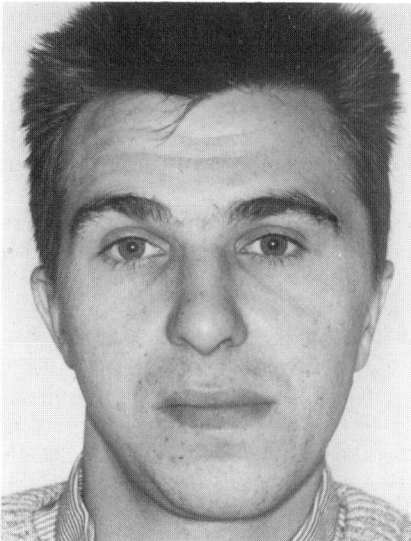

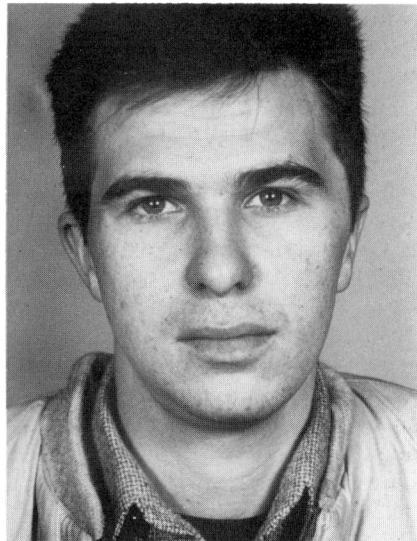

a

b

c

d

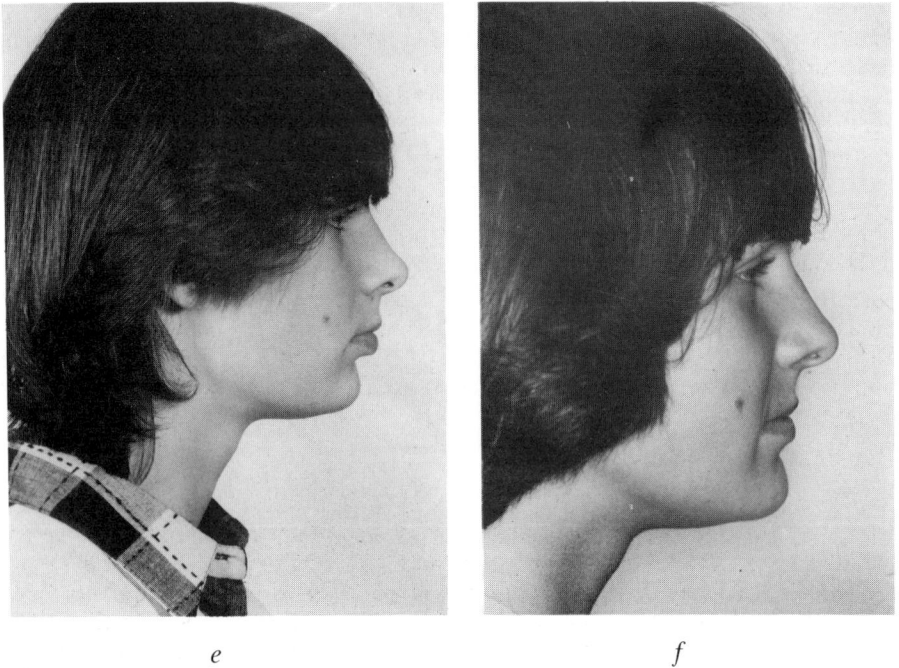

e   f

Fig. 19.4. *a*, High Obwegeser osteotomy cuts for classic sagittal split technique. *b*, Dal Pont modification of Obwegeser sagittal split. *c*, *d*, Pre- and postoperative views of asymmetrical prognathism with asymmetry corrected by Obwegeser 'high' sagittal split bilaterally with push-back and rotation. *e*, *f*, Pre- and postoperative profile where orthodontic treatment combined with Dal Pont modification sagittal splits were used to advance the body of the mandible.

Sagittal Split Techniques

The original Obwegeser[4] method, in the ramus, has great merit for push-back procedures. It is sparing of damage to the inferior dental nerve and is a particularly versatile procedure, allowing the correction of asymmetry and crossbite and occasionally closure of small degrees of anterior open bite (*Fig.* 19.4).

The Dal Pont[5] modification of Obwegeser's technique is widely used for mandibular advancement: it provides a large area of bony contact, but has the disadvantage of greater inferior dental nerve morbidity. It is probably the most widely used method of correction of prognathism and mandibular retrusion in the United Kingdom and Europe. Rare instances of severe haemorrhage and postoperative VIIth nerve paresis have been reported but these are the exception. The absence of facial scars and the relative stability of the procedure have enhanced the reputation of the sagittal split method as the operation of first choice whenever case assessment indicates the possibility of this approach to treatment.

Vertical Subsigmoid Osteotomy

This technique can be used from either an extra-oral or an intra-oral approach. It is very popular from the intra-oral route in the United States of America, because of the low incidence of paraesthesia of the inferior dental and lingual nerves when the method is used to correct prognathism. The technique also produces an aesthetically pleasing angle to the previously obtuse mandible, though care should be taken not to run the risk of a hamster-like flare of the lower third of the face in those patients with a square or oval facial type.

The procedure is not suitable for mandibular advancement and the degree of mandibular retrusion achieved may be constrained by the width of the ramus posteriorly or the impaction of the coronoid process on the temporal aspect of the zygomatic arch. Coronoidectomy may be necessary in some instances, but is associated with trismus. The procedure is performed very rapidly, with little postoperative swelling, especially in the pharynx. Although necrosis of the tip of the distal segment has been reported, this is not a common problem and the incidence of complications is extremely low.

The surgical approach to the ramus, in the intra-oral technique, involves exposure of the lateral aspect of the ramus only. Retractors in the sigmoid notch above, and under the angle below, provide adequate access and visibility for sectioning of the ramus vertically, behind the anti-lingula, by means of an oscillating saw. Once the mandible has been sectioned by an oblique cut from the notch above to the lower border, the posterior fragment is overlaid on the lateral aspect of the ramus and the wound is closed. In the hands of the experienced operator the whole procedure takes less than one hour and the patient is usually discharged from hospital the following day. Fixation is maintained for 8 weeks (*Fig.* 19.5).

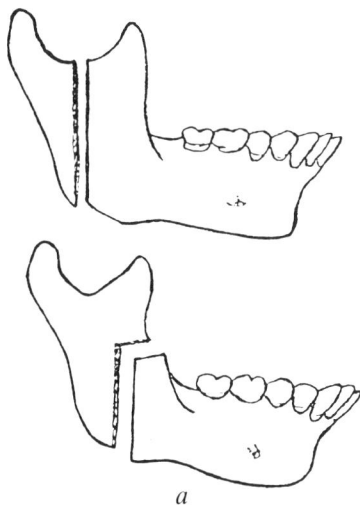

a

Fig. 19.5. *a*, Diagrams showing classic and L-modification vertical subsigmoid bone cuts used for correction of prognathism. *b*, *c*, *d*, *e*, Pre- and postoperative views of mandibular prognathism treated by classic intra-oral vertical subsigmoid procedure. The arch-bar fixation provides good visual repositioning of occlusal surfaces with reasonable aesthetics and minimum inconvenience to the patient.

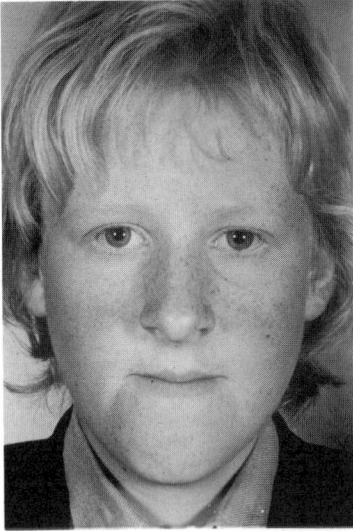

b

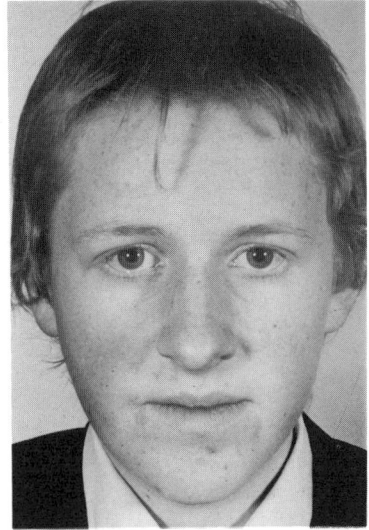

c

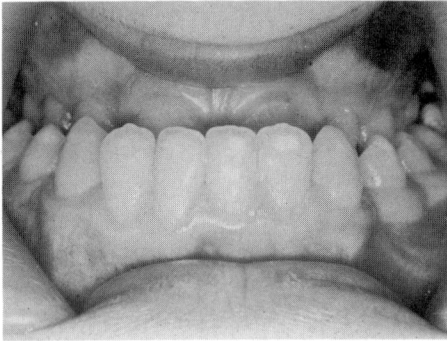

d

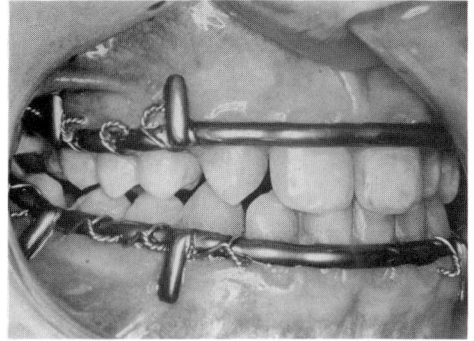

e

Post-condylar Cartilage Grafts

Trauner[6] and, later, Poswillo[7] described these procedures for the correction of distocclusion in the adolescent who could posture forwards into an acceptable incisal relationship. Using bilateral pre-auricular incisions, blocks of autogenous or lyophilized cartilage are anchored to the root of the zygoma above, extra-articularly, between the posterior aspect of the head of the condyle and the bony auditory meatus. These blocks hold the whole mandible forwards in the anticipated position of intercuspation (*Fig.* 19.6). Although postoperative fixation with functional appliances has been used, it is not mandatory. Viability of the cartilage is maintained by tissue fluid perfusion. Forward movement by this technique is usually limited to the width of one premolar tooth. Long-term follow-up reveals that remodelling in the condyle and fossa produce permanent changes in the relationship of the mandible to the base of the skull. The function of the temporomandibular joint is not impaired and the correction of distocclusion and the associated retrognathism are not compromised by relapse.

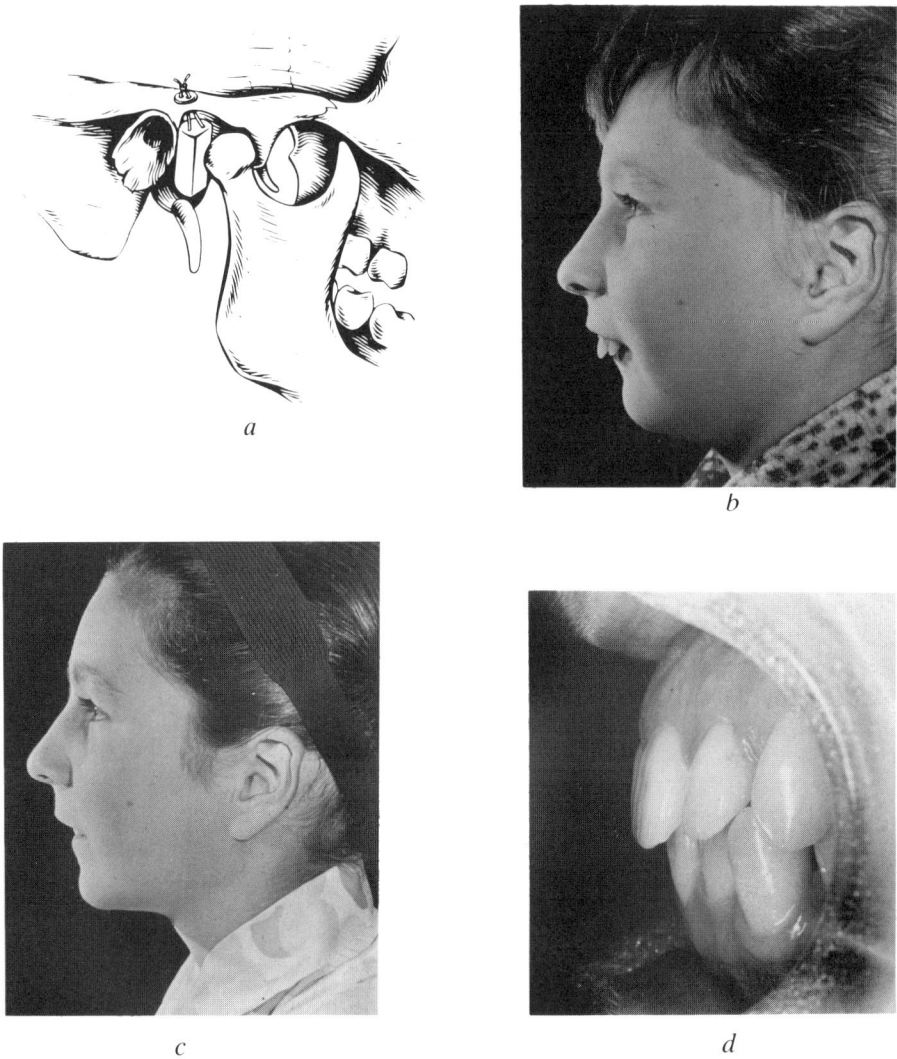

Fig. 19.6. *a,* Diagram of post-condylar cartilage graft technique. *b, c,* Pre- and 1-year postoperative views of corrected distocclusion following this procedure. *d,* Lateral view of anterior occlusion of the same patient 15 years after post-condylar cartilage grafts for mandibular advancement.

The procedure has been favoured by some authors because of lack of interference with the periosteum of the ramus of the mandible. Where the choice of advancement lies between sagittal split procedures or post-condylar grafts and the extent of the advance is not more than one premolar unit, the latter procedure may be preferred for the patient in the late mixed dentition. Early surgical correction of retrognathism by this method permits further functional catch-up growth of the retruded mandible.

Correction of Micrognathia and Retrognathia

While both micrognathia and retrognathia are often loosely used to describe
anterior mandibular deficiency, these terms are not synonymous. Micrognathia
refers to abnormal smallness of the jaw; a localized form of this is microgenia,
where the chin is deficient. Retrognathia implies a retruded position (associated
with Angle Class II, or distocclusion) of the mandible without diminution in size.

In surgical terms, correction of micrognathia is more difficult than the
correction of prognathism for two principal reasons. First, it is more difficult to
augment the mandible than to reduce it; and secondly, when the mandible is
small the investing soft tissues are correspondingly reduced. Expansion of the
soft tissue envelope by elongation of the jaw may fall short of that which is
adequate or desirable.

Ideally, surgical techniques for correction of micrognathia should provide an
adequate Class I occlusion, overall aesthetic improvement, including restoration
of the chin prominence, a satisfactory gonial angle and minimal disruption to the
contents of the mandibular canal or lingual nerve. Innumerable operations have
been described, many of which, while technically feasible, have fallen from
regular use because of problems associated with relapse. The C osteotomy and
the sliding L osteotomy previously referred to have been used with a degree of
success, as have modifications of the sagittal split procedure. A combination of
the L technique with sagittal splitting of the body portion of the mandible,
described by Hayes,[8] has probably been the most successful procedure for
elongation of the micrognathic mandible (*Fig.* 19.7). The method appears to
satisfy all the criteria mentioned above, with few, if any, of the disadvantages of
the L osteotomy or sagittal split procedures when used alone. The results in the
short term, as described by Byrne and Hinds,[9] would suggest that relapse is not
severe and may be further reduced by the application of a sliding graft of cortical

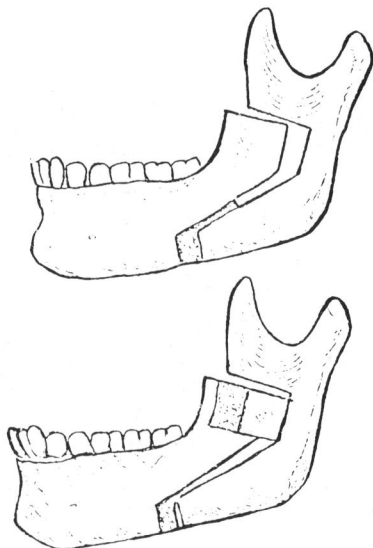

Fig. 19.7. Hayes modified L sagittal split used to advance mandibular body. The onlay
bone bridge is obtained from the split margin of mandibular bone, thus eliminating an
additional operation to 'harvest' bone.

bone which extends from the anterior portion of the ramus, below the coronoid process, back to the bone cut in the posterior section of the ramus, so that the osteotomy gap is bridged and stabilized.

Microgenia and Genioplasty Techniques

While osteotomy procedures and post-condylar grafts are frequently used to extend the body of the mandible forwards into a more acceptable occlusion and a better aesthetic position, compromise procedures may occasionally produce equally acceptable results with less morbidity.

When the occlusion is acceptable and all that is required is improvement in the appearance of the chin, augmentation genioplasty may be the procedure of choice. The simplest method of augmentation is the implantation of a contoured wedge of Proplast into a pocket of periosteum over the chin point. Adjustments to the shape of the alloplastic material permit the correction of small degrees of asymmetry of the chin.

The major disadvantages of alloplastic augmentation of the chin, in the past, have been the degree of bone resorption that subsequently occurs beneath the implant and the migration of the onlays from the position in which they were originally placed. These problems have been most obvious when cartilage or Silastic have been used. It is anticipated, on the basis of short-term experience, that these difficulties may not arise when Proplast or Interpore is used; neverthe-

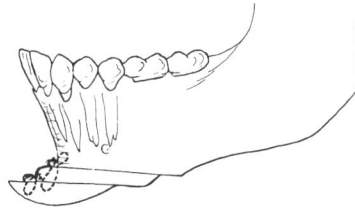

a

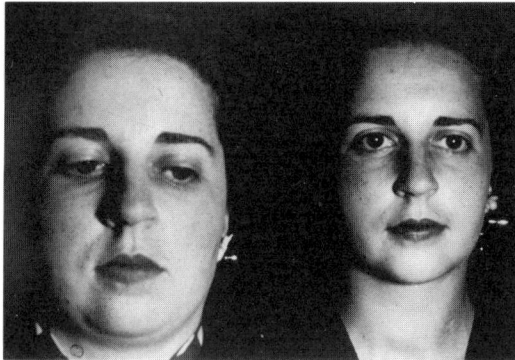

b

Fig. 19.8. *a*, Diagram of two layer chin advancement by genioplasty. *b*, Pre- and postoperative views showing chin contour enhanced by sliding genioplasty.

less most alloplastic augmentation techniques have their limitations.

The procedure which has best stood the test of time in the field of enlargement of the chin has been the anterior lower border osteotomy procedure suggested by Obwegeser.[10] This is a modification of Hofer's[11] original method; by an intra-oral approach, the anterior mandible is degloved and single or even double section horizontal sliding osteotomy cuts are made. The bone sections are pulled forwards, rotated and contoured, as occasion demands, and the forward-sliding grafts are then fixed by transosseous wires. Slight overcorrection is used; lateral portions of the osteotomy segment which project slightly in the mental region are not usually contoured at the time of initial surgery in order to prevent undue rounding of the chin as remodelling proceeds (*Fig.* 19.8).

A similar technical procedure has been used to reduce chin prominence, often in association with upward movement of the lower border of the mandible in the long face syndrome. Instead of advancing the upper sliding section in a two-section genioplasty, it is removed, thus reducing the depth of the chin and allowing aesthetic repositioning of the chin point and lower border. This flexible technique of genioplasty has been found to provide long-term stability when used both for chin augmentation and reduction. It is infinitely superior to onlay techniques in which autogenous bone grafts are used.

Condylar Hyperplasia and Mandibular Hypertrophy

Developmental hyperplasia of the mandibular condyle usually appears about the time of the adolescent growth spurt. The result is excessive growth of the ramus and condyle on the affected side, leading to asymmetric prognathism.

The most rapidly effective surgical treatment is excision of the condyle, through the condylar neck, on the affected side. This technique, timed as soon as opportunity arises after the condition is diagnosed, rapidly restores symmetry of growth and form to the affected side. Within 6–12 months of condylar excision a new condyle has regenerated. The phenomenon of excessive elongation of the condylar head and neck has not been observed in the condyle that appears *de novo*; thus long-term stability is achieved by an uncomplicated surgical pro-

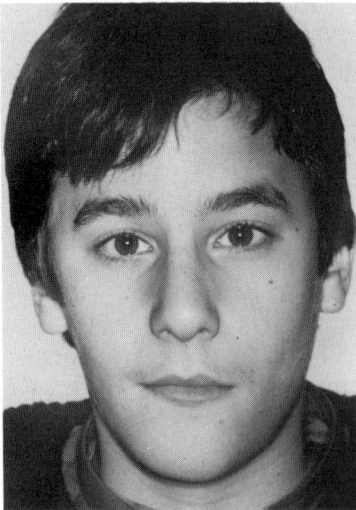

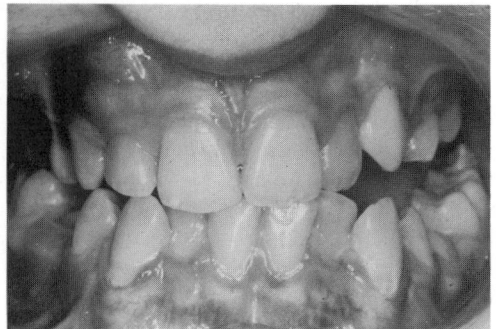

a   *b*

d

c

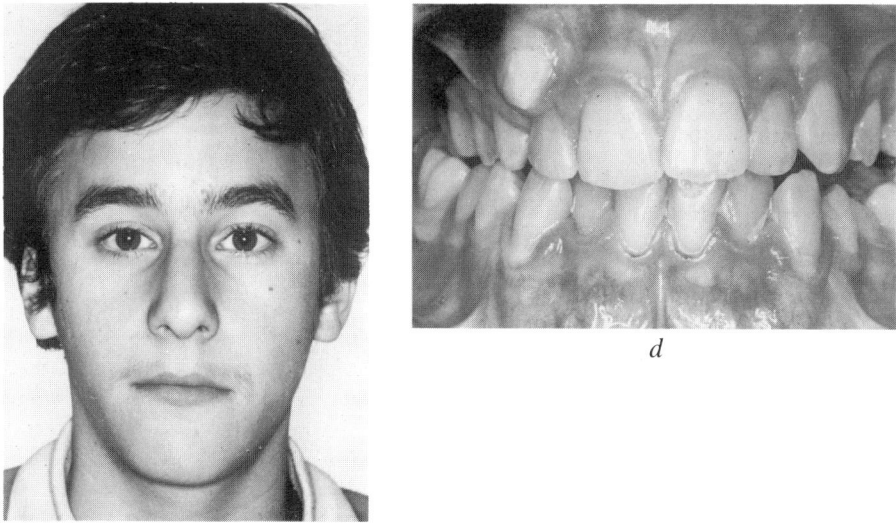

Fig. 19.9. Full face (*a*) and dental view (*b*) show left-sided asymmetry and open bite associated with left condylar hyperplasia. Full face (*c*) and dentition (*d*) prior to definitive orthodontic treatment, 1 year after left total condylectomy.

cedure in a condition which, if untreated, results in severe lateral open bite, or crossbite, with marked facial asymmetry (*Fig.* 19.9). Occasionally orthodontic assistance is required to align the arches on the affected side, after condylectomy, and to facilitate the closure of lateral open bite.

If the developmental deformity is not observed until after the cessation of growth, and lateral shift of the mandible has resulted in severe crossbite and prognathism, a sagittal split osteotomy on the affected side, with or without condylotomy on the contra-lateral side (depending on the degree of rotation of the jaw likely to be required for the correction of acquired cross bite) is the procedure of choice.[12]

In mandibular hemihypertrophy there may be a lowering of the occlusal plane on the affected side with aesthetically unacceptable down-growth of the lower border of the mandible. This produces a form of asymmetry which is difficult to mask without removal of excess basal bone from the lower border of the affected side of the mandible (*Fig.* 19.10).

The presence of the mandibular canal and its contents further complicates surgical approaches to lower border reduction. The optimal procedure, which allows some shortening of the ramus, reduction of open bite (if it exists) and trimming of excess basal bone, is a sagittal split operation extending from above the lingula on the lingual side to the mental foramen labially. Once the mandible is split and the contents of the mandibular canal are dissected free, lower border reduction can be done to the appropriate level on both labial and lingual plates; the ramus may be shortened, and finally, the nerve placed in the soft tissues below the resected border of the mandible before wound closure and skeletal fixation.

Collaboration with the orthodontist in the planning stages, when model

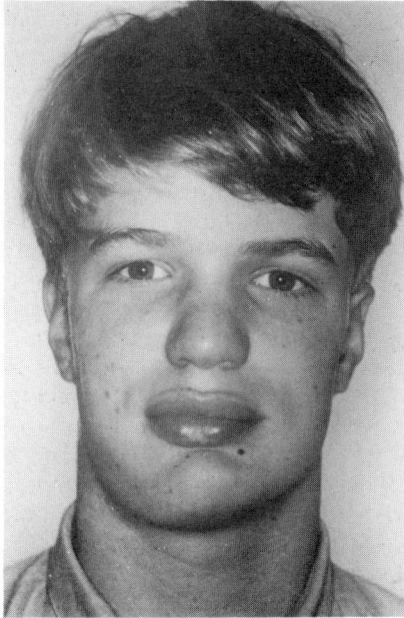

a

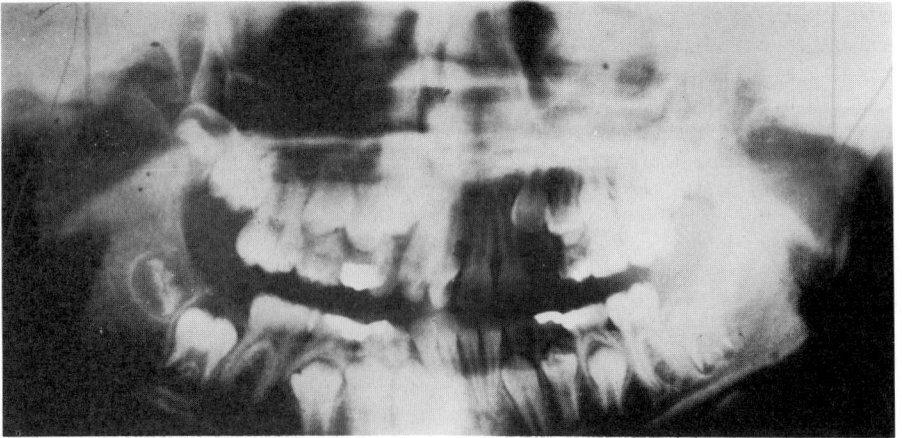

b

Fig. 19.10. *a*, Full face in right hemi-hypertrophy of mandible prior to orthognathic correction. *b*, Orthopantomogram showing increased size of mandible and permanent check teeth on affected side.

surgery on a plaster or acrylic mandible is undertaken, can be of invaluable assistance to the surgeon when planning definitive treatment of these complicated asymmetrical cases. It is generally unwise to proceed to surgical correction of this condition until adolescent growth is complete. In males this may mean deferring final assessment until the early twenties, by which time the third molars will also be in place and their future status may be considered prior to completion of the treatment plan.

Maxillary Osteotomy Procedures

Repositioning of the entire maxillary alveolar process has advanced dramatically in recent years. More than any other orthognathic operation the 'down-fracturing' modification of the earlier Le Fort 1 osteotomy has permitted access and visibility in areas of the maxilla which were previously unknown territory in the field of orthognathic surgery (*Fig.* 19.11). Access to the superior surface of the maxillary fragment has permitted a wide range of variations in the original one-piece repositioning procedure. Bell[13] and others have made numerous important contributions to technique and it is now common for the maxilla to be surgically segmented into numerous parts, which permit optimal positioning of tooth-bearing segments. With adequate illumination, good haemostasis and a substantial palatal pedicle to provide viability to the segments, the range of adjustments to the tooth-bearing maxilla is almost unlimited (*Fig.* 19.12).

Maxillary surgery has permitted greater attention to discrepancies in facial height (e.g. in the long-face and short-face syndromes and vertical maxillary excess), rotational anomalies (e.g. open bite), and anteroposterior deficiencies, especially maxillary hyperplasia. One of the outstanding advantages of this flexible approach has been the ease with which palatal expansion, elevation or lowering may be achieved. By improving the space available for the tongue, incisor stability is enhanced. These new maxillary techniques have involved, more than ever before, the collaboration of the orthodontist in the preparation of cases for orthognathic surgery.

All cases should be planned with an eye to excellent arch matching prior to surgery; such preparation greatly reduces the need for surgical arch levelling and re-angulation of individual small segments. Sectional orthodontic arches are sometimes used to facilitate the definitive correction of occlusal irregularities by multiple step sectioning of the maxilla; and after repositioning, no further

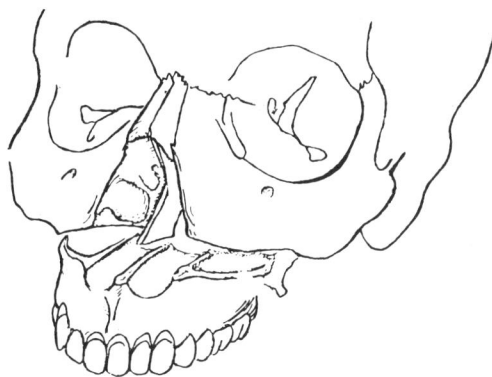

Fig. 19.11. Diagram showing principle of 'down-fracture' for Le Fort I maxillary osteotomy.

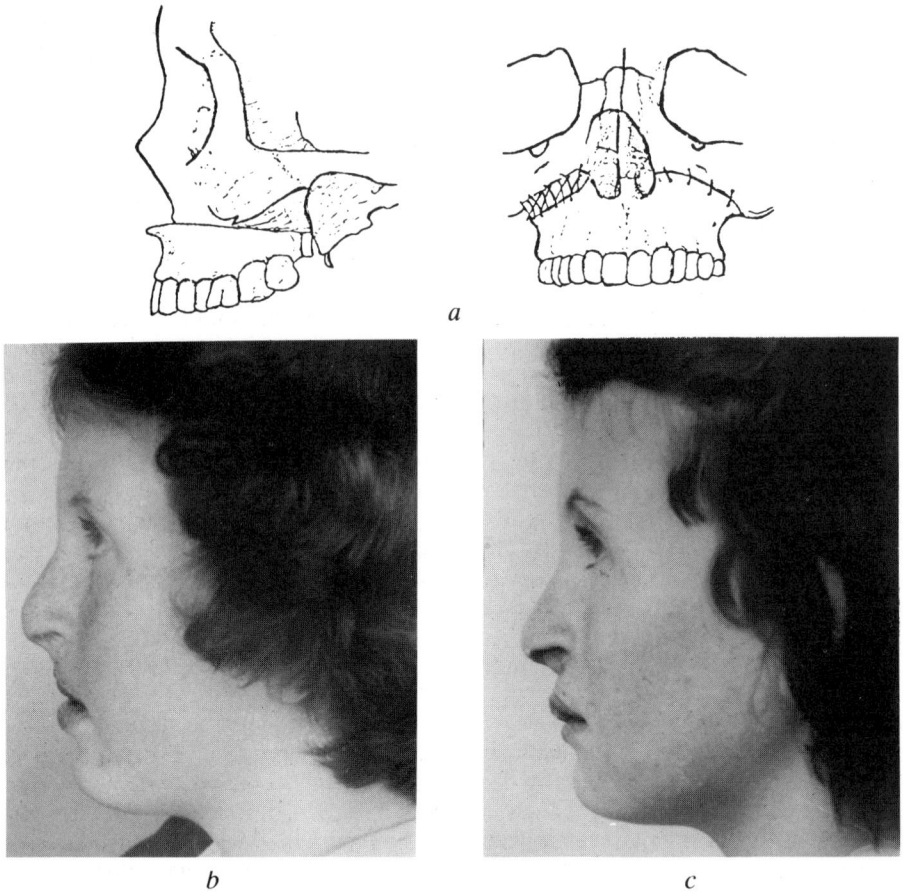

Fig. 19.12. *a,* Diagrammatic view of anterior repositioning of maxilla in Le Fort I osteotomy and asymmetrical adjustment of vertical facial height. The right side shows a stabilizing onlay rib graft technique and the left, direct wire fixation. *b, c,* Pre- and postoperative profile photographs of Le Fort I maxillary advancement in the secondary surgical correction of a cleft lip and palate defect.

orthodontic correction is required.

The technique of maxillary down-fracture involves a vestibular incision, preferably with a cutting diathermy, from one malar buttress to the other. This is followed by osteotomy cuts above the apices of the teeth. The nasal septum, lateral nasal walls and pterygoid plates are separated with appropriate chisels. By leverage, the maxilla is mobilized, appropriate bone cuts are made in the maxilla proper or in the attached bones above, in order to realign the tooth-bearing segments, or move the maxilla upwards, forwards or backwards as the case demands. Bone grafts, while not mandatory, are frequently used to stabilize the segments and promote union. Various methods of fixation, by external rods or internal wires and/or plates, may be used to support the maxilla in the correct relationship to the mandible below and the cranial base above, for periods of up to 12 weeks.

While this short description of technique would suggest that the procedure is usually simple and uncomplicated, it is not always so. Occasionally, maxillae tethered by scar tissue are exceedingly difficult to mobilize. This is especially true of the post-traumatic injury. Haemorrhage may be brisk and tedious to arrest. Fixation is not always a simple procedure. When orthodontic collaboration has been provided preoperatively, it is prudent to use the bands and fixed sturdy arch wires (to which cleets for wires or elastics have been attached) for definitive intermaxillary fixation. A thin cast silver wafer may be placed in the desired position of intercuspation to augment fixation and ensure ideal cuspal interdigitation and stability.

After removal of the intermaxillary wires, attention should be paid by the orthodontist to any minor irregularities in the position of the teeth before fixed orthodontic appliances are removed. These finishing touches are of the greatest assistance to the oral surgeon in the pursuit of excellence in orthognathic surgery.

It may be observed, in cases where multiple small segments of maxilla have been repositioned, that teeth do not respond to clinical vitality tests for long periods after operation. While teeth on smaller segments may be compromised to a greater or lesser degree by postoperative ischaemia, studies have shown that pulp viability, as distinct from vitality, is usually maintained. In the fullness of time, ingrowth of sensory nerves from the adjacent periodontal tissues provides a degree of recovery of traditional pulpal vitality.[14]

Bimaxillary Orthognathic Surgery

Some cases of dentofacial deformity are sufficiently severe to warrant surgical repositioning of both maxillary and mandibular tooth-bearing segments. Where anteroposterior movements of greater than 1·2 cm are needed, or where, for example, the maxilla must be elevated and the mandible advanced, it is desirable to carry out procedures on both jaws at the one operative intervention.

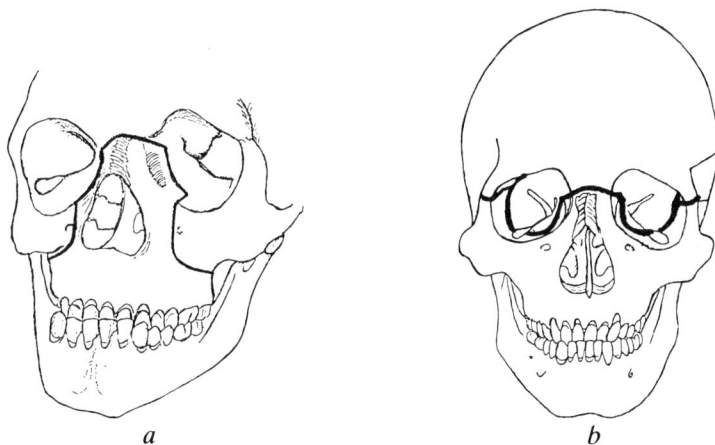

a   *b*

Fig. 19.13. *a*, Surgical bone cut lines used for Le Fort II osteotomy. *b*, Bone cuts in Tessier I Le Fort III osteotomy.

The bimaxillary approach has the considerable advantage of permitting the surgeon to reposition the total maxilla–mandible complex in a new position with respect to the cranial base. The jaws may be advanced, raised, lowered, rotated or asymmetrically moved in order to achieve the planned position. Maxillary osteotomies, while usually carried out at the Le Fort 1 level, may be at any other level, and in general, the entire dental arches of both maxilla and mandible are mobilized and repositioned (*Fig.* 19.13).

Technically, the basic procedures of mandibular and maxillary osteotomies (previously described) are carried out sequentially; the surgeon will decide which jaw is to be repositioned first. While stable internal fixation can be applied after bimaxillary procedures it is common to use external rods attached to cranial fixation. When fixed orthodontic appliances are utilized for intermaxillary fixation, external rods may be fitted by special heavy attachments to the molar bands and arches. The complexities of the fixation and the degree of acceptability of each alternative method should be discussed with the patient before completion of the treatment plan.

The lengthy surgical procedure involved in bimaxillary correction produces additional burdens on patient and surgeon: blood transfusions may be required; bone grafts (with the added morbidity of a donor site) may be necessary; the period of intermaxillary fixation may be prolonged; the risk of injury to peripheral sensory nerves is greater; and the chances of incorrect surgical repositioning are increased, as is a higher rate of relapse. All these matters should be discussed with the candidate for bimaxillary surgery when informed consent to the procedure is sought.

The versatility of combined maxillary and mandibular procedures makes possible the correction of almost any conceivable deformity that may present to the orthodontist and his surgical colleague. The results will depend less on the imagination of the experts than on the degree of care which is taken with the case assessment and preoperative planning and the ability with which the essential technical procedures are carried out.

Surgical Correction of Open Bite

There are numerous ways to close anterior or posterior open bite. The choice of procedure is determined by the results of clinical and cephalometric analysis. Attention should be paid to the pattern of rotational development of the face, the relationship between the skeletal bases, anteriorly and posteriorly, the angles of the maxillary and mandibular occlusal planes, and the anterior and posterior facial heights. Measurements should be made of the relationship between the nasolabial angle, the upper lip and the upper incisors. The aim of the procedure is to produce lip competence and incisor control, an aesthetic nasal tip and pleasing nasolabial and labiomental curves. The orthodontist provides invaluable preoperative assistance by flattening the dental arches and realigning the incisors in such a way that an ideal interincisal angle may be achieved after surgery.

While there are many technical options, including upper and lower segmental procedures, Le Fort 1 maxillary repositioning and anteromandibuloplasty, the choice will ultimately be made on the results of case analysis. Simple rotation of the mandible seldom produces a stable result. Similarly, intrusion of the upper

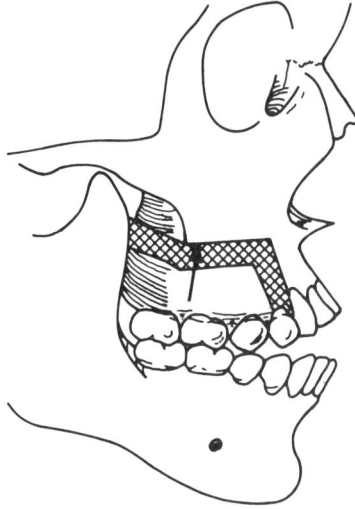

Fig. 19.14. Schuchardt upper buccal segment repositioning procedure. Cross-hatched area represents excised bone.

buccal segments by a Schuchardt[15] procedure is seldom successful unless it is combined with a mandibular sagittal osteotomy (*Fig*. 19.14). While the Schuchardt technique may be suitable when there is a convenient step in the maxillary arch, the technique may have to be varied considerably when the maxillary dental arch is well aligned. In general, the upper buccal segment is intruded more than the anterior segment, by any suitable maxillary procedure, and the mandible is then rotated forwards and upwards. If chin retrusion remains a problem, it may be corrected by combined advancement and reduction genioplasty.

Finally, the role of the tongue in the maintenance of open bite is very much a matter for consideration by the orthodontist during the planning of procedures to close, permanently, an anterior open bite. When abnormal tongue function cannot be controlled, a surgically closed anterior open bite almost invariably relapses. Lip competence and optimal interincisal angulation does much to reduce this problem, but it cannot always be eliminated. Anticipation is the best method of avoiding this form of relapse.

Segmental Osteotomies

As early as 1849, Hullihen[16] described the first anterior mandibular segmental osteotomy. In 1942 Hofer[17] used a similar intra-oral approach to accomplish a forward movement of the anterior maxillary segment. Since these early descriptions, a plethora of small osteotomy procedures, carried out by an intra-oral approach, have been described for the correction of severe malposition of the teeth, all on the same segment, when the basal bone is in a relatively satisfactory position. These techniques have the advantage over conventional orthodontic alignment in that the teeth can be moved a considerable distance, upwards, downwards, laterally or obliquely, by a one-stage surgical repositioning with little likelihood of significant relapse. The anterior maxillary and mandibular segmental osteotomies rapidly produce the refinements of lip contour and anterior occlusion that orthodontic treatment might be hoped to provide, but with less likelihood of idiopathic root resorption, especially in adults.

The anterior maxillary osteotomy of Wassmund[18] is a one-stage procedure to alter, to a more acceptable aesthetic and functional position, the premaxillary segment which is protruded (*Fig.* 19.15). The segment to be treated may include the premolar teeth bilaterally and all the anterior teeth on any of the various segments within these limits. The midline of the premaxilla may also be split to move the two halves independently and close a diastema between the incisors. The anterior maxillary arch may be recontoured, moved superiorly or inferiorly, rotated or even advanced (utilizing an interpositional graft) by this well-established technique.

Originally, the method involved vertical incisions in the midline and premolar regions which enabled, by a tunnelling approach, bone cuts to be made in predetermined sites so that the premaxilla could be separated from the maxilla without depriving it of essential blood supplies. On the palatal aspect, gingival margin and midline incisions enabled tunnels to be created, giving access to burs and chisels with which adequate bone was removed to effect the desired new position of the segment. After detachment from the nasal septum the

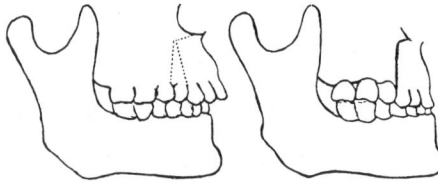

a

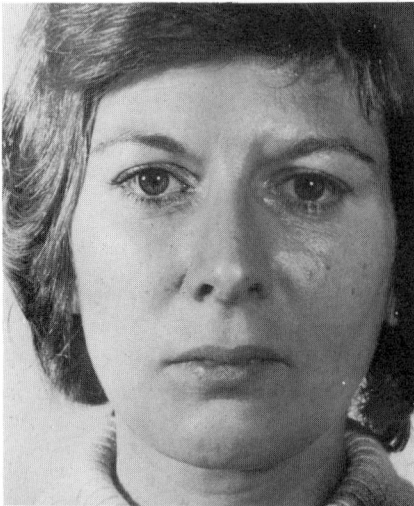

b

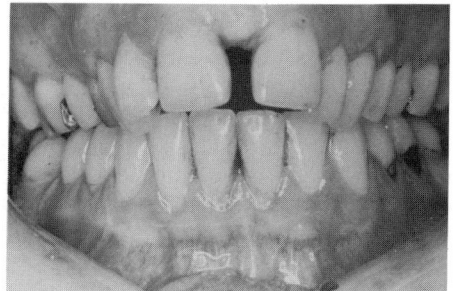

c

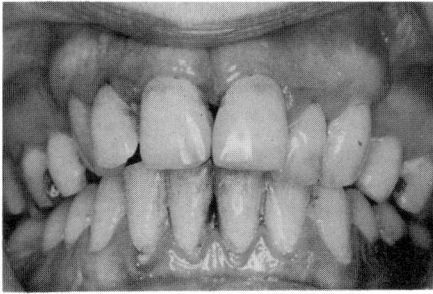

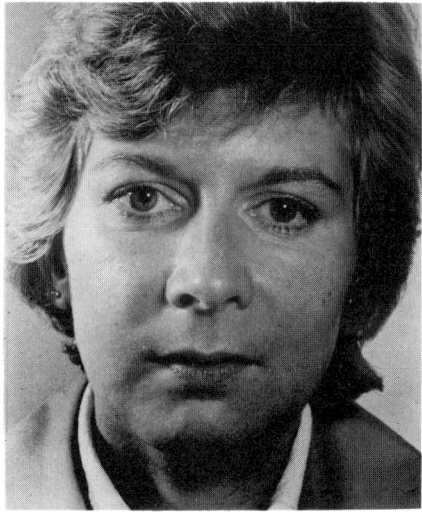

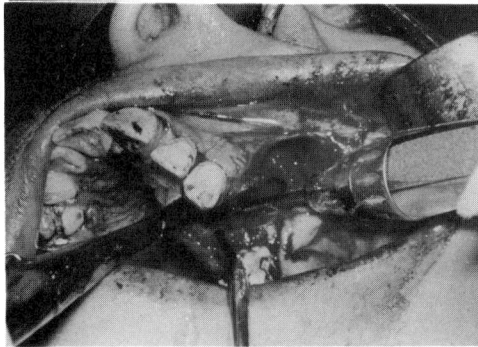

Fig. 19.15. a, Posterior repositioning of maxillary anterior segment by Wassmund technique. b, c, d, e, Pre- and postoperative views of face and teeth where orthodontic treatment with removable appliances in adolescence had not been successfully completed. The residual aesthetic and occlusal problems were corrected by a compromise procedure of Wassmund repositioning with sagittal splitting of the premaxilla to close the diastema. Preservation of the anterior nasal spine has maintained columella prominence. f, surgical tunnelling to divide palatal bone prior to splitting premaxilla.

premaxillary segment was moved to the new position and fixed with an arch bar constructed on the surgically corrected models.

Numerous variations of the technique permit the surgery to be carried out from a palatal approach (Wunderer)[19] or by a down-fracture of the anterior maxilla. The principal advantage of the premaxillary osteotomies is that they can reduce maxillary excess in the adult who has a reasonable nose and mandible, in circumstances where orthodontic treatment may not be acceptable. Occasionally the procedure is valuable in the realignment of upper incisors that are suffering severe gingival stripping on the palatal aspect. Rarely, anterior open bite may be corrected by this technique.

One serious disadvantage of the anterior maxillary osteotomy by the classic

Wassmund[18] or the down-fracture approach is the loss of the anterior nasal spine during sectioning of the anterior nasal rim. When this happens a flat, ugly lip, with loss of nasolabial angle, develops. This so-called Wassmund lip is seldom observed by the patient, but it mars the appearance in profile of the patients, who otherwise may be considered to have a satisfactory result. This complication can be avoided by careful dissection of the nasal rim, permitting bone cuts that free the anterior maxilla without detachment of the nasal spine. Attempts to restore the lost nasal spine by small bone grafts are doomed to failure through rapid resorption of the onlay.

Following the Wassmund-type procedure the teeth on the premaxillary segment may remain unresponsive to sensory stimuli for periods of a year or more. Careful radiological review of such teeth is essential, for the incidence of pulp death, followed by periapical infection, is higher in this procedure than in many other orthognathic operations.

The posterior maxillary osteotomy of Schuchardt[15] is used for the treatment of posterior maxillary excess, the long-face syndrome and, occasionally, anterior open bite. By intruding the buccal segments upwards into the space provided by the maxillary sinus, the occlusal plane can be levelled both anteroposteriorly and laterally, and the anterior face can be shortened. Where much of the beneficial effect results from autorotation of the mandible, as mentioned in the discussion of open bite (p. 286), results are disappointing because of the frequent tendency to early relapse.

The surgical technique usually involves a one-stage procedure in which a buccal approach is made to the lateral and palatal walls of the posterior osseous segment. Removal of the precise amount of bone from the lateral wall with an oscillating saw allows access to the alveolar and palatal bone on the deep aspect. Sectioning is completed by the use of a curved osteotome or bur, and the maxillary segment is finally separated from the pterygoid plates with a fine curved osteotome. The freed segment is positioned exactly and fitted into a prefabricated cap splint. Additional fixation is provided by a circumzygomatic wire attached to a loop on the splint. If mandibular surgery has been carried out at the same time, the circumzygomatic wire may be attached to the mandibular arch.

The complications from this procedure are few. As with all alveolar osteotomies in the maxilla, union of the fine bones may be slow. Rarely, an oro-antral fistula may appear. The principal reason for the waning popularity of this technique is the unpredictable nature of the relapse, which has so frequently dogged the method.

The lower labial segment repositioning procedure of Köle[20] is frequently used to reduce excessive anterior mandibular height, flatten the labiomental curve and drop the occlusal plane with a reverse curve of Spee. Occasionally it is used to correct anterior open bite or realign proclined mandibular incisors.

Technically, the procedure is relatively simple. The reflection of the labial tissues permits a direct approach to the bone cuts. The vascular pedicle of the genial muscles nourishes the segment from the lingual side. Before surgery begins the operation must be planned to the last millimetre by model surgery. Critical attention must be given to the intercanine width and the feasibility of fitting the repositioned lower arch into an appropriate relationship within the curve of the upper arch. Changes in lower facial height must be calculated with

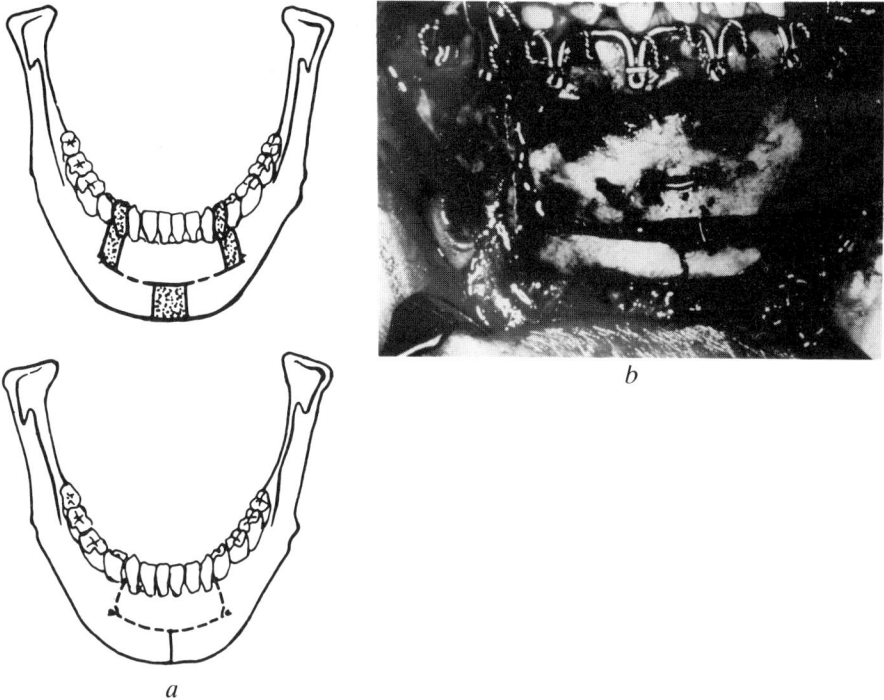

Fig. 19.16. a, Technical stages in Sowray–Haskell anterior mandibuloplasty. b, Intra-oral operative view after removal of central section of lower border of mandible, retrusion and intrusion of lower labial segment and stabilization by direct bone wiring and lower arch wiring.

care: avoiding damage to the roots of teeth can often be a difficult exercise, The sulcus tissues must be closed in layers with great care to avoid seepage of fluid and subsequent infection.

This procedure, when performed with meticulous attention to detail, alone or in combination with other orthognathic procedures, can be of the greatest value to the oral surgeon and orthodontist. Under optimal circumstances the complications of numbness of the lip and devitalization of the teeth are only transitory problems. Rarely, infarction and loss of the whole segment has occurred. This is a very high price to pay for what is, in the final analysis, aesthetic dentofacial surgery.

The Sowray–Haskell[21] technique incorporates the lower labial segmental osteotomy with a step-excision of basal bone at the lower border (Fig. 19.16). If a block of basal bone is excised in the midline and the margins are pulled together, lateral crossbite and mild prognathism can be reduced. Removal of bone sections unilaterally permits correction of asymmetry. As with the Köle[20] procedure, great care must be taken to obtain precise measurements of anticipated movements of segments at the model planning stage. The method is occasionally used to advantage in correcting mandibular discrepancies in the cleft palate patient. The principal advantage of this technique, and other anteromandibuloplasties, over the Köle procedure, is that there is a greater opportunity to control chin prominence and minor asymmetry while varying the height and inclination of the lower labial segment.

The complications associated with these procedures are those previously described for lower labial segment repositioning. Most difficulties can be prevented by careful model surgery and good preoperative radiological assessment of the position of the roots of the teeth and the location of the mental nerves.

Guidelines for Orthodontic and Oral Surgical Collaboration

Joint procedures between orthodontists and oral surgeons are more successful when there is early agreement on the likelihood of surgical intervention. Appropriate arrangements can then be made for clinical and radiological examinations and joint consultations throughout the preoperative treatment period. Decisions can be taken, during combined clinics, on such vital factors as the amount of arch expansion or decompensation, the optimal interincisal angulation and the ultimate lip levels required to achieve competence and aesthetics.

Collaboration at the stage of profile planning permits the development of an ideal orthodontic prescription. Decisions can be made on the method and extent of surgery. If bimaxillary surgery appears likely, the associated orthodontic constraints, if any, can be determined.

Regular reviews of the progress of orthodontic treatment by both surgeon and orthodontist enable final technical details to be decided. Arrangements can be made concerning the type of fixation to be used, modifications needed in the fixed appliances can be discussed and arranged, and the patient can be advised of all likely events, orthodontic and surgical, that should be expected during the postoperative period.

The attendance of the orthodontist during the final stages of the orthognathic surgical procedure is of great assistance to the surgical team. Definitive decisions can then be made jointly on such matters as the suitability of the position of the dento-alveolar segments and the load imposed on the orthodontic appliances by the surgical fixation; agreement can be reached on individual responsibilities for continuing care of the patient during the recovery period. Finally, mutual understanding between orthodontist and surgeon creates a climate for innovation and research, which is essential for the development of the art and science of craniomaxillofacial reconstruction. The pioneers of surgical orthodontics would agree that Blair's[22] classic comment in 1909 that the mandible 'is a hoop of bone capable of almost any kind of adjustment' is more relevant and realistic now than ever before. One suspects that his comment today to the orthodontists and their surgical collaborators would be to ask: 'Are there any restrictions on the timing or technique of orthognathic surgery; and if so, what are you doing to overcome them?'

REFERENCES

1. Obwegeser H. and Trauner R. (1957) The surgical correction of mandibular prognathism and retrognathism with consideration of genioplasty. *Oral Surg.* **10**; 677.
2. Bell W. H., Proffitt W. R. and White R. P. (1980) *Surgical Correction of Dentofacial Deformities*. Philadelphia, W. B. Saunders.

3. Henderson D. and Poswillo D. (1985) *A Colour Atlas of Orthognathic Surgery*. London, Wolfe.
4. Obwegeser H. (1964) The indications for surgical correction of mandibular deformity by the sagittal splitting technique. *Br. J. Oral Surg.* **1**; 157.
5. Dal Pont G. (1961) Retromolar osteotomy for the correction of prognathism. *J. Oral Surg.* **19**; 42.
6. Trauner R. (1954) Die retrokondylare implantation eine operationsmethode zum vorbringen des unterkiefer beim distalbiss. *Dtsch. Z. Mund. Kieferh.* **21**; 391.
7. Poswillo D. (1968) The aetiology and surgery of cleft palate with micrognathia. *Ann. R. Coll. Surg. Engl.* **43**; 61.
8. Hayes P. A. (1973) Correction of retrognathia by modified 'C' osteotomy of the ramus and sagittal osteotomy of the mandibular body. *J. Oral Surg.* **31**; 682.
9. Byrne R. P. and Hinds E. C. (1974) The ramus 'C' osteotomy with body split. *J. Oral Surg.* **32**; 259.
10. Obwegeser H. (1961) Vorteile und moglichkeiten des intraoralen vorgehens bei der korrektur von unterkieferanomaliess. *Fortschr. Kieferh. Gesichtschir.* **7**; 159.
11. Hofer O. (1942) Operation der prognathie und microgenie. *Dtsch. Z. Mund. Kieferh.* **9**; 121.
12. Poswillo D. (1964) The surgery of orofacial deformity. *Aust. Dent. J.* **9**; 345.
13. Bell W. H. (1975) Le Fort 1 osteotomy for correction of maxillary deformities. *J. Oral. Surg.* **33**; 412.
14. Poswillo D. (1972) Early pulp changes following reduction of open bite by segmental surgery. *Int. J. Oral Surg.* **1**; 87.
15. Schuchardt K. (1961) Experiences with the surgical treatment of some deformities of the jaws: prognathia, micrognathia, and open bite. In: Wallace A. B. (ed.) *Transactions of the 2nd Congress of the International Society of Plastic Surgeons*, London, 1959. Edinburgh, Livingstone, p. 73.
16. Hullihen S. P. (1849) Case of elongation of the underjaw and distortion of the face and neck 1965. Zurich, Swiss Society of Plastic and Reconstructive Surgeons.
17. Hofer O. (1942) Die vertikale osteotomie zur verlangerung des einseitig verkurtzen aufsteigenden unterkieferastes. *Oest. Z. Stomat.* **34**; 286.
18. Wassmund M. (1935) *Lehrbuch der Praktischen Chirurgie des Mundes und der Kiefer*, vol. 1. Leipzig, Barth.
19. Wunderer S. (1965) Surgical correction of the profile by operation on the maxilla. *Proceedings of the 2nd Meeting of the Swiss Society of Plastic and Reconstructive Surgeons*, Zurich, November· 1965. Zurich Swiss Society of Plastic and Reconstructive Surgeons.
20. Köle H. (1970) In: Reichenbach E., Köle H. and Bruckl H. *Chirurgische Keiferorthopadie*. Leipzig, Barth.
21. Sowray J. H. and Haskell R. (1968) Osteotomy at the mandibular symphysis. *Br. J. Oral Surg.* **6**; 97.
22. Blair V. P. (1909) Underdeveloped lower jaw with limited excursion. *JAMA* **53**; 178.

Chapter 20

Craniofacial Anomalies

Alan C. Campbell and David Poswillo

CLEFTS OF THE LIP AND PALATE

Clefts of the lip and palate are the most common congenital facial deformity affecting the head and neck. The incidence varies according to the type of cleft, racial group and sex: cleft lip with or without cleft palate—CL(P)—ranges from about 3·6 per 1000 births for Indians to 0·5 per 1000 for Negroes, with an incidence of about 1 per 1000 for Caucasians.[1] The reported frequency varies, however, even within racial groups. Some of these differences may be due to variations in methods and efficiency of recording facial deformity. In Caucasians at least, CL(P) is more common in males (about 70 per cent) and unilateral clefts occur more often on the left side. Isolated cleft palate is less common, occurring about once in 2000 births, and more often in females.

The aetiology of clefts of the lip and palate is still a matter of debate. Certain types of cleft have a family history and so there is sometimes a genetic predisposition to clefting which may be triggered by environmental factors. This hypothesis is supported by the results of studies in animals. Some strains of mice, for example, are particularly susceptible to clefting of the palate, which occurs spontaneously in a proportion of the offspring, but the frequency can be increased greatly by a variety of drugs and other environmental insults at critical periods in development.[2] However, the role of such teratogenic influences is not clearly established in man.

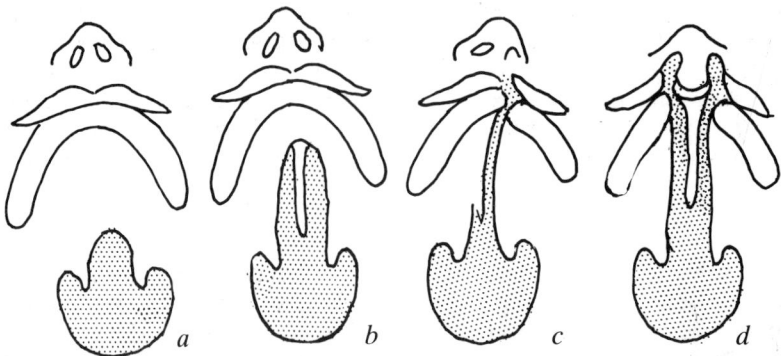

Fig. 20.1. Veau's classification: *a*, cleft involving the soft palate only; *b*, cleft of the soft palate and the hard palate as far forward as the incisive foramen; *c*, unilateral complete cleft of lip and palate; *d*, bilateral complete cleft of lip and palate.

294

Classification

Clefts can vary in severity from minor notching of the lip or a bifid uvula, to complete bilateral clefting of lip and palate. A number of different methods of classification have been proposed. Veau's classification[3] was one of the earlier and is most widely known (*Fig.* 20.1).

Kernahan and Stark[4] introduced a more comprehensive classification, based upon the embryology of the deformity. The incisive foramen is regarded as the demarcation between primary and secondary palates.

Clefts of the primary palate: These vary from notching of the upper lip to clefts of the lip and alveolar process as far as the incisive foramen.

Clefts of the secondary palate: Clefts of the soft and hard palate as far as the incisive foramen.

Clefts of the primary and secondary palates: These may be complete or incomplete, unilateral or bilateral.

Embryology

The embryology of facial development is complex and is still not fully elucidated.[5] The embryonic median nasal processes, give rise to the tip of the nose, columella, philtrum of the upper lip and primary palate. At between 7 and 8 weeks in utero (i.u.), mesodermal invasion results in a merging of the lateral and medial nasal process with the maxillary processes to form the upper lip. Failure of adequate mesodermal migration can result in complete or incomplete clefting of the lip.

The soft palate and that part of the hard palate posterior to the incisive foramen are formed from the palatal shelves which develop from the inner surfaces of the maxillary processes during the 6th week in utero. Because the tongue fills the oronasal cavity at this stage, the palatal shelves are bent down at its sides. By the 8th week, the stomatodeal chamber has enlarged so that the tongue descends, allowing the palatal shelves to swing up and achieve contact with one another, with the primary palate anteriorly and the nasal septum above. The epithelium at the sites of contact breaks down and these processes fuse at between 8 and 12 weeks in utero. Lack of elevation of the palatal processes at the critical time, or failure to contact, or inadequate epithelial breakdown, gives rise to a cleft of the secondary palate. A submucous cleft can arise if mesodermal invasion is inadequate, and this can cause poor soft palate control and defective speech.

Facial Growth

The studies that have been conducted into the facial characteristics in adults with unrepaired clefts of the lip and palate[6] demonstrate remarkably little interference with facial growth (*Fig.* 20.2). The upper face is often rather wide, but whether this has been an aetiological factor, or arises as a result of the structural discontinuity, is not yet clear.

In many children with surgically repaired clefts of lip and palate, maxillary growth is affected, and in some cases to a serious extent (*Fig.* 20.3). There are

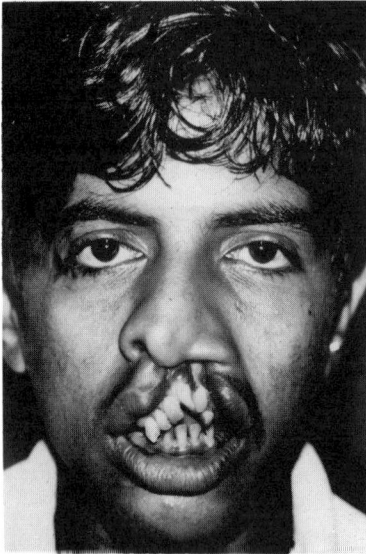

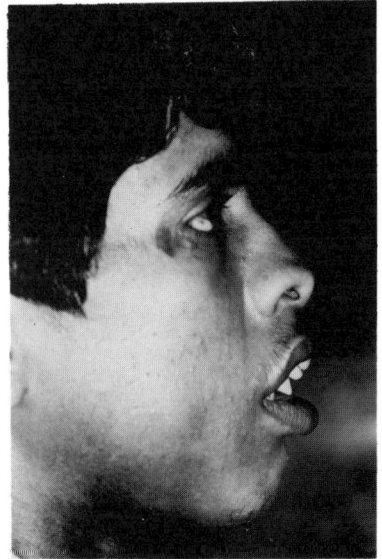

a   *b*

Fig. 20.2. *a*, A young adult with an unrepaired complete unilateral cleft of lip and palate. *b*, Note how the midface is not retruded.

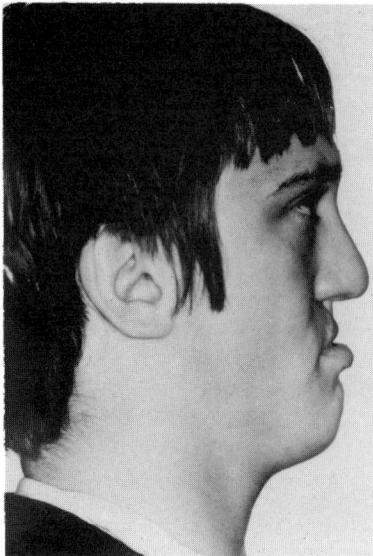

Fig. 20.3. A young adult with fairly severe midface retrusion associated with a repaired unilateral complete cleft of the lip and palate.

several reasons for this. The repaired lip may be very scarred and tight, and this not only restrains the upper incisor teeth but could restrict forward growth of the entire maxilla. In some surgical procedures for repair of the palate, the mucoperiosteum is undermined extensively and scar tissue in the pterygomaxillary suture area could interfere with growth. The type of surgical

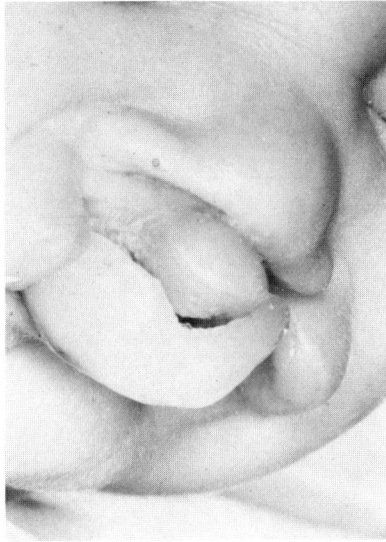

Fig. 20.4. A feeding plate in a child with a bilateral cleft of lip and palate.

procedure and the skill of the surgeon are important factors influencing the severity of growth deficiencies. It must also be acknowledged that in many cases of cleft lip and palate, tissue is deficient from the start, and if the cleft is closed, the maxilla must be narrowed.

THE CHILD WITH A CLEFT OF LIP AND PALATE

Parents are generally very distressed when they learn that their child has a facial cleft. At an early stage, the general implications and management of the problem should be discussed and it can be helpful to illustrate the points in broad terms, with photographs of a child who had a similar type of cleft (*see*, for example, *Figs*. 20.11, 20.12). It is important to be realistic and to use an illustration of a typical rather than an outstandingly good result, otherwise expectations may be unreasonably high.

Some infants with clefts of the lip and palate have other congenital deformities and if they are serious, their management takes precedence.

Feeding can be a problem but the difficulties should not be exaggerated. Most infants can be bottle-fed by the mother, if a large teat with an enlarged hole is used. Some need to be spoon-fed. A feeding plate (*Fig.* 20.4) can be helpful.

Respiratory and middle ear infections are particularly common in cleft palate children, due to regurgitation of food and saliva into the nasopharynx, and inadequate drainage of the Eustachian tubes. This is a serious matter in that any hearing loss exacerbates the difficulties with speech development and, if unrecognized, interferes with educational progress.

Table 20.1. A guide to timing treatment for children with clefts of lip and palate

Age	Plastic surgery	Orthodontics	General dental care	ENT	Speech therapy	Oral surgery
Birth	Evaluation and counsel parents	Records/feeding plate and/or orthopaedic appliance	Advice to parents on dental care, prevention of carries			
3 mths–2 yr	Lip repair Palate repair		Regular checks continuing until adult	Regular checks until adult	Observation. Evaluate speech at 2–3 yr Speech therapy	
5–12 yr	Minor lip revision	Simple correction of instanding incisors. Arch expansion if required prior to alveolar bone graft Definitive orthodontic treatment				Alveolar bone graft at about 10 yr
12–14 yr						
15–18 yr	Nose revision		Bridge and denture work			Maxillofacial surgery to correct skeletal malrelationships if required

Supervision of the Cleft Palate Clinic

The child with a cleft of lip and palate will require the services of a number of experts, including plastic and maxillofacial surgeons, ear nose and throat specialists, speech therapists, paediatricians, orthodontists and dental practitioners. It is very important that the different specialists work together as a team, one of whose members will coordinate their activities and maintain contact with the child and parents throughout the period of growth. Because of the need for extended supervision of facial growth and occlusal development, the orthodontist is often well placed to accept the responsibility as coordinator.

It is not possible to describe here the comprehensive management of the child with cleft lip and palate. The typical timing of different contributions is indicated in *Table* 20.1, but of course individual needs vary. In the interests of clarity, surgical and orthodontic management and the role of the dental practitioner are discussed separately, but of course these have to be coordinated with one another and with the other specialities.

General Management

Isolated Clefts of the Lip and Alveolar Process

The orthodontic problems are usually quite minor. Even when the cleft does not extend to the alveolar process, the lateral incisor may be diminutive, missing or divided (*Fig.* 20.5). Where the cleft involves the alveolar process, the central

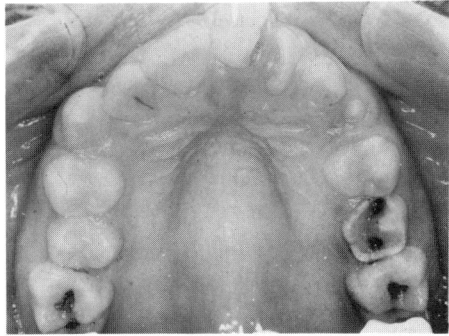

Fig. 20.5. Dental irregularities associated with a unilateral cleft of the lip: the central incisor is rotated and there is a supernumerary lateral incisor.

incisor may be rotated, dilacerated and hypoplastic, possibly as a consequence of the surgical repair of the defect within 3 months of birth. There may be a localized open bite affecting the central incisor and canine on either side of the cleft, possibly as a result of reduced alveolar bone growth. These local features may, of course, be superimposed upon other types of malocclusion.

Isolated Clefts of the Palate (*Fig.* 20.6)

The palate is normally repaired at between 9 and 18 months. There may be problems with speech if the palate is not long and mobile enough to prevent a nasal escape of air. Where surgery has involved extensive flap mobilization with scar tissue formation in proximity to sutures, maxillary growth may be restrained, so that a Class III malocclusion develops. The upper arch is often

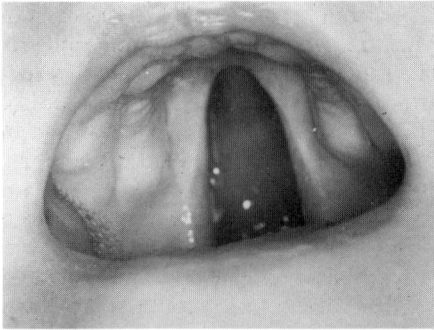

Fig. 20.6. A cleft of soft and hard palate but not extending beyond the incisive foramen.

narrow following repair of the hard palate, so that there is a crossbite. In general, the orthodontic problems can be treated by conventional appliances.

Complete Clefts of the Lip and Palate

The magnitude of the deformity varies greatly, depending on the severity of the original tissue deficiency, the interference with growth and on any underlying skeletal malrelationship. The problems are more serious in a child who has a basic tendency to a Class III skeletal pattern than when the skeletal pattern is Class II.

Primary Surgical Management

The lip is repaired at 6–12 weeks and the alveolar process cleft is usually closed at the same time when access is good. The exact timing and surgical procedure depend on the practice of the surgeon and on the health of the infant. If presurgical orthopaedic alignment of the maxillary segments is undertaken (see p. 303, the lip is usually repaired at about 3 months.

Many different procedures can be used to repair the lip. The objective is to produce a lip of adequate length, that is not tight and that is functionally satisfactory. The mucosa, muscle and skin are sutured separately. It is now recognized that in a cleft lip the orbicularis oris is abnormally inserted into the bony margins at the cleft and these attachments need to be detached and sutured together otherwise the lip will not function well. A good vermilion border is important, and this may need later revision.

Attempts have been made to close the bony defect in the alveolar process by bone grafting at the time of the primary lip repair. The results were generally disappointing and primary bone grafting has been abandoned in most centres.[7]

The optimal timing of closure of the secondary palate is a subject of fierce debate. There are strong arguments for closing the palate by 18 months to obtain more normal function before speech is established, and to reduce the problems of regurgitation into the nasopharynx. The potential disadvantage of early repair is the risk of interference with maxillary growth. Postponement of hard palate repair until 5 years or even later, following earlier closure of the soft palate, is advocated by a number of authorities.[8] No convincing evidence is available to support the view that facial growth is superior in these cases, but adequate comparative studies are lacking.

A number of surgical procedures for palate closure are currently used. In all of these, the nasal mucosa, muscle and oral mucosa are closed in separate layers. The extent of the deficiency and the need to lengthen the soft palate are factors that influence the approach. It is important to obtain adequate soft palate function in order to minimize nasal escape during speech and swallowing. In some patients a pharyngoplasty is undertaken later to improve the velopharyngeal seal.

A variety of secondary surgical procedures may be required: revision of nose or lip to improve the appearance; delayed bone grafting to stabilize the maxillary segments; closure of palatal fistulae; and maxillofacial surgery to correct skeletal malrelationships (see p. 308). Repeated surgical intervention should be avoided; it can result in extensive scarring and is a continuing strain on the patient and family. Most secondary surgical procedures should be deferred until the mid to late 'teens, when they can be undertaken in a comprehensively planned and definitive manner.

Delayed bone grafting, however, is undertaken prior to eruption of the permanent canines.[9] Bone chips from the iliac crest are inserted into the bony defect in the alveolar process, following elevation of the soft tissues to form a suitable pocket for the graft which is then covered by a flap of alveolar or oral mucosa. The bone graft stabilizes the maxillary segments and provides bone into which the canine can erupt and which supports other teeth adjacent to the cleft (Fig. 20.7). Other benefits are that closure of oronasal fistulae in this region is facilitated, and the contour of the alveolar process is restored so that lip support is improved.

Orthodontic Management

The orthodontist should see the infant soon after birth and will continue to review facial growth and occlusal development throughout the period of growth.

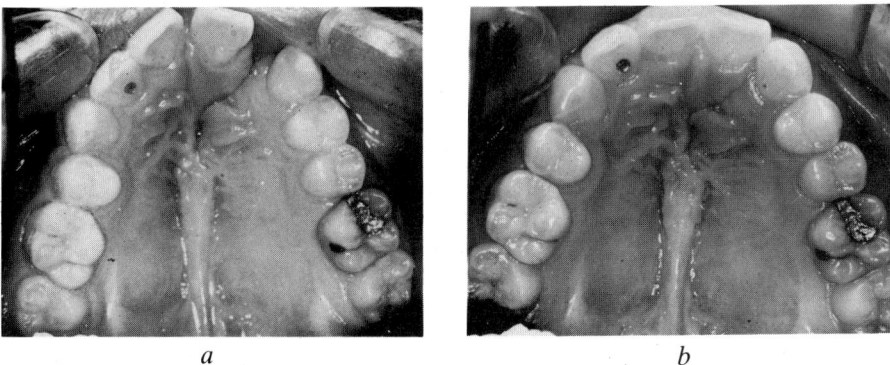

a   b

Fig. 20.7. Secondary bone graft. a, A unilateral cleft of lip and palate. The lateral incisor adjacent to the cleft was malformed and has been removed. Orthodontic closure of the space would not be possible because there is no bone in the cleft into which teeth could be moved. b, Following bone grafting, orthodontic treatment with a fixed appliance has closed the space by moving the canine into the bone graft. Where the bone graft is inserted slightly earlier, the canine has the opportunity of erupting into the graft.

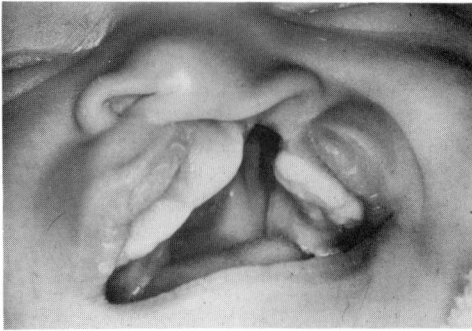
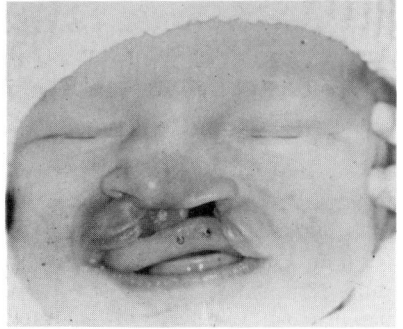

a   *b*

Fig. 20.8. *a*, An infant with a unilateral cleft of the lip and palate; *b*, wearing an orthopaedic alignment plate.

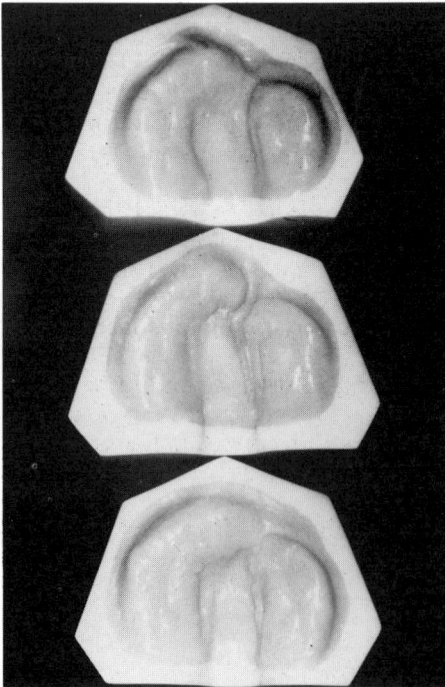

Fig. 20.9. Models of a child with a unilateral complete cleft of lip and palate, showing the improvement of alignment of the segments and reduction in the size of defect as a result of presurgical orthopaedic treatment.

Almost all children with clefts of lip and palate require orthodontic intervention at some stage. Because of the continuity of supervision, the orthodontist is often the most appropriate member of the cleft palate team to coordinate treatment and to counsel the child and parents. He should also take this opportunity to emphasize the importance of good oral hygiene and to ensure that the child receives regular dental and preventive attention.

Presurgical Orthopaedic Treatment (Figs. 20.8, 20.9)

Lacking structural continuity, the segments of the maxilla become displaced even before birth. This can complicate surgical repair of the lip and alveolar process, and presurgical alignment may facilitate the surgery.

Presurgical orthopaedic treatment was initiated by McNeil[10] and was developed by Burston.[11] McNeil believed it was possible to stimulate closure of a cleft by appliances, but this does not happen. A number of studies have indicated that the arch form is better in children who have had presurgical orthopaedic alignment, but there have been few adequately controlled long-term studies. The long-term benefits are not universally accepted, at least in unilateral cases; and it is difficult to compare results from different centres because of differences in surgical technique. On balance, presurgical ortho-paedic treatment can be justified where the surgeon considers it will help him to achieve a better result. It should be recognized that the need for frequent visits to a hospital during the first 3 months places an additional burden on the family.

UNILATERAL COMPLETE CLEFTS OF LIP AND PALATE (*Fig.* 20.8)

The major segment is generally rotated to the non-cleft side, while the lesser segment may be well-related to the lower arch or displaced laterally. If the segments are not greatly displaced, presurgical alignment will not be required. Quite often simple extra-oral elastic strapping is sufficient to approximate the segments. If displacement is greater, presurgical alignment with an appliance is helpful.

The first impression is taken within 48 hours of birth. The initial appliance is usually passive and is worn as an obturator for the first 2 weeks. This can help with feeding. A further impression is obtained at that stage and the model is sectioned and realigned to improve the relations between the segments, which should not be moved by more than 3–4 mm. An acrylic plate is made on the adjusted model (*see Fig.* 20.8). This is worn full time and the wings are strapped to the cheeks with Micropore tape or tied to a bonnet in order to prevent the appliance from being displaced. If appropriate, the strapping is applied under tension to help to align the segments. The parent is instructed in the application of the strapping and within a few weeks the segments should be aligned accord-ing to the activation of the plate. Where the segments need to be aligned by a substantial amount, a series of plates is made in this way with progressively improved segmental relationships. In some centres an adjustable split plate with a hinged screw is used.

BILATERAL COMPLETE CLEFTS OF LIPS AND PALATE (*see Fig.* 20.10)

The premaxillary segment is displaced anteriorly on the nasal septum while the lateral segments are often in quite a good relationship with the lower arch, but they may be contracted. Alignment of the segments is particularly useful in bilateral cases to facilitate surgery.

Many different approaches to arch alignment have been proposed. Some surgeons repair the lip in two stages, separated by some weeks, so that lip pressure restrains the premaxilla. However, this can lead to asymmetries and can make a really good lip repair difficult. Surgical repositioning of the premaxil-

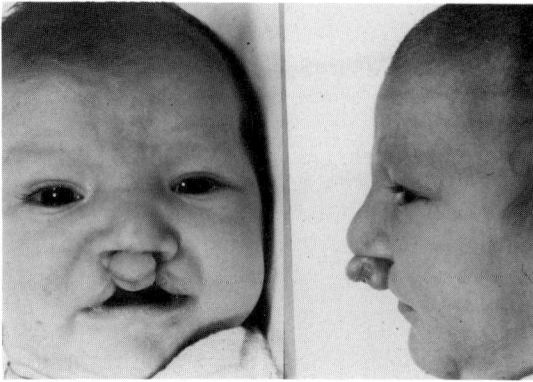

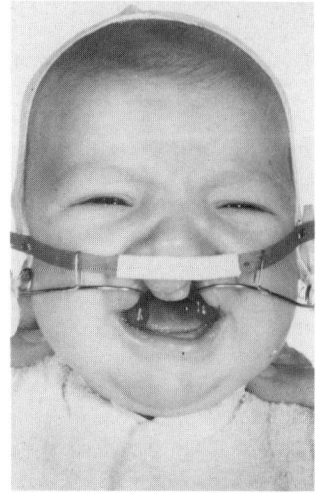

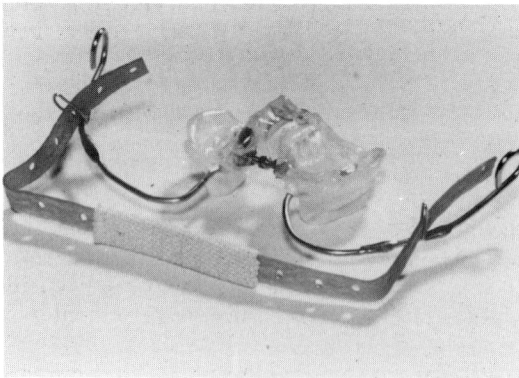

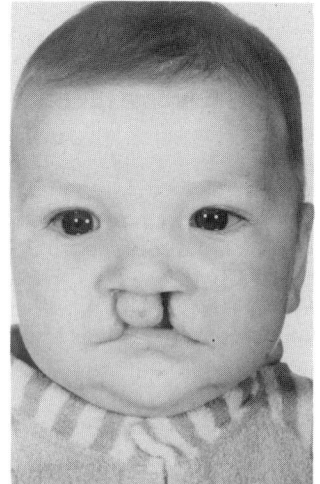

Fig. 20.10. *a*, A child with a bilateral complete cleft of lip and palate. *b*, Wearing an alignment plate and with strapping to reduce the prominence of the premaxillary segment. *c*, The alignment plate. *d*, The prominence of the premaxillary segment has been reduced.

lary segment following removal of part of the vomer and nasal septum has also been undertaken in severe cases, but there is the risk of serious interference with growth leading to maxillary retrusion in the long term. Alignment can be achieved with plates that hold the lateral segments apart while the premaxilla is retracted with the strapping (*Fig.* 20.10). The general principles of their use are similar to those for unilateral cases.

Orthodontic Treatment (*Figs.* 20.11, 20.12)

These cases will almost always require orthodontic treatment in the permanent dentition. It is most important not to burden these children with interim treatment of questionable long-term benefit. Thus, although appliance treatment in the deciduous dentition has been advocated by some authorities, it has little if any advantage in the long term and should be avoided. If the upper incisors are in lingual occlusion in the early mixed dentition and a stable correction of the overjet can be obtained, this should be done. However, active orthodontic treatment should be kept to a minimum. Secondary bone grafting is frequently indicated at about 9–10 years of age (*see* p. 301).

Treatment planning in the late mixed and early permanent dentition stages should involve the restorative dentist and maxillofacial surgeon where appropriate so that a comprehensive approach can be agreed. In many cases there are problems in all three dimensions. The maxillary arch is retruded and narrow and there may be local or general deficiencies in vertical development. If there is mandibular overclosure due to deficient vertical development of the maxilla, the true extent of mandibular protrusion will be exaggerated when the patient occludes the teeth, and so treatment must be planned with the mandible in the rest position.

If surgical correction of the maxillary position and skeletal pattern is required, orthodontic treatment is planned to achieve an arch form that will be appropriate for the corrected jaw relationship. In milder cases an acceptable result can be obtained by orthodontic treatment alone.

Fixed appliances are generally required and the edgewise technique is often the most suitable because heavy arches can be used in the later stages to help control the segmental relationships.

Dental Management

Cleft palate patients frequently have inadequate plaque control, in part because of poor self-cleansing in some areas and in part because they are often resentful of the amount of treatment they require and tend to neglect oral hygiene. Retention of a healthy dentition is of the greatest importance to the patient with a cleft of the palate.

It is essential that from an early stage the parents are informed of the necessity for good dental care and of the need for preventive measures. Fluoride supplements should be given where the fluoride level in the water supply is deficient, and the child must have regular dental inspections. The provision of routine dental care for these patients is often a demanding task but the dental practitioner has the responsibility of providing the care and encouragement they require.

The central incisor on the side of the cleft may be hypoplastic or deformed, possibly as a result of early surgery; and the lateral incisor is often absent or pegshaped. The provision of a bridge or denture has a number of problems: the tooth crowns may be short and the maxillary segments may be slightly mobile. This is a difficult task that is best undertaken by a practitioner with special expertise in the treatment of patients with clefts of the palate.

CLEFT LIP AND PALATE: SECONDARY TREATMENT

The primary repair of cleft lip and palate has, for years, often failed to satisfy the ideal criteria outlined by pioneers such as Skoog[12] and Millard.[13]

The deleterious effect of lip tension and bands of scar tissue on growth and development of the maxilla has been a most difficult problem to resolve. Prodigious efforts on the part of orthodontists have failed to achieve optimal results in the areas of occlusion and aesthetics, and only recently has it been

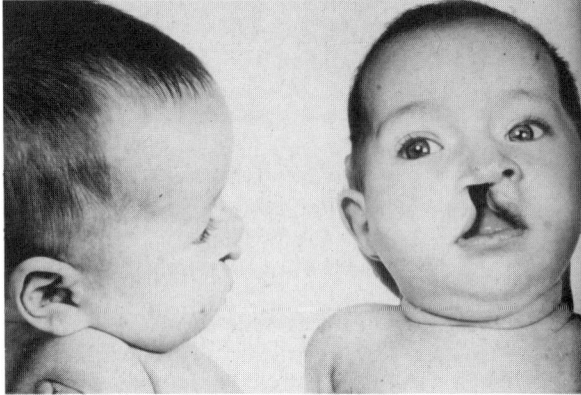

a

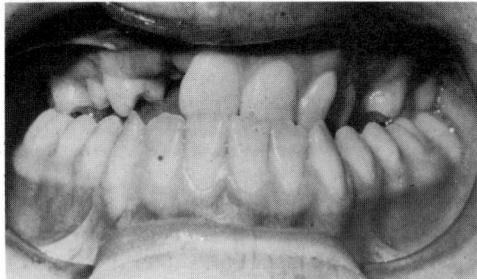

b

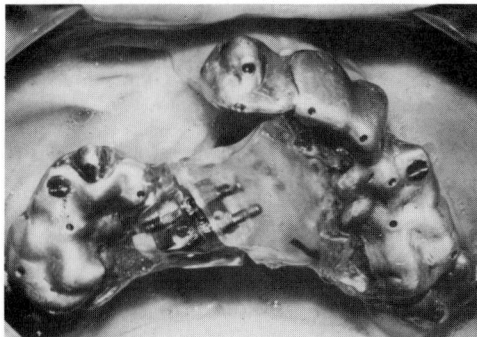

c

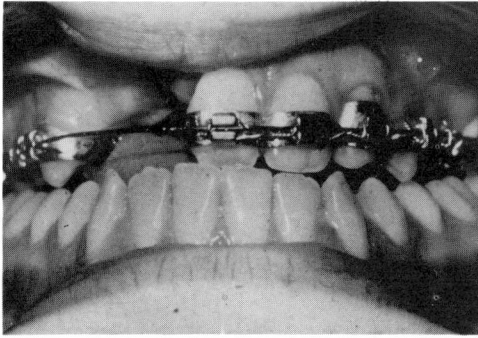

d

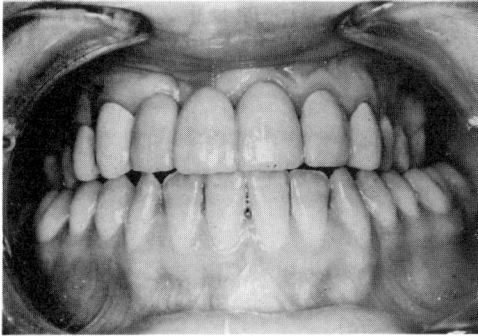

e

Fig. 20.11. *a*, A child with a unilateral complete cleft of lip and palate. *b*, In the early permanent dentition, the upper arch is short and narrow: the upper incisors are in lingual occlusion and there is a unilateral crossbite. *c*, A rapid expansion splint. *d*, A fixed orthodontic appliance is used to complete alignment of the teeth as far as is necessary to provide a bridge. *e*, Bridge in place.

recognized that the vast number of small surgical procedures which have developed over the years to deal with separate aspects of the problem are better replaced by an overall reconstructive procedure at the appropriate age.

From a surgical point of view the specific areas to be considered are the lip and associated scars, the alignment and function of the orbicularis muscle, the asymmetry of the nose and alar bases, anterior palate fistulas, when present, and the position of the maxilla proper and each maxillary segment with regard to each other and to the face as a whole.

For effective treatment in the adolescent or adult, the problems require precise presurgical delineation and a plan which leads to simultaneous correction of all the surgical deficiencies.

Technical Surgical Procedures

The most severe cases of maxillary hypoplasia and retrusion, often accompanied by anterior oronasal fistula and collapse of the dental arch, require a Le Fort 1 osteotomy with expansion of the upper arch, repositioning of the major and minor segments and closure of the oronasal fistula. Surgery to the mandible is

Fig. 20.12. *a, b,* A patient with a bilateral complete cleft of lip and palate. *c,* Expansion of the upper arch with a quad helix. *d,* A fixed appliance is used to align the teeth. *e,* Orthodontic treatment has obtained alignment of the upper teeth but the anterior open bite remains. This could be treated by surgery.

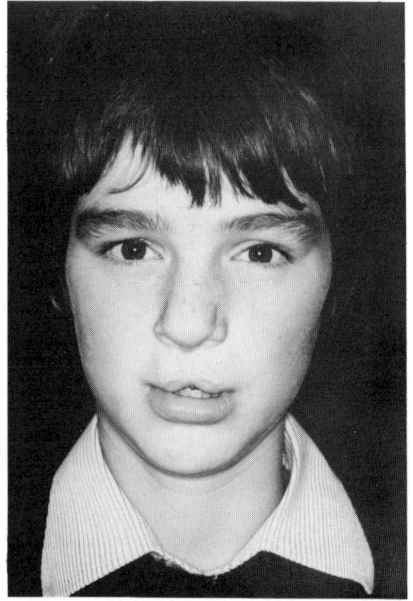

a

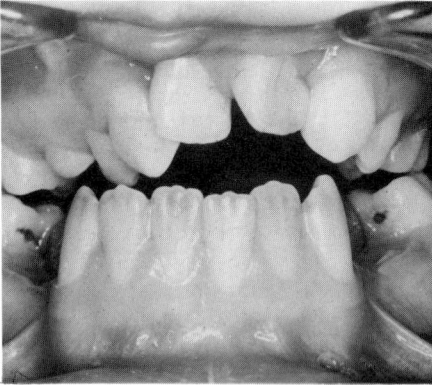

b

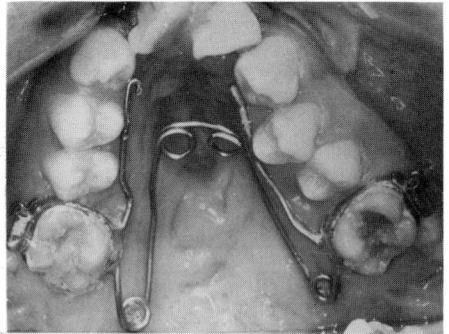

c

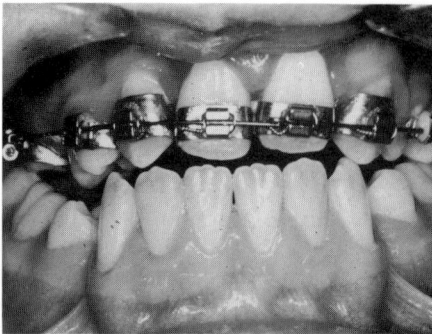

d

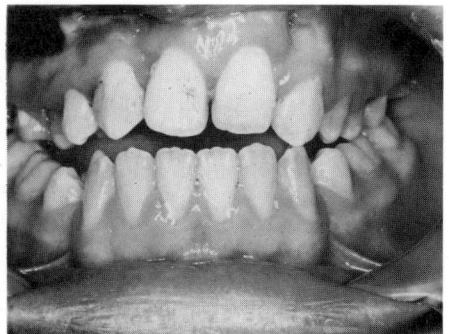

e

usually avoided where there is a maxillary deformity: it invariably results in an unsatisfactory profile. Where lip and palate scarring is marked, particularly in bilateral cleft lip and palate, good mobilization is difficult to obtain. In order to obtain a good stable postoperative occlusion, without the disaster of relapse, overcorrection of the maxillary segments is usually essential. Bone grafts from the iliac crest, ribs or calvarial bones to the osteotomy sites, as buttresses or onlays, are usually required. The period of fixation must be extended to about 12 weeks if relapse is to be avoided. Forward movement of the maxilla may, by traction, pull the tight soft palate forwards, recreating speech problems. When these arise, they should be investigated by direct nasendoscopy and treated by an appropriate pharyngoplasty or posterior pharyngeal wall augmentation. These are late procedures and should be deferred until the maxillary surgical and orthodontic procedures have been completed.

Occasionally, the anatomical problems of a severely hypoplastic cleft maxilla will make a Le Fort II osteotomy the procedure of choice. This is most appropriate when more of the maxilla and nose need to be brought forward. Only rarely should a Le Fort III osteotomy be contemplated for the cleft patient: it is the lower half of the midface which requires repositioning and the Le Fort III procedure brings infra-orbital margins, which are often appropriately situated, too far forwards in the reconstruction of the usual case of maxillary hypoplasia associated with primary cleft lip and palate repair.

The approach to lip revision will depend on the soft tissue defects revealed at the assessment stage. Although some types of primary lip repair make it extremely difficult for a standard rotation advancement revision of the tight scarred lip, the majority of cases are best treated by the standard Millard[14] advancement repair. Henderson and Jackson[15] have described a combined lip revision, anterior fistula closure and maxillary osteotomy, done as a one-stage reconstruction, which is felt to meet the demands of most problems in this area.

A fixed bridge may need to be constructed after all orthodontic treatment has been completed. The last stage in aesthetic reconstruction is a standard cosmetic rhinoplasty with the addition of a septal cartilage strut for nasal tip support.

CRANIOFACIAL MICROSOMIA AND MANDIBULOFACIAL DYSOSTOSIS

The first and second branchial arch syndromes, so called, comprise a variety of asymmetrical and symmetrical congenital deformities which involve the eyes, ears, midface and mandible. The most common of these is hemifacial microsomia, more recently renamed craniofacial microsomia because the defects extend from the cranium above to the mandible below.

The incidence of this birth defect is about 1:3500 live births. Research in animal models [16] suggests that a spontaneous haemorrhage of the developing cranial stapedial artery (the precursor of the external carotid system) destroys and disorganizes, in a haphazard manner, the differentiating mesechyme which ultimately provides soft tissues and skeleton between the temporal bone and the lower border of the mandible.

Because of this extraordinary and uncontrolled mechanism of malformation, a very wide range of craniofacial abnormalities may be present. These vary from simple ear tags and pre-auricular sinuses, to gross clefting defects affecting the whole side of the face. In severe forms of this deformity there is

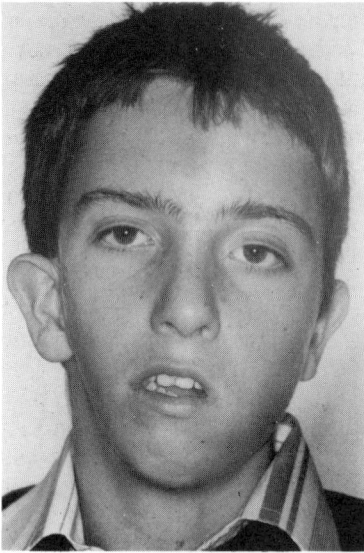

Fig. 20.13, *a, b,* Asymmetrical growth of face and dentition in right-sided craniofacial microsomia during adolescent growth spurt and prior to surgical reconstruction

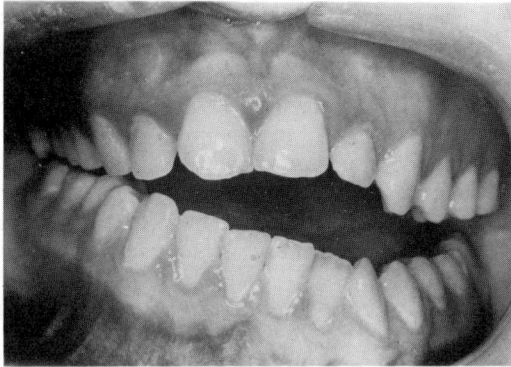

a

b

a gross shortage of soft tissue, notably masticatory muscles and overlying skin, and a three-dimensional failure of growth because of the destruction of the functional periosteal matrix. Occasionally, the deformity at birth may appear relatively mild; but as growth proceeds and the domino effect of one deformed structure interacts with another component of facial growth, the disparity between the two sides of the face becomes worse. The unaffected, or less affected side, may overgrow, without normal restraint, adding to the overall deformity.

In the Goldenhar variant, clefts of the upper eyelid (coloboma) and intrabulbar dermoids may add severe ophthalmological problems to the procedures of facial reconstruction.

Craniofacial microsomia is almost invariably asymmetrical; while both sides of the craniofacial complex are disadvantaged by the embryonic mechanism of malformation in only about 30 per cent of cases, there cannot be symmetrical growth in any patient afflicted with hemifacial microsomia (*Fig.* 20.13). This problem adds very considerably to the difficulties of treatment. In the most severe cases, most, if not all, of the craniofacial tissues are affected: the masseter, medial pterygoid and temporal muscles, the parotid gland and the external and middle ears may be totally or partially absent.

Attitudes towards the timing of reconstruction have begun to crystallize in recent years, using techniques of tissue replacement which have developed with the extended use of the operating microscope in facial reconstructive surgery. While it is agreed that reconstruction of the frontal, zygomatic and temporal bones may be begun at about 10 years of age in order to rebuild the orbital rim, malar prominence and glenoid fossa, expanding the tight covering integument in the process, rebuilding the lower third of the face is best left until late adolescence.

Attempts are being made to introduce new growing tissue, such as free composite grafts, into the growing face; but to date, these concepts have failed to produce the expected benefits. Better use of vascularized grafts comprising skin, fat, muscle and bone, sutured to functioning vessels and nerves, as appropriate, by microvascular and microneural methods, may eventually overcome the fundamental problems caused by tissue deficiency. Experience to date has shown that simple onlay bone grafting with lengthening of the mandible on the most affected side is doomed to failure unless the soft tissue envelope of the face is increased in volume. Where attempts to achieve this have involved extensive mobilization of soft tissues, late scar tissue contraction has produced total resorption of the tissues used for augmentation.

Where there exists a rudimentary or absent condylar head and ramus of mandible, reconstruction of the temporomandibular articulation may be necessary. Obwegeser[17] has described a definitive two- or three-stage reconstructive procedure in which the malar, orbital rim and articular fossa are reconstructed by split rib and rib–cartilage grafts in the first intervention. The second surgical stage involves reconstruction of the temporomandibular joint by the use of a costochondral graft to build a condylar head and establish the normal vertical facial height. The final stage, which may be combined with stage two or perfomed later, involves mobilization of the maxilla by down-fracture at the Le

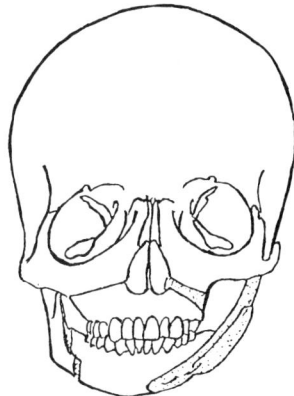

Fig. 20.14. Obwegeser-style diagram of right sagittal split, left ramal reconstruction of mandible and Le Fort I maxillary osteotomy with vertical repositioning Combinations of these procedures are most suitable for reconstruction of craniofacial microsomia after the completion of active growth.

Fort I level, alignment of the maxilla to the new position of the mandible and establishment of mid-line facial symmetry (*Fig.* 20.14).

Harvold[18] has promoted the use of activator orthodontic appliances prior to reconstruction of the mandible and in the intervals between the progressive reconstructive procedures. It is suggested that the stimulus to the defective growth mechanism, provided by the functional appliance, increases the growth potential of the compromised tissues and facilitates full functional rehabilitation.

While definitive assessment of these methods cannot yet be made, current experience in many centres would strongly support the concept of active orthodontic appliance therapy concurrent with phased surgical reconstruction. These techniques, it is believed, may permit earlier surgical intervention with less fear of the devastating relapse which had been experienced previously in the early static reconstruction of craniofacial microsomia by onlay and interpositional bone grafting of the affected mandible.

Mandibulofacial dysostosis, or Treacher Collins syndrome, is an autosomal dominant craniofacial malformation with 100 per cent penetrance and variable expressivity. A proportion of new cases arise as mutant conditions. Unlike craniofacial microsomia, mandibulofacial dysostosis is generally symmetrical. This symmetry extends to the soft tissue deformity of the ears, the antimongoloid slope of the eyes, malar hypoplasia, mandibular ramal underdevelopment and coloboma (notching) of the lower eyelids. The accompanying conductive deafness is due to maldevelopment of the ossicles of the middle ear. The nose is usually beak-like, with an obtuse frontonasal angle; the mandibular angle is also

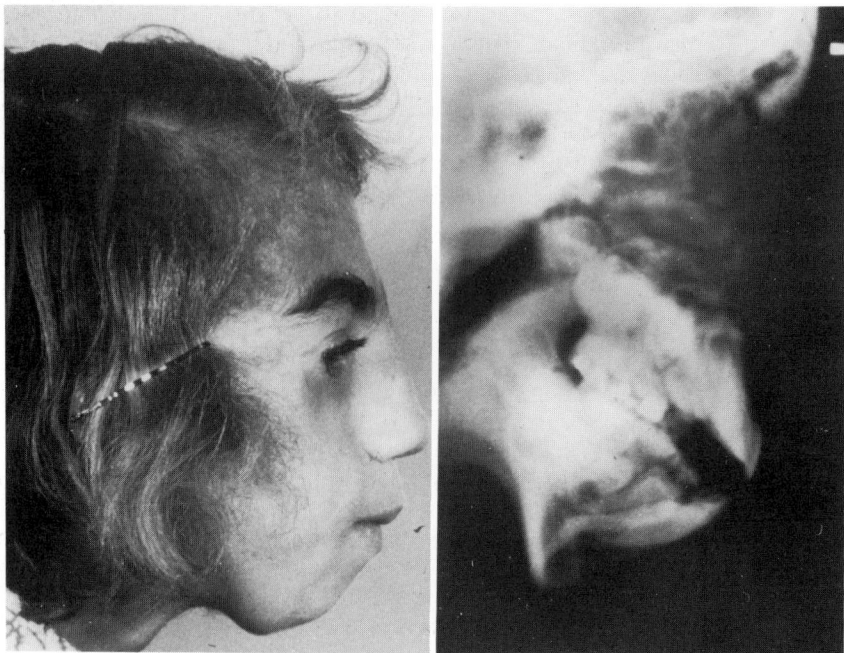

Fig. 20.15. Characteristic facial and radiological appearance in mandibulofacial dysostosis.

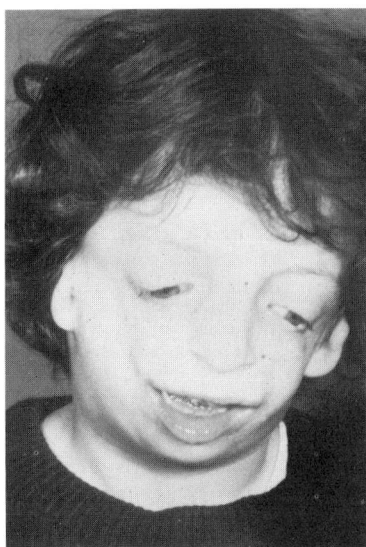

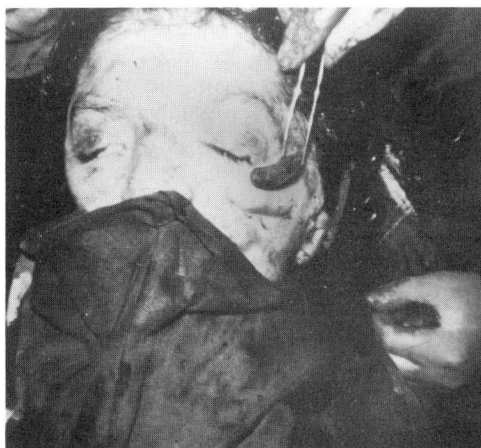

Fig. 20.16. *a*, Classic mandibulofacial dysostosis. *b*, Insertion of white Proplast tissue expanders to augment lateral orbital margin and malar eminences. *c*, Post-augmentation photograph. Final osseous reconstruction will attend to mandibular retrusion by sagittal split advancement together with advancement genioplasty.

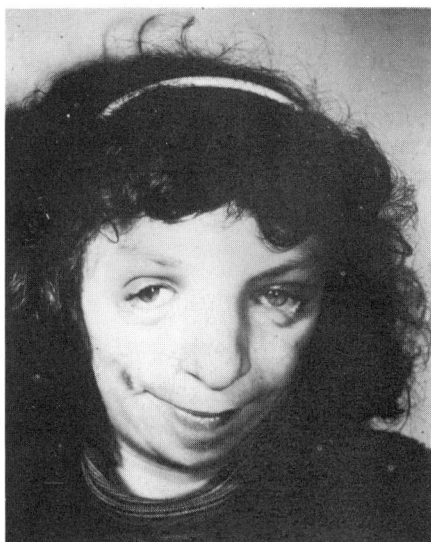

obtuse, the chin receding severely, and the palate is cleft in one-third of patients. Another unusual facial feature is a tongue of hair which extends downward and forwards from the temple to the cheek (*Fig.* 20.15).

Correction of these facial deformities, to date, has begun with reconstruction of the malformed ears and lower eyelids. This has been followed, at between 10 and 12 years of age, with expansion of the tight soft tissues of the cheek by implants of Proplast or bone which reconstruct the form of the lateral and inferior orbital rims (*Fig.* 20.16). Finally, the mandible is lengthened by C or L osteotomy with interpositional bone grafts after the adolescent growth spurt in the lower third of the face. Where chin retrusion is severe, it may be corrected by a one- or two-layer sliding genioplasty. When anterior open bite is severe, and not amenable to orthodontic correction, anterior segmental osteotomies of maxilla and mandible have been carried out. While these procedures have done much to improve the facial appearance of mandibulofacial dysostosis, they have not always produced stable reconstruction or results that have come up to the expectations of the reconstructive surgeon. Poswillo[19] has described the fundamental muscle defects in this condition, which compromise many attempts to restore normal mandibular morphology and function.

Recent advances in the use of a cranio-orbital approach to facial reconstruction have led to proposals for earlier correction of mandibulofacial dysostosis, starting about the age of 4 years. Tessier (personal communication) has proposed that combined intracranial and facial surgery now enable the orbits to be advanced and rotated, the malar and orbital deficiencies to be corrected by onlay bone grafts, and canthal dystopia, eyelid deficiencies and other soft tissue defects to be corrected simultaneously. Finally, mandibular advancement and genioplasty are carried out to complete, in one stage, total reconstruction. Orthodontic treatment is commenced, when necessary, in the mixed dentition stage and is completed after eruption of the second molars. While time alone will demonstrate the stability of one-stage total reconstruction, the results in a small series of patients are most impressive. It is likely that this type of procedure, which can be carried out before the social problems of the facial deformity become of great consequence to the affected child, will be widely adopted in future. The psychological effects of craniofacial deformity on the patient and the family are greatly diminished when reconstruction is seen to be a matter of urgency rather than a programmed period of review and delay as growth and social awareness proceed.[20]

Crouzon and Apert Syndromes

Craniofacial dysostosis is a loose term applied generally to patients with craniostenotic syndromes such as Crouzon and Apert syndromes and plagiocephaly. It can be applied to many patients who exhibit abnormal growth of the skull and face.

It is suggested, on slim evidence,[21] that most, if not all, of these deformities of the cranial vault arise because of premature fusion of the cranial sutures.

Ideally, these craniosynostoses should be detected in infancy, when the fused sutural margins are released and severe deformity of the skull is prevented. The early diagnosis and treatment is beyond the scope of this chapter: those wishing further information on the role of the orthodontist in the craniofacial team concerned with the management of these cases should consult a modern text[22] on the subject.

Late treatment of these birth defects is that which commences after the first year of life. The timing of surgery then depends on the age of the patient and the severity of the defect. Where hydrocephalus and exorbitism are a major concern, as may occur in Crouzon and Apert syndromes, treatment is needed urgently. It should be remembered that the eye grows to adult size by 6 years; if anterior growth of the orbital rims does not keep pace with eye growth, anterior dislocation of the eye and acute blindness may happen in as short a time as 20 minutes.

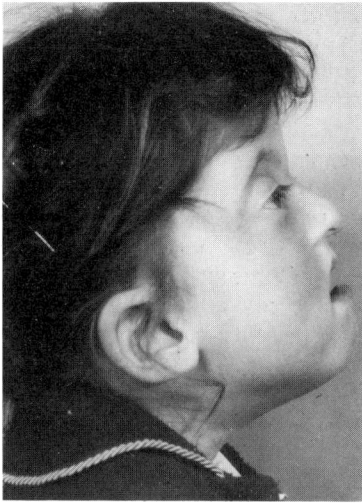

a

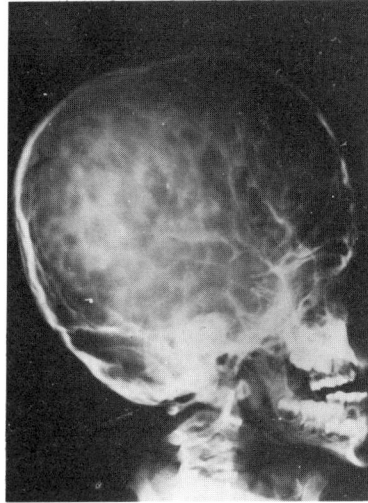

b

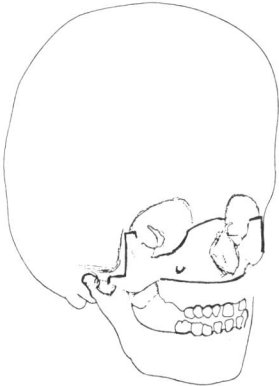

c

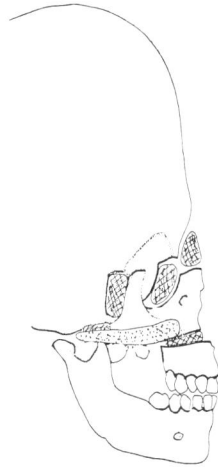

d

Fig. 20.17. *a, b,* Profile photograph and radiograph of classic Crouzon orbito-midfacial retrusion, to be corrected by frontomaxillary advancement prior to eruption of permanent buccal segment dentition. *c,* Lines of bone cut for combined Le Fort I and III advancement of nose and maxilla in Crouzon syndrome. *d,* Stabilization of advanced segments by iliac crest and split-rib bone grafts. (After David D. J., Poswillo D. and Simpson D. (1983) *The Craniosynostoses.* Berlin, Springer–Verlag.)

Principles of Treatment

The maxilla may be hypoplastic from birth in many of these syndromes. If surgical procedures on the cranial vault, carried out in infancy, do not release the maxilla to grow forwards, then it must be overcorrected by an osteotomy which will provide a Class II dental relationship (*Fig.* 20.17). Surgery to advance the maxilla 15 mm, when performed at 5 years of age, equals the advancement by normal maxillary growth to 10 years of age. Opinion remains divided on the optimal time for late total reconstruction of those with craniostenotic deformities. Ortiz–Monasterio[23] and Tessier[24] have proposed that early (2 years) reconstruction produces excellent results. Others believe that the long-term results of surgery before 8 years of age are likely to be devastatingly bad. Prospective studies in major craniofacial centres will provide some information on these matters in the next 5 years.

Leaving aside the respective claims for early and late delayed surgical reconstruction, it should be stated that the general medical state of the patient, the motivation and the psychological and emotional states must all be analysed before the decision to treat is made. Surgery of this kind, which involves the mobilization and rotation of the orbits, advancement of the forehead by a 'floating forehead' bone flap, release of the maxilla by a Le Fort osteotomy and stabilization and augmentation of all bone cuts by bone grafts, requires the team approach more than any other type of surgery. The disciplines of neurosurgery, plastic surgery and maxillofacial surgery are all involved when combinations of midface and intracranial surgery are required.

In many cases the separation of neurosurgical procedures from those of the midface reduces the risk of life-threatening meningeal infection. Compromises are seldom successful, and masking procedures help only where the bony superstructure is more or less in the optimal position with only minor irregularities of contour present.

REFERENCES

1. Gorlin R. J., Cervenka J. and Pzuzansky S. (1971) In: Bergsma D. (ed.) *Facial Clefting and its Syndromes*. (Third conference on the clinical delineation of birth defects. Part XI: Orofacial structures.) Baltimore, Md., Williams and Wilkins.
2. Loevy H. (1962) Developmental changes in the palate of normal and cortisone treated strain A mice. *Anat. Rec.* **142**; 375–90.
3. Veau V. (1931) *Division Palltaie*. Paris, Masson.
4. Kernahan D. A. and Stark R. B. (1958) A new classification for cleft lip and cleft palate. *Plast. Reconst. Surg.* **22**; 435.
5. Sperber G. H. (1976) *Craniofacial Embryology*. Bristol, Wright.
6. Ortiz–Monasterio F., Serrano A., Barrera G. et al. (1959) A study of untreated adult cleft palate patients. *Plast. Reconst. Surg.* **24**; 53–61.
7. Jolleys A. and Robertson N. R. (1972) A study of the effects of early bone grafting in complete clefts of the lip and palate: a five year study. *Br. J. Plast. Surg.* **25**; 229–37.
8. Schweckendiek W. (1978) Primary veloplasty. Long term results without maxillary deformity: a 25-year report. *Cleft Palate J.* **15**; 268–74.
9. Turvey T. A., Vig K., Moriarty J. et al. (1984) Delayed bone grafting in the cleft maxilla and palate: a retrospective multidisciplinary analysis. *Am. J. Orthodont.* **86**; 244–56.
10. McNeil C. L. (1964) In: Hotz R. (ed.) *Orthopaedic Principles in the Treatment of Lip and Palate Clefts*. (International symposium on early treatment of cleft lip and palate.) Berne, Huber.
11. Burston W. R. (1958) The early treatment of cleft palate conditions. *Dent. Pract.* **9**; 41–52.
12. Skoog, T. (1969) Repair of unilateral cleft deformity; maxilla, nose and lip. *Scand. J. Plast. Reconstr. Surg.* **3**; 109.
13. Millard D. R. (1960) Complete unilateral clefts of the lip. *Plast. Reconstr. Surg.* **25**; 595.
14. Millard D. R. (1968) Extensions of the rotation advancement principle for wide unilateral cleft lips. *Plast. Reconstr. Surg.* **42**; 535.

15. Henderson D. and Jackson I. T. (1975) A combined cleft lip revision, anterior fistula closure and maxillary osteotomy: a one-stage procedure. *Br. J. Oral Surg.* **13**; 33.
16. Poswillo D. (1973) The pathogenesis of the first and second branchial arch syndrome. *Oral Surg.* **35**; 302.
17. Obwegeser H. (1974) Correction of skeletal anomalies of otomandibular dysostosis. *J. Max-fac. Surg.* **2**; 72.
18. Harvold E. (1974) *The Activator in Interceptive Orthodontics.* St Louis, Mosby.
19. Poswillo D. (1974) Otomandibular defects: pathogenesis as a guide to reconstruction. *J. Max-fac. Surg.* **2**; 64.
20. Clifford E. (1979) Psychologic aspects of craniofacial anomalies. In: Converse J. M., McCarthy J. G. and Wood–Smith D. (ed.) *Symposium on Diagnosis and Treatment of Craniofacial Anomalies.* St Louis, Mosby, pp. 117–22.
21. Poswillo D. (1986) Experimental investigations into the aetiopathogenesis of syndromes of the head and neck. *J. Irish Coll. Phys. Surg.* **15**; 3.
22. David D. J., Poswillo D. and Simpson D. (1982) *The Craniosynostoses: Natural History, Diagnosis and Management.* New York, Springer.
23. Ortiz–Monasterio F. and Fuente del Campo A. (1979) Reconstructive surgery for Crouzon's disease and Apert's syndrome. In: Converse J. M., McCarthy J. G. and Wood–Smith D. (ed.) *Symposium on Diagnosis and Treatment of Craniofacial Anomalies.* St Louis, Mosby, pp. 370–84.
24. Tessier P. (1976) Recent improvements in treatment of facial and cranial deformities of Crouzon's disease and Apert's syndrome. In: Tessier P., Callahan A., Mustarde J. C. et al. (ed.) *Symposium on Plastic Surgery in the Orbital Region.* St Louis, Mosby, pp. 271–303.

INDEX

Numbers in *italic* refer to figures

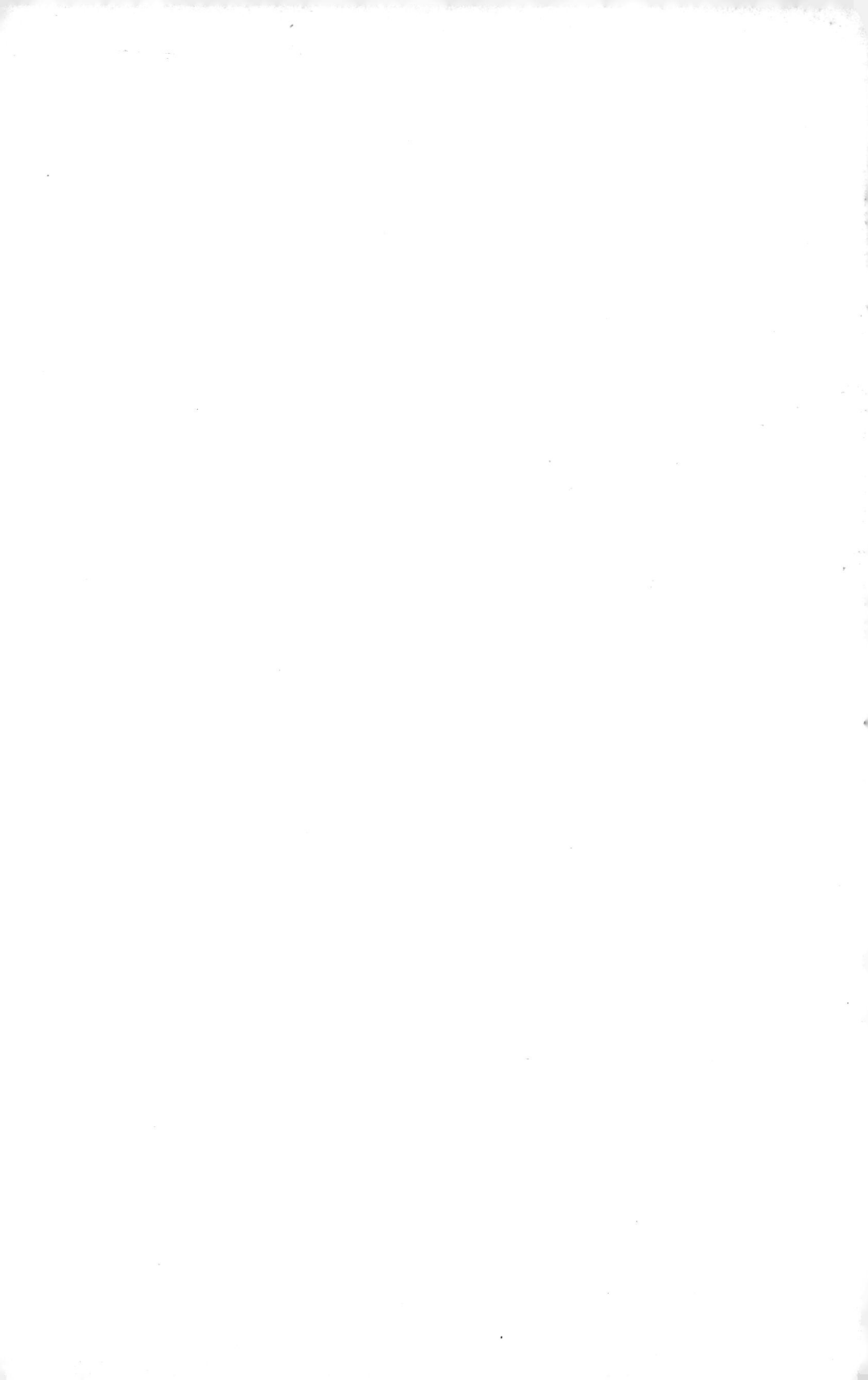